Theory and Practice of Chinese Medicine

Theory and Practice of Chinese Medicine

Editor: Harriet Schmidt

www.callistoreference.com

Callisto Reference,
118-35 Queens Blvd., Suite 400,
Forest Hills, NY 11375, USA

Visit us on the World Wide Web at:
www.callistoreference.com

ISBN: 978-1-64116-294-4 (Hardback)

Printed in China.

Cataloging-in-Publication Data

Theory and practice of chinese medicine / edited by Harriet Schmidt.
p. cm.
Includes bibliographical references and index.
ISBN 978-1-64116-294-4
1. Medicine, Chinese. 2. Alternative medicine--China. 3. Medicine--China. I. Schmidt, Harriet.
R601 .T44 2020
610.951--dc23

Table of Contents

Preface

In my initial years as a student, I used to run to the library at every possible instance to grab a book and learn something new. Books were my primary source of knowledge and I would not have come such a long way without all that I learnt from them. Thus, when I was approached to edit this book; I became understandably nostalgic. It was an absolute honor to be considered worthy of guiding the current generation as well as those to come. I put all my knowledge and hard work into making this book most beneficial for its readers.

Chinese medicine is an ancient medical practice which includes various forms of therapies including acupuncture, massage, dietary therapy, herbal medicine and exercise. It primarily focuses on the functions of the body like breathing, temperature maintenance and digestion. Chinese medicine is generally used as an alternative medicine approach and its philosophy is based on yinyangism. The diagnosis in Chinese medicine is majorly based on the methods of inspection, olfaction, inquiry, auscultation and palpation. Face, tongue, body odor, and other symptoms such as chills, fever, perspiration, taste, pain, sleep and menses, all are examined for diagnosis. The topics included in this book on Chinese medicine are of utmost significance and bound to provide incredible insights to readers. This book will also provide interesting topics for research which interested readers can take up. It will help the readers in keeping pace with the rapid changes in this field.

I wish to thank my publisher for supporting me at every step. I would also like to thank all the authors who have contributed their researches in this book. I hope this book will be a valuable contribution to the progress of the field.

Editor

1

Electroacupuncture for the prevention of postoperative gastrointestinal dysfunction in participants undergoing vascular laparotomy under general anesthesia

Meng-yue Liu[1†], Cheng-wei Wang[1†], Zhou-peng Wu[2] and Ning Li[1*]

Abstract

Background: Postoperative gastrointestinal dysfunction (PGD) is a common complication following laparotomy under general anesthesia (GA). Abdominal distension occurs in 8–28% of surgeries within 24 h postoperatively. The present study aimed to analyze the efficacy of electroacupuncture (EA) for the prevention of PGD by applying preoperative EA stimulation of PC6 (*Neiguan*), ST36 (*Zusanli*), and ST37 (*Shangjuxv*) bilaterally twice within 24 h prior to surgery, compared with no acupuncture treatment.

Methods: The study participants were assessed and selected from participants undergoing vascular laparotomy under GA at the Liver and Vascular Surgery Unit in West China Hospital of Sichuan University. The selected participants were randomly allocated to two groups: routine-treatment (RT) and EA group receiving EA at PC6, ST36, and ST37. A computer-generated list of random numbers was used to determine the allocation of the participants, with numbered opaque sealed envelopes containing the randomization schedule. Eligible participants were all adults aged 18 years or above who were scheduled to undergo vascular laparotomy under GA within 24 h and had no history of EA treatment. The exclusion criteria included participants with serious systemic disease and history of EA treatment. While the RT group received standard treatments, the EA group received additional EA treatments. During each treatment session, EA stimulation was performed for a duration of 20 min at a frequency of 15 Hz with a continuous wave. All such participants received two EA treatments within 24 h before surgery. The outcomes were measured in three metrics: incidence and degree of abdominal distension; first times of flatus and defecation; and duration of hospitalization.

Results: Forty-three participants were recruited, of whom 42 participants successfully completed the study. Each group contained 21 participants. The incidence of abdominal distension (42.8, 76.2%) and degree of abdominal distension were significantly reduced in the EA group ($P = 0.03$ and $P = 0.03$, respectively). In comparisons of the first times of flatus (3.05 ± 0.58, 3.29 ± 0.42 days) and defecation (2.81 ± 0.51, 3.20 ± 0.55 days) and duration of hospitalization (5.33 ± 0.68, 5.75 ± 0.66 days), the EA group was superior to the RT group to some extent ($P = 0.13$, $P = 0.02$, and $P = 0.04$, respectively).

*Correspondence: zhenjiuhuaxi@163.com
†Meng-yue Liu and Cheng-wei Wang contributed equally to this work
[1] Department of Integrated Traditional Chinese and Western Medicine, West China Hospital of Si-chuan University, Chengdu, Sichuan, China
Full list of author information is available at the end of the article

Conclusions: Preoperative EA at PC6, ST36, and ST37 might be useful for preventing PGD, thereby improving gastrointestinal function recovery.

Background

Postoperative gastrointestinal dysfunction (PGD) is a complication in participants undergoing major surgical procedures under general anesthesia (GA) [1]. Opioid-induced gastrointestinal dysfunction is as high as 81% in the United States [2]. Abdominal distension within 24 h of surgery occurs in 8–28% of all operations [3]. PGD causes longer hospital stays, greater medical cost [4], and higher risks for other complications, such as infections. In China, the rate of PGD remained the same between 1974 and 2011 [5]. In Japan, the rate increased by 10% over a 5-year period at the turn of the twenty-first century [6]. Internationally, an analysis was conducted on the records of more than 5000 participants undergoing major vascular surgery in 206 National Surgical Quality Improvement Program hospitals from 2008 to 2009 [7]. The results showed that >25% of participants with endovascular treatment, regardless of severity, suffered from postoperative complications, postoperative intestinal obstruction, and other gastrointestinal dysfunctions within 30 days of surgery. Although the 30-day survival rate of thoracoabdominal aortic operations was 92% [8], gastrointestinal dysfunction was ranked 4th among the causes for death [9].

Currently, there are four major methods of treatment for PGD: diet and nutritional support, drug treatment, operative procedure, and complementary medicine. Most of these treatments are open-label treatment trials with small samples [10]. Acupuncture is widely used in obstetrics and gynecology [11], gastrointestinal surgery [12], and orthopedics [13].

As a potential alternative therapy, acupuncture has gradually gained acceptance from physicians following the demonstration of its efficacy in clinical and basic research. For example, a 165-patient clinical study demonstrated that electroacupuncture (EA) reduced the duration of operative ileus [14]. Another small-sample-size trial found EA useful for postoperative recovery of abdominal distension [15], and a similar study showed that acupressure improved the recovery of stomach distension [16]. Animal experiments identified the factors contributing to PGD, including reduction in the number of interstitial cells of Cajal and atrophy of their structure [17], activation of the sympathetic nervous system and postoperative inflammatory cytokines [18], and leukocyte cell-induced nitrous oxide release, which restrained gastrointestinal peristalsis and causes intestinal inflammation [19]. Other animal studies showed that acupuncture ameliorated PGD by regulating these pathological changes [20].

The present study aimed to analyze the efficacy of EA for preventing PGD by applying preoperative EA stimulation of PC6 (*Neiguan*), ST36 (*Zusanli*), and ST37 (*Shangjuxv*) bilaterally twice within 24 h prior to surgery, compared with no acupuncture treatment.

Methods

Ethics approval

This study was approved by the Ethics and Research Committee of West China Hospital of Sichuan University (WCHSU), China [No. 2013 (105); Additional file 1]. The Ethics and Research Committee of WCHSU is an ethical approval committee organized by leading professors in their own fields. The study strictly followed the principles for medical ethics outlined in the Declaration of Helsinki [21]. The study was registered with the Chinese Clinical Trial Registry: ChiCTR-TRC-13003649. All participants were provided with information regarding the study and signed a written consent form in advance (Additional file 2). The Chinese Cochrane Center was responsible for the whole trial including the randomization, blinding, statistical analyses, and data management. The study was performed according to the CONSORT 2010 checklist (Additional file 3).

Trial design

This was a single-center, single-blind, pragmatic randomized controlled study. With balanced randomization (1: 1), the participants were assigned to two groups: EA group and RT group (routine-treatment group).

Participants

All participants were recruited from the WCHSU, China, after meeting the eligibility criteria and signing the informed consent forms. Chengdu is a major business city in the west of China, with a population of 14,047,600, and WCHSU is the primary health care provider in the west of China. Eligible participants were all adults aged 18 years or above who were scheduled to undergo vascular laparotomy under GA within 24 h and had no history of EA treatment.

The exclusion criteria were as follows: participants undergoing endovascular surgery; participants with a history of hypothyroidism, hyperthyroidism, cardiopulmonary disease, diabetes, or psychological disorder; participants with a history of EA treatment; participants with a cardiac pacemaker; participants in the menstruating phase of the menstrual cycle; participants who refused to accept acupuncture; participants who were unconscious before surgery; participants with inability to communicate; participants participating in another clinical trial that could interfere with the primary endpoint of the study; participants with a bleeding disorder (hemophilia or fibrinogenemia); participants with serious systemic disease (AIDS or sepsis); participants with initial body temperature of above 38.0 °C or below 36.0 °C; participants with a known history of alcohol or substance abuse; participants requiring systemic sedation for other reasons; participants needing emergency procedures; participants who were pregnant or lactating women.

The withdrawal criteria were as follows: at the patient's own request or at the request of their legal representative; if, in the opinion of the investigator or the specialized physician performing the acupuncture or examination, continuation of the trial would be detrimental to the patient's wellbeing (e.g. strong pain at insertion points, allergic reactions, other independent acute health problems).

Interventions

For prevention of PGD by EA, three acupuncture points, PC6 (*Neiguan*), ST36 (*Zusanli*), and ST37 (*Shangjuxv*), were selected.

The participants receiving EA therapy were treated bilaterally at the above three distal acupuncture points. PC6 is an acupuncture point of the pericardium meridian, which is located between the palmaris longus tendon and the flexor carpi radialis muscle tendon, 2 cun above the rasceta (Fig. 1). ST36 in a point between the tibialis anterior and extensor digitorum longus, which is located on the anterolateral side of the lower leg, 3 cun below *Dubi* and one finger width lateral of the anterior border of the tibia. ST37 is a point in the tibialis anterior, which is located 3 cun below ST36 (Fig. 2). The anterior tibial artery and anterior tibial vein are present around both ST36 and ST37, while there are the lateral sural cutaneous nerve and cutaneous branch of the saphenous nerve. The locations of these acupuncture points are described in *The National Standards for Acupoint Location* [22].

The participants in EA group were given the following EA treatment. After each insertion site was disinfected with 75% alcohol, sterile single-use 0.25 × 38-mm needles (Wuxi Jiajian Medical Instrument Co. Ltd., Jiangsu, China) were inserted vertically to a depth of 4–10 mm. At the appropriate depth, the acupuncturist manipulated the needles for *Deqi* sensation, defined as a feeling of heaviness around the acupoint [23], and then bilaterally connected a Nerve and Muscle Stimulator (Suzhou Medical Appliance Factory, Suzhou, China) to PC6 (positive electrode) and ST36 (negative electrode) on the ipsilateral limbs. In each treatment session, EA stimulation was performed for a duration of 20 min at a frequency of 15 Hz with a continuous wave. The participants received two EA treatments within 24 h before surgery, one at 10:00 a.m. and another at 16:00 p.m.

All participants in 2 groups received similar routine treatments after surgery, including gastrointestinal

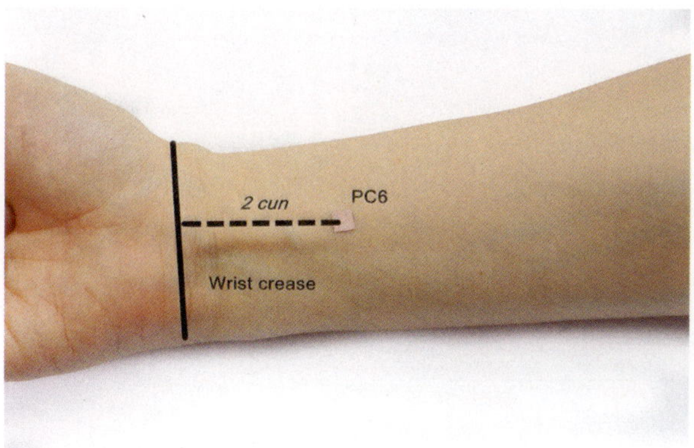

Fig. 1 Location of PC6

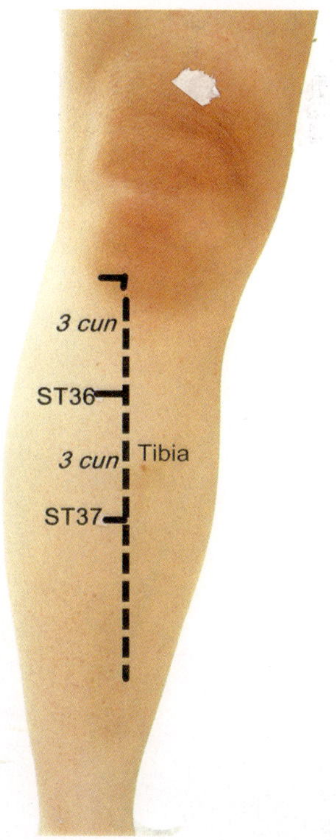

Fig. 2 Locations of ST36 and ST37

decompression, maintenance stabilization of homeostasis (especially maintenance of electrolyte balance), routine nursing care, and early walking, with no further EA treatments in EA group. The only combination therapy received by all participants was 1500 mL of physiological saline with 1.5 g Potassium Chloride Injection (China Otsuka Pharmaceutical Co. Ltd., Tianjin, China) for 2 days postoperatively.

All participants underwent preoperative and postoperative supervision and evaluation of curative effects by a blinded observer at 10:00 a.m. daily, until they were discharged. A third party performed all data treatments and analyses. The study was performed as shown in the flowchart (Fig. 3).

The participating acupuncturist had more than 2000 h of acupuncture training before participating in the trial and received their diploma 6 years ago. The physician had applied acupuncture in practice for more than 6 years and had treated about 1000 participants with acupuncture in the year before the trial.

Outcomes

A blinded observer obtained the postoperative data including the degree of abdominal distension, times of first flatus and defecation, and duration of hospitalization after surgery. As a subjective sensation, abdominal distension was measured by a Likert-type scale (Table 1) [24]. Postoperative abdominal distension was defined as a postoperative gastrointestinal motility change leading to invalid transfer of gastrointestinal contents [25], caused by intraoperative wound traction, abdominal adhesions, or lack of visceral perfusion [2]. In this study, the incidence and degree of abdominal distension after surgery were the main outcome indicators, while the times of first flatus and defecation and duration of hospitalization were secondary outcomes. The study focused on the prevention of PGD; therefore, the incidence of PGD was the primary endpoint.

Table 1 Presentation of the Likert-type scale

Score	Explanation
0	I feel no abdominal distension at all
1	I feel a little of abdominal distension
2	I feel abdominal distension but I can bear
3	I feel obvious abdominal distension that I cannot bear but it doesn't affect my life
4	I feel horrible abdominal distension and need it addressed

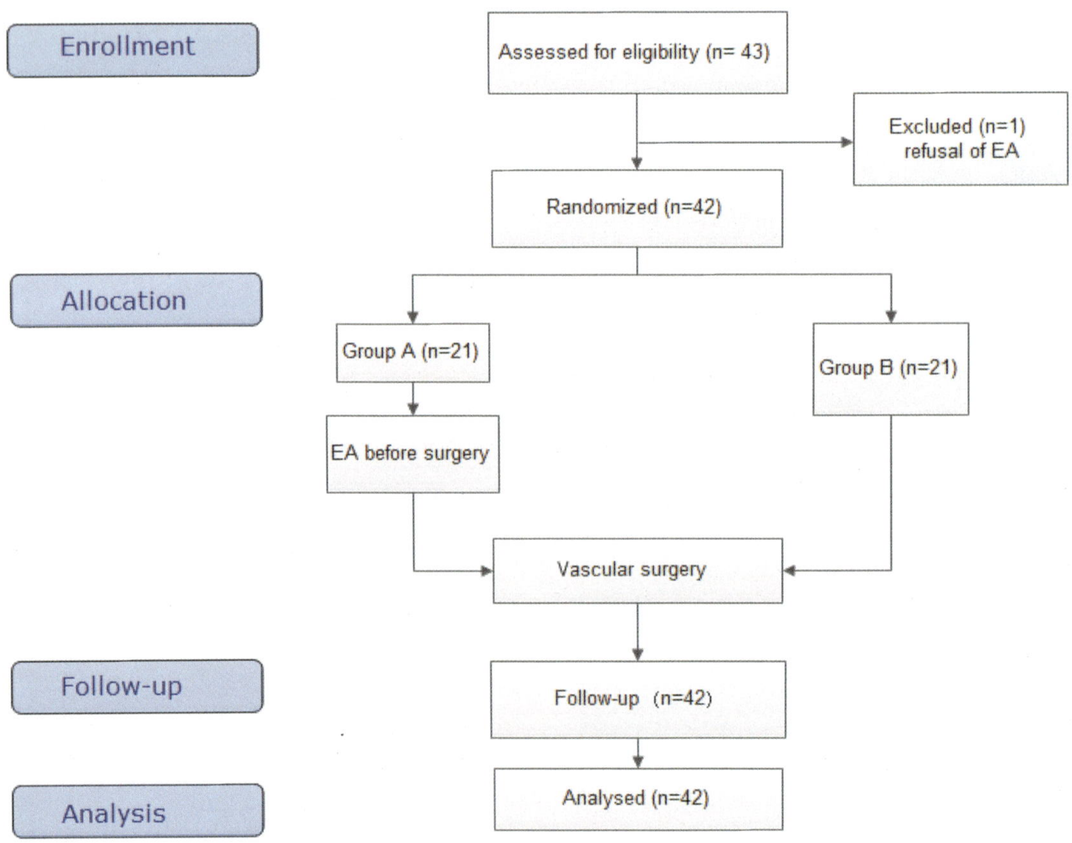

Fig. 3 Flowchart of the study

The study included a period from 24 h preoperatively to 7 days postoperatively. A graduate student, who did not participate in patient management, recorded the treatment details, including demographic data, anesthesia time, surgery duration, and dosage of opioids. The demographic data collected included: age; sex; race; marital status; job status; educational background; weight; and telephone number. Considering that the type of intravenous fluid given during and after surgery is a factor in postoperative recovery, we specified that all participants enrolled in the study were only under GA perioperatively and that all of their postoperative routine treatments, especially the combination therapy, were the same to avoid any bias conferred by administration of a different intravenous fluid.

Sample size calculation

Owing to a lack of previous reports on PGD-related acupuncture and vascular surgery, the study was designed to include a minimum of 20 cases [26] in each group following the minimum sample-size requirements. With consideration of selecting an appropriate sample size, controlling random errors, and achieving a certain effect, the lower limit of the sample size was set at 20 cases (20–30 cases per group stipulated by the China Food and Drug Administration, 20–50 cases in the European Union, 20–80 cases in the United States [26]).

Randomization and blinding

All participants were randomly assigned to the two groups on the basis of a concealed allocation approach using statistical analysis PROCPLAN statements (SAS 9.4; World Headquarters SAS Institute Inc., Cary, NC, USA). A computer-generated list of random numbers was used to determine the allocation of the participants, with numbered opaque sealed envelopes containing the randomization schedule. The envelopes were kept by an investigator who was not an assessor in the study, and who was informed of the outcomes at the end of the study. The researchers recording the outcomes and those making the conclusions were all blinded to patients' assessments.

Statistical analysis

All continuous data, including the incidence of abdominal distension, all secondary outcomes, and some of the baseline data, were expressed as mean ± standard deviation (SD). For these data, a t test used to compare normally distributed data between the two groups, while the Wilcoxon rank sum test applied for non-normally distributed data. Nominal variables, including the degree of abdominal distension and the remaining baseline data, were presented as frequency and percentage and analyzed using the Chi square (χ^2) test. Values of $P < 0.05$ were considered statistically significant. All the efficacy and safety analyses were performed using the intent-to-treat population. A third person performed blinded estimation and statistics of the curative effect.

Adverse events

All adverse events, such as hematoma, stuck needle, and fainting, were reported. In participants with serious adverse events, the experimental intervention was ceased immediately, and proper treatments were provided.

Results

Selection of participants

Recruitment for the study began on 10 February 2014 and finished on 14 July 2014, while follow-up was completed on 17 July 2014. During the 8-month-study, 43 participants were recruited, and 42 participants completed the study, with 21 participants in each group. One participant was excluded because of refusal to receive EA. The baseline demographic data and clinical characteristics of the two groups did not differ significantly and were comparable (Table 2). The mean morbidity age

Table 2 Demographic data for all participants

	EA group (N = 21)	RT group (N = 21)	t	χ^2	P
Age (years), mean ± SD	56.0 ± 11.31	56.8 ± 12.16	0.221		0.826
Gender (F), %	23.8%	23.8%	–	0.130	0.641
Race (Han), %	90.5%	85.7%	–	0.000	0.500
Married, %	95.2%	100%	–	0.000	0.235
Retirement, %	23.8%	23.8%	–	0.000	0.280
Illiteracy/yes, %	4.8%	19.0%	–	0.980	0.472
Weight (kg), mean ± SD	65.6 ± 2.56	64.7 ± 1.16	1.467	–	0.150
Anesthesia time (h), mean ± SD	4.03 ± 0.35	4.19 ± 0.38	1.419	–	0.164
Surgery duration (h), mean ± SD	3.52 ± 0.28	3.43 ± 0.31	0.987	–	0.329
Opioids' dosage (g), mean ± SD	0.86 ± 0.48	0.67 ± 0.66	1.067	–	0.292

EA electroacupuncture, *RT* routine treatment

was 56.40 ± 11.61 years, and the participants comprised 23.8% women and 76.2% men.

Outcomes and estimations

Primary endpoints

As shown in Table 3, there were significant differences in the incidence and degree of abdominal distension between the two groups ($P = 0.03$ and $P = 0.03$, respectively). The percentage of participants suffering from abdominal distension was 42.8% in EA group and 76.2% in RT group. The number of participants who could not stand the distension was 14.3% in EA group and 33.3% in RT group, as well as 28.6% in EA group and 37.9% in RT group were with sustainable abdominal distension which don't need any pharmacotherapy.

Secondary endpoints

As shown in Table 4, the time of first defecation (2.81 ± 0.51, 3.20 ± 0.55 days) and duration of hospitalization (5.33 ± 0.68, 5.75 ± 0.66 days) showed significant differences between the two groups ($P = 0.02$ and $P = 0.04$, respectively), while the time of first flatus (3.05 ± 0.58, 3.29 ± 0.42 days) showed no significant difference ($P = 0.13$). Among the three items, the reduction in first defecation time was most noticeable (12.18%), while the time of first flatus, showing the beginning of gastrointestinal function recovery, was reduced by 7.29% and the duration of hospitalization was shortened by 6.98%.

Table 3 Outcomes for incidence and degree of abdominal distension

	EA group (N = 21)	RT group (N = 21)	*t*	Z	*P*
AD's incidence	9 (42.8%)	16 (76.2%)	4.842		0.029
AD's degree				−2.109	0.035
0	12 (57.1%)	5 (23.8%)			
1	0 (0%)	2 (4.6%)			
2	6 (28.6%)	7 (33.3%)			
3	3 (14.3%)	4 (19.0%)			
4	0 (0%)	3 (14.3%)			

Data are shown as *n* (%)

EA electroacupuncture, *RT* routine treatment, *AD* abdominal distension

Table 4 Outcomes of the secondary endpoints

	EA group (N = 21)	RT group (N = 21)	*t*	*P*
First time flatus (d)	3.05 ± 0.58	3.29 ± 0.42	1.536	0.132
First time Defecation (d)	2.81 ± 0.51	3.20 ± 0.55	2.383	0.022
Hospitalization (d)	5.33 ± 0.68	5.75 ± 0.66	2.031	0.049

Data are shown as mean ± SD

EA electroacupuncture, *RT* routine treatment, *AD* abdominal distension

Table 5 Descriptions of the four common methods of sham-acupuncture

Advantages	Limitations	Indications
Sham-acupuncture		
Fine masking	Not suitable	Insistent estimation
Low stimulation	For all acupoints	Without EA history
		Acupoints on back
Non-acupoints		
Fine masking	Can't avoid	Different ganglion segment
Better feasibility	Physiological effect	Without EA history
		Study on acupoints' specificity
Shallow acupuncture		
Better masking	Narrow indication	Study on depths of needling
Low stimulation		
Non-disease-related acupuncture		
Better masking	Low feasibility	Without EA history
Lowest bias		Study on acupoints' specificity

Adverse events

There were no participants with needle breakages, unbearable pain, and other acupuncture-related adverse events during the study.

Discussion

This study was carried out to determine whether a preventive intervention program can reduce PGD after vascular surgery under GA. In WCHSU, gastrointestinal decompression or early walking is usually used for treatment of PGD, and these methods were applied to all study participants. For prevention of PGD, a previous study stated that EA should be applied from anesthesia induction to surgery completion [27]. However, application of EA was chosen during the 24-h period before surgery for four reasons: research purposes; safety; easy isolation of control and treatment groups; and efficacy. As a pre-validation study, the present study focused on whether this preventive intervention had an impact on PGD, while rehabilitation or acupuncture is often prescribed after surgery. In addition, this study used EA, which may interfere with other equipment used intraoperatively, such as an electric knife. In traditional Chinese medicine theory and human research [28], *Deqi* is a prerequisite for effective treatment. During or after surgery, GA and postoperative incision pain can cause a needling sensation, resulting in reduced levels of patient compliance.

The anesthetic items for both groups were compared, and only laparotomy was included to mitigate the experimental bias caused by different operative methods and anesthetic concentrations, especially opioids [29]. As the anesthetic concentration was proportional to weight, and there was no significant difference in weight between the two groups, the anesthetic dosages for both groups were comparable.

All secondary outcomes, used extensively for evaluating functional recovery, indicated that EA could accelerate the rehabilitation program for PGD. Among the three endpoints, the reduction of first defecation time showed the largest effect. Studies in the literature have used varying endpoints, such as bowel sounds, flatus, and bowel movements [30, 31]. Among these three endpoints, bowel movements are the most reliable endpoint [32].

To mitigate the potential bias among consenting participants induced by the Hawthorne effect, many studies have required inclusion of a sham acupuncture group. There are four methods in common use [33], as shown in Table 5. However, researchers rarely use placebo-controlled trials when comparing interventions with general routine therapy [34]. Acupuncture treatments are complex, multicomponent interventions. In sham-controlled trials that attempt to control only certain potentially therapeutic acupuncture-specific components, such as location, insertion depth, stimulation, needle size, and number [35], the moderately large nonspecific effects of sham acupuncture can decrease the reliability and the usefulness of the test results [36].

The incidence and degree of abdominal distension determined that EA was useful for preventing PGD and helped in the drawing of accurate conclusions. The Likert-type scale was used to measure the degree of abdominal distension, and the sustainable uncomfortable, which don't influent sleep, is 1′–2′ and the uncomfortable need pharmacotherapy is 3′–4′. In our study, EA could alleviate abdominal distension more. However, the Likert-type scale is only a rough estimation, although there is no specialized abdominal-distension personnel. Therefore, regarding validity of the findings, a comparison of objective parameters is necessary in a future study. The latest animal and human studies have demonstrated that not only a leukocytic pathway and subsequent injury-specific local inflammatory responses [37, 38], but also secondary lymphoid organs 0, are involved in the progression of postoperative ileus. It is indispensable to add an inflammatory cytokine test to a future study. There is also a necessity for a comparison of abdominal circumference as an objective factor 0.

There is a bias to the present study that cannot be ignored, namely that EA group had more doctor–patient contact hours and might experience placebo effects, even though the acupuncturist was not their surgeon. Considering that the acupuncturist performed EA only twice, the acupuncturist was recommended to get in contact with the participants in RT group in a future study.

Conclusions

Preoperative EA at PC6, ST36, and ST37 might be useful for preventing PGD, thereby improving gastrointestinal function recovery.

Abbreviations

EA: electroacupuncture; GA: general anesthesia; PGD: postoperative gastrointestinal dysfunction; WCHSU: West China Hospital of Sichuan University.

Authors' contributions

MYL, ZPW and NL designed the study. CWW performed the data analysis. MYL and CWW wrote the manuscript. All authors read and approved the final manuscript.

Author details

[1] Department of Integrated Traditional Chinese and Western Medicine, West China Hospital of Si-chuan University, Chengdu, Sichuan, China. [2] Department of Liver and Vascular Surgery, West China Hospital of Si-chuan University, Chengdu, Sichuan, China.

Acknowledgements

We must give our acknowledgement to Qian Wen, Physician-in-charge of WCHSU, for her performing the experiment and Jianghua Yan for data collection. We would like to thank Yu Zhao and Jian-Qin Lv from the Department of Integrated Traditional and Western Medicine, WCHSU, Chengdu, China for their support in designing the study. We also need to thank Si-jia Li, Maryland University, and Sha wang, National University of Singapore for their greatly help in language issues.

Competing interests

The authors declare that they have no competing interests.

References

1. Steinbrook RA. Epidural anesthesia and gastrointestinal motility. Anesth Analg. 1998;86:837–44.
2. Bell TJ, Panchal SJ, Miaskowski C. The prevalence, severity, and impact of opioid-induced bowel dysfunction: results of a US and European Patient Survey (PROBE 1). Pain Med. 2009;10:35–8.
3. Gu KM, Zeng M, Liu M. Comparison of several methods in treating postoperative abdominal distension. Harbin Yi Yao. 2007;27:22–3.
4. Eappen S, Lane BH, Rosenberg B. Relationship between occurrence of surgical complications and hospital finances. JAMA. 2013;309:1599–608.
5. Sheng DJ, Jun DY, Fang L. The development situation and tendency of vascular surgery in China. Hebei Med J. 2002;24:397–402.
6. Nowygrod R, Egorova N, Greco G. Trends, complications, and mortality in peripheral vascular surgery. J Vasc Surg. 2006;43:205–12.
7. Ma X, Yuan QH, Yu ZX. Efficacy comparison between endovascular aneurysm repair versus open surgery for patients with abdominal aortic aneurysms: a meta-analysis. Zhonghua Xin Xue Guan Bing Za Zhi. 2012;40:878–86.
8. Yamamoto H, Yamamoto F, Ishibashi K. Long-term outcomes of open surgical repair for ruptured iliac artery aneurysms. Ann Vasc Surg. 2011;25:740–8.
9. Girotti ME, Ko CY, Dimick JB. Hospital morbidity rankings and complication severity in vascular surgery. J Vasc Surg. 2013;57:158–67.

10. Svensson LG, Crawford ES, Hess KR, Coselli JS, Safi HJ. Experience with 1509 patients undergoing thoracoabdonimal aortic operations. J Vasc Surg. 1993;17:357–68.
11. Zerbino DD. Kuzyk lul. Aortic dissecting aneurysms: clinical masks, differential diagnosis. Klin Med. 2002;80:58–62.
12. Van Noord BA, Roffey P, Thangathurai D. Abdominal compartment syndrome following opioid-induced postoperative ileus. J Clin Anesth. 2013;25:146–54.
13. Camilleri M, Parkman HP, Shafi MA. Clinical guideline: management of gastroparesis. Am J Gastroenterol. 2013;108:18–20.
14. Wan Q. Auricular-plaster therapy plus acupuncture at zusanli for postoperative recovery of intestinal function. J Tradit Chin Med. 2000;20:134–42.
15. Kexin L. One hundred and forty-six cases of postoperative abdominal distention treated by electroacupucnture. World J Acu Mox. 2009;19:60–1.
16. Wanting H, Yichuan C, Meiling Y, et al. Acupressure improves the postoperative comfort of gastric cancer patients: a randomized controlled trial. Complement Ther Med. 2015;23:339–46.
17. Forster J, Damjanov I, Lin Z. Absence of the interstitial cells of Cajal in patients with gastroparesis and correlation with clinical findings. J Gastrointest Surg. 2005;9:102–7.
18. Kalff JC, Carlos TM, Schraut WH. Surgically induced leukocytic infiltrates within the rat intestinal muscularis mediate postoperative ileus. Gastroenterology. 1999;117:378–87.
19. Kalff JC, Schraut WH, Billiar TR. Role of inducible nitric oxide synthase in postoperative intestinal smooth muscle dysfunction in rodents. Gastroenterology. 2000;118:316–27.
20. Senna-Fernandes V, França DL, Souza D. Acupuncture at "Zusanli" (St.36) and "Sanyinjiao" (SP.6) points on the gastrointestinal tract: a study of the bioavailability of (99 m)Tc-sodium pertechnetate in rats. Evid Based Compl Alt. 2011;2011:823941.
21. Allen TK, Habib AS. P6 stimulation for the prevention of nausea and vomiting associated with cesarean delivery under neuraxial anesthesia: a systematic review of randomized controlled trials. Anesth Analg. 2008;107:1308–14.
22. Ouyang MW, Qin ZS, Lin CS. Prophylactic effect of acupuncture on nausea and vomiting after laparoscopic operation. Zhongguo Zhen Jiu. 2009;29:915–24.
23. Molsberger A. Acupuncture in orthopedics. ORTHOPADE. 2012;41:100–1.
24. General administration of quality supervision, inspection and quarantine of the People's Republic of China, standardization administration of the People's Republic of China. Nomenclature and location of acupuncture points. (GB/T 12346-2006).
25. Langevin HM, Churchill DL, Fox JR. Biomechanical response to acupuncture needling in humans. J Appl Physiol. 2001;91:2471–8.
26. Xuezhong Z, Xuerui T, Hongxing P. The sample size of clinic trials. Shi Jie Hua Ren Xiao Hua Za Zhi. 2006;14:1339–40.
27. Klaus L, Karin N, Antonius S, et al. How large are the nonspecific effects of acupuncture? A meta-analysis of randomized controlled trials. BMC Med. 2010;8:75–6.
28. Andrew L, Edward L, Yvette T. Mechanisms and treatment of postoperative ileus. Arch Surg. 2003;138:206–14.
29. Lee A, Chan S. Acupuncture and anesthesia. Best Pract Res Clin Anaesthesiol. 2006;20:303–12.
30. Chen TY, Zhou J, Wang K, Xu JJ, Ma W, Wu YY. Electroacupuncture intervention combined with anesthetics for analgesia and post-surgical gastrointestinal recovery in pneumectomy patients. Zhen Ci Yan Jiu. 2015;40:461–4.
31. Huanqin L, Huilin L, Cunzhi L. Effect of "Deqi" during the study of needling "Wang's Jiaji" acupoints treating spasticity after stroke. Evid Based Compl Alt. 2014;2014:715351.
32. Helene M, Langevin L, Peter M. Paradoxes in acupuncture research: strategies for moving forward. Evid Based Compl Alt. 2011;2011:180805.
33. Oh DS, Jung SY, Kim AR. A crossover clinical trial to determine the effect of Siguan (four gates) points on gastrointestinal motility suppressed by loperamide administration. J Korean Oriental Med. 2008;29:1–6.
34. Schmidt J, Stoffels B, Chanthaphavong RS. Differential molecular and cellular immune mechanisms of postoperative and LPS-induced ileus in mice and rats. Cytokine. 2012;59:49–58.
35. Yin J, Chen JD. Gastrointestinal motility disorders and acupuncture. Auton Neurosci. 2010;157:31–7.
36. Koscielny A, Engel D, Maurer J. The role of lymphoid tissue in the attenuation of the postoperative ileus. Am J Phys. 2012;304:401–12.
37. Van Bree SHW, Cailotto C. Systemic in flammation with enhanced brain activation contributes to more severe delay in postoperative ileus. Neuro-Gastroent Motil. 2013;25:540–50.
38. Magalhães FJ, Mendonça LB, Rebouças CB. Risk factors for cardiovascular diseases among nursing professionals: strategies for health promotion. Rev Bras Enferm. 2014;67:394–7.

2

In silico approach in reveal traditional medicine plants pharmacological material basis

Fan Yi[1,2,3*], Li Li[1,2], Li-jia Xu[3], Hong Meng[1,2], Yin-mao Dong[1,2], Hai-bo Liu[3*] and Pei-gen Xiao[3]

Abstract

In recent years, studies of traditional medicinal plants have gradually increased worldwide because the natural sources and variety of such plants allow them to complement modern pharmacological approaches. As computer technology has developed, in silico approaches such as virtual screening and network analysis have been widely utilized in efforts to elucidate the pharmacological basis of the functions of traditional medicinal plants. In the process of new drug discovery, the application of virtual screening and network pharmacology can enrich active compounds among the candidates and adequately indicate the mechanism of action of medicinal plants, reducing the cost and increasing the efficiency of the whole procedure. In this review, we first provide a detailed research routine for examining traditional medicinal plants by in silico techniques and elaborate on their theoretical principles. We also survey common databases, software programs and website tools that can be used for virtual screening and pharmacological network construction. Furthermore, we conclude with a simple example that illustrates the whole methodology, and we present perspectives on the development and application of this in silico methodology to reveal the pharmacological basis of the effects of traditional medicinal plants.

Keywords: Traditional medicinal plants, Virtual screening, Network pharmacology, Medicinal plants information analytics, Pharmacological basis

Background

Over three quarters of the world's population relies mainly on plants and plant extracts for health care. World Health Organization (WHO) report indicated that over 30% of all plant species have at one time or another been used for medicinal purposes [1]. The scientific study of traditional medicinal plants is of great importance for human health.

Identifying and predicting the pharmacological basis of the activity of traditional medicinal plants are important for the goal of modernizing their use [2]. Because the chemical constituents of medicinal plants are complex and varied, clarifying the specific chemical components in such plants and their major biological functions is a complex task.

The traditional model of medicinal plant research can usually be divided into the following steps: first, the extraction of compound monomers or fractions, followed by their qualitative and quantitative identification and then a variety of pharmacological experiments such as in vitro experiments and injection or feeding these solution in animal then performing effective measurement [3]. In general, the whole research process is time consuming and expensive. However, several parts of this common approach can be modified to improve the efficiency. At present, the chemistry of the most widely used medicinal plants, such as *ginseng* and *licorice*, has been studied quite thoroughly. Hundreds of chemical compounds have been extracted from these medicinal herbs. However, most of these compounds have not to be studied whether they have potential no biological activity. It would be a vast and time-consuming project to systematically evaluate the activities of these ingredients by conventional methods.

*Correspondence: fantasyee@btbu.edu.cn; wavingsea2008@gmail.com
[1] Key Laboratory of Cosmetic, China National Light Industry, Beijing Technology and Business University, No. 11/33, Fucheng Road, Haidian District, Beijing 100048, People's Republic of China
[3] Institute of Medicinal Plant Development, Chinese Academy of Medical Sciences, Peking Union Medical College, Beijing, 151 Malianwa North Road, Haidian District, Beijing 100193, People's Republic of China
Full list of author information is available at the end of the article

In recent years, with an increasingly in-depth understanding of the structure and function of compounds, a series of new technologies and methods have been applied to the development of medicinal plants [4]. If we can establish a quick and convenient pathway by which to first accurately predict a large number of chemical compounds and then, based on these results, perform in vivo and in vitro pharmacological experiments for verification, this procedure will significantly improve the efficiency of evaluating the chemical activities of medicinal plants [5]. Back to 1950s, Artemisinin, the most famous antimalarial drug, was also obtained through large-scale screening from herbs. After that, several FDA approved drugs were developed from natural herbs or animal through the in silico approaches. The first case use enzyme-inhibitor structure to develop drug was the Angiotensin converting enzyme inhibitor-Captopril in 1970s [6]. And the first FDA approved HIV-1 enzyme inhibitor—Saquinavir also developed by in silico approaches [7]. Nowadays, with the continuous advancement of computer science, successful examples of finding drugs from natural products using computer-aided drug design methods have become more frequently, such as Dozamide (Approved by FDA in 1995), Imatinib (Approved by FDA in 2001), Dasatinib (Approved by FDA in 2006), and Ponatinib (Approved by FDA in 2012) [8]. With the continuous maturation of computer technology, the in silico approach of utilizing a computer platform to calculate the combinations of simulated compounds and targets has become increasingly accurate. In addition, the development of network pharmacology technologies has enabled the rapid elucidation of the complex relationships between compounds and their various activity targets [9]. Traditional Chinese medicine (TCM) involves a highly complex system of chemical substances. Its complexity is not only reflected in the composition of the chemical constituents but also embodied in the network of relationships between the prescription and the human body and the exertion of pharmacological effects through multiple channels, multiple targets and the overall regulatory mechanism [10].

Regarding the implications of Chinese medicine informatics, the application of modern informational technology to study TCM must address information on a variety of characteristics of the medicines themselves, as well as the interactions between TCMs and the human body [11]. The definition of Chinese medicine informatics is as follows: an interdisciplinary science that applies information science theory and computer technology to study the regulation and process of TCM information flow and investigates the views of TCM practitioners for the purpose. The definition of network pharmacology is as follows: a new discipline based on systems biology theory, in which the network analysis of biological systems is used to select the characteristics of signal nodes for multi-target small molecular drug design [12]. Therefore, we can treat a single medicinal plant with the same complexity as TCM, utilizing technical means from TCM informatics and network pharmacology to explore the chemical composition and the potential pharmacological foundation of the plant's effects. In this paper, we elucidate the methodology in detail (Fig. 1).

Design of the methodology

In this paper, we elucidate the methodology in detail (Fig. 1). Considering the medicinal plant as the object and virtual computational screening as the central

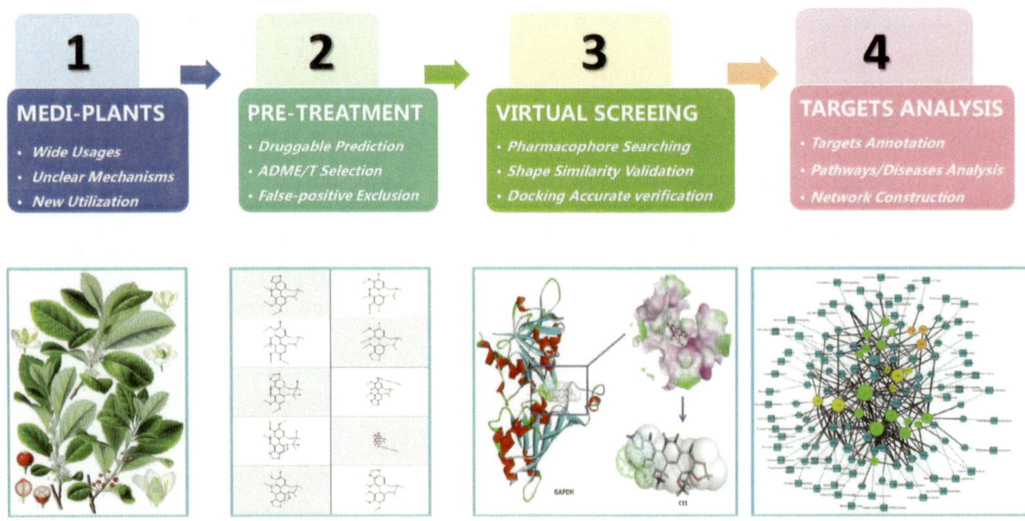

Fig. 1 The overall design of the methodology

methodology within Chinese medicine informatics, and using network pharmacology as the technical means, we have employed a set of effective and accurate methods to reveal the pharmacological basis of the effects of medicinal plant materials and predict the potential bioactivity of their compounds. The approach proceeds from the selection of the plant compounds to virtual screening and evaluation of the targets, related signalling pathways and disease networks. Techniques from virtual computational screening, Chinese medicine informatics and network pharmacology are used to construct a complete technical routine for this methodology. The first step is to confirm the research significance of the plants. These medicinal plants can be organized into three categories: (1) common herbs with a more complex mechanism than that of other herbs; (2) herbs with a long history of traditional usage but fewer studies on their phytochemistry and pharmacology; and (3) herbs with a history of traditional usage but now with a new utilization. The second step is the organization and collection of the natural products to construct the natural products database. The third step is the pre-treatment of these compounds, including drug-like analysis, ADME/T (absorption, distribution, metabolism, excretion and toxicity) prediction and the exclusion of false-positive compounds. The fourth step is the core technique of this methodology, the in silico virtual screening. We designed this step by combining three different theoretical bases: the first is virtual target fishing based on pharmacophore theory; the second is dual validation based on small molecule shape similarity theory; and the third is compound-target analysis based on docking. The fifth step is the analysis of the set of targets identified. By utilizing the technical methods of network pharmacology and different protein information databases and websites, we can analyse the relationships of signalling pathways, pathological pathways and related diseases with potential targets. Finally, we construct the network of relationships among medicinal plants, natural compounds, biological targets, signalling pathways, and diseases. We thereby elucidate the mechanistic basis of the effects of the natural compounds in medicinal plants and predict their potential pharmacological activities.

Confirmation of the objective

At present, the pharmacological mechanisms of numerous single compounds extracted from herbs have been elucidated. However, herbs contain diverse and complex compounds that are involved in multiple biological pathways and that correspond to different diseases. Therefore, investigating the different types of medicinal plants and their chemical constituents is a task with both broad and specific significance. We have recommended three categories of herbs that are suitable for the use of the in silico approach to unveil their chemical mechanisms. The first type of medicinal plants can be described by "common usage, but their mechanism is more complicated", such as *Panax notoginseng* (Burk.) F. H. Chen (Notoginseng), which is mainly cultivated in Yunan, China [13]. The medicinal part of notoginseng is its dry roots, and their main clinical activity is "scattered blood stasis, swelling pain". The noteworthy point is that notoginseng can not only promote blood circulation but also stop bleeding. The common theory regarding this two-way regulatory function is that the notoginseng saponins can invigorate the circulation of blood, while dencichine performs a haemostatic function [14]. Therefore, it is necessary to identify the pharmacological basis of the effects of the constituents of these herbs. The second type of medicinal plants is ones that "have a long history of traditional usage, but their study is in the early stages and not yet mature". Several medicinal plants in different regions have a history of more than 1000 years of traditional usage, such as "Peruvian ginseng" *Lepidium meyenii* Walp (maca), which is mainly distributed in the Andean mountains in the south of Peru at an altitude greater than 3000 m. The local people have consumed the subterranean part of maca to enhance their energy, improve their fertility and sexual function, or treat menopausal syndromes, rheumatism, depression, and anaemia for more than 1000 year [15]. However, pharmacological research on such plants only began in the last decade, so research on these medicinal plants is particularly important and urgent. The third category of medicinal plants are those that have new and different uses. To shorten the development cycle of new drugs, reduce risk and improve the success rate, new uses of traditional herbs in other diseases are often proposed. Berberine, also known as puerarin, is mainly extracted from *Coptis chinensis* Franch and has anti-bacterial activity. In vitro experiments show broad-spectrum anti-bacterial activity, which is mainly used clinically to treat digestive system infections such as acute gastroenteritis and dysentery. Interestingly, in recent years, researchers have found that berberine has an excellent effect in the treatment of cardiovascular disease [16]. Artemisinin, extracted from *Artemisia annua* L., was the most efficient anti-malarial drug in use for decades. Researchers have recently found that it can also counteract tuberculosis, diabetes, and trauma, treat systemic lupus erythaematosus and perform other pharmacological functions [17].

Research on the development and utilization of three types of medicinal plants is particularly likely to be valuable. Once the objectives (medicinal plants) have been selected for study, we can perform the next step, the collection of their compounds.

The acquisition of chemical compound information

A thorough understanding of the effective compounds in medicinal plants is the key to the research and development of medicinal plants. Therefore, the collection of constituent information and the construction of the compound database are highly important for their application. The construction of a compound database can effectively manage the large quantities of compounds found in medicinal plants.

Collection of chemical compound information

The information contained in a medicinal plant is the initial raw material for determining the basis of the herb's pharmacological properties. Compound information was mainly collected from the following sources: (1) separation and purification of the compounds in a local laboratory; (2) literature reports; and (3) small molecule compound databases. Among these three information-gathering pathways, the extraction of compounds in a local laboratory is the most direct and convenient method and can provide samples for later experimental studies. When a single compound is purified from herbs, the relevant information such as its recording number, CAS number, name, source plant, extractive fraction and structure information such as the SMILES code or InChiKey must be recorded. The compounds obtained from the laboratory are doubtless the best research objects; however, these compounds are often either relatively simple or difficult to obtain intact as constituents of a given herb. Therefore, the literature and various databases may offer a simple way to collect information on a set of different compounds from our herb of interest. To use these resources, relevant information such as the name, structure, classification and plant source must be recorded. With the continuous upgrades to virtual screening technology, the online large-scale direct search database has become a quicker and more convenient approach. At present, various research institutions, laboratories, government agencies and pharmaceutical enterprises have developed and constructed a number of small molecule compound databases reporting different characteristics and functions (Table 1).

Software and database of medicinal plant compounds

Many commercial or access-restricted software programs or websites can satisfy the needs of constructing a medicinal plant compound database. Different software programs focus on specific functions embodied in diverse storage formats, for instance, the accdb format of Microsoft Company, the MDB format within the MOE software, and the SDF format from Accelary Discovery Studio. A complete medicinal plant compound database must provide at least the following descriptors: (1) compound storage number; (2) compound name and CAS (Pubchem) ID; (3) sources of plant information (Latin name and extractive fraction); and (4) compound structure (SMILES code, InChiKey). In addition, several software programs can also calculate the relative molecular weight, the lipid partition coefficient (AlogP), the number of rotatable bonds, the number of hydrogen donors/receptors and other physical and chemical properties of compounds. The combination of all this relatively trivial information can make follow-up work requiring transparency and data processing more convenient.

Pre-treatment of chemical compounds

The number of compounds collected from medicinal plants is very high; however, the majority lack pharmacological potency. To enhance the efficiency of screening, the first step is to remove these non-potential compounds and refine the included compounds.

Prediction of drug-like properties

Drug-like characteristics are a qualitative concept used in drug design for a compound's utility with respect to factors such as bioavailability, which is estimated based on the molecular structure characteristics [31]. Certain structure properties indicate that a compound has a higher likelihood of becoming a successful drug. In the past, research on these properties of a drug has been among the most important components of downstream drug development. In recent years, it has become imperative to integrate the study of drug properties during the early stages of drug discovery. Pharmacologists are interested in the following properties of the drugs, among others: (1) structural characteristics: hydrogen bonding, polar surface area, lipophilicity, shape, molecular weight, and acid dissociation constant (*pKa*); (2) physicochemical properties: solubility, pH value, permeability and chemical stability; (3) biochemical properties: metabolism, protein binding affinity and transport ability; and (4) pharmacokinetics and toxicity: half-life, bioavailability, drug interactions and half lethal dose, LD50. According to Lipinski's proposal [32], a small molecule suitable for development as a drug needs the following properties (Lipinski's rule of five, RO5): (1) no more than 5 hydrogen bond donors (the total number of nitrogen–hydrogen and oxygen–hydrogen bonds); (2) no more than 10 hydrogen bond acceptors (all nitrogen or oxygen atoms); (3) a molecular mass less than 500 Daltons; and (4) an octanol–water partition coefficient logP not greater than (5) Small molecules that satisfy the RO5 criteria have higher bioavailability in the metabolic process of the organism and therefore are more likely to become oral medications. In 2002, Veber and his group presented

Table 1 Common small molecular databases overview

Databases	Development organizations	Websites	Overview	References
Alkamid Database	Ghent University, Belgium	http://www.alkamid.ugent.be	Provided the source of plants, biosynthetic pathways and pharmacological information of *N*-alkyl amides compounds in traditional medicinal plants	[18]
Asian Anti-Cancer Materia Database	Institute of East-West Medicine, USA	http://www.asiancancerherb.info/herbList/list_s.htm	Summarizes 700 kinds of anti-cancer drug information from Asia, which 80% is derived from medicinal plants. Afford the commonly used Chinese medicine name, Latin name, medicinal properties, the major compounds and other information	[19]
Chem-TCM	Institute of Pharmaceutical Science at King's College, UK	http://www.chemtcm.com	Contains more than 350 TCMs and their more than 9500 compounds. Record their compounds related plants, chemical properties, common target activities and other information	[20]
Chinese National Compound Library	National Health and Family Planning Commission of the People's Republic of China	http://www.app.cncl.org.cn	A library of small molecule compounds consisting of core libraries and satellite libraries. Contains nearly 2 million small molecules of the physical and chemical information	[20]
CHMIS-C (A Comprehensive Herbal Medicine Information System for Cancer)	University of Michigan Medical School, USA	http://www.sw16.im.med.umich.edu/chmis-c	Provided 527 anti-cancer herb prescriptions, 937 components and 9366 small molecule structures for the clinical treatment of different types of cancer, combined a reference database and a molecular target aided database	[21]
CNPD (Chinese Natural Products Database)	Shanghai Institute of Materia Medica, Chinese Academy of Sciences, China	http://www.neotrident.com/product/detail.aspx?id=16	The CNPD database currently collects more than 57,000 natural products from 37 categories, of which 70% of the molecules are drug-like molecules. The relevant data include the CAS number, name, molecular formula, molecular weight, melting point and other physical and chemical properties of natural products	[21]
KEGG Compound Database	Kyoto University, Japan	http://www.genome.jp/kegg/compound	Contains the name, molecular formula, relative molecular mass, structural formula, CAS number and corresponding chemical reaction or metabolic pathway of more than 17,000 metabolites and other small molecule compounds in the KEGG database	[22]

Table 1 (continued)

Databases	Development organizations	Websites	Overview	References
NAPRALERT (Natural Products Alert)	College of Pharmacy University of Illinois at Chicago, USA	http://www.napralert.org	A natural product relationship database according to more than 200,000 references which including pharmacology, biochemical information and data in various experiments (in vivo, in vitro, clinical, etc.)	[23]
NCI	National Cancer Institute, USA	https://cactus.nci.nih.gov/download/nci/	Database contains the chemical properties of compounds, such as the molecular formula, CAS number, and other common physical and chemical properties; anti-HIV activity and other related biological activity prediction value	[24]
TCM Database@Taiwan	China Medical University, Taiwan	http://www.tcm.cmu.edu.tw	Including 443 Traditional Chinese medicine and 20,000 kinds of ingredients, for the physical and chemical properties and 3D structure. Support the complete contents of the compounds from Chinese medicine and related references	[25]
TCMID (Traditional Chinese medicine Integrated Database	East China Normal University, China	http://www.megabionet.org/tcmid	Provide information on all aspects of Chinese medicine, including formula, herbal and herbal ingredients. Also collected information on drugs that are studied in depth by modern pharmacology and biomedical science	[26]
TCMSP	Center for Bioinformatics, College of Life Science, Northwest A&F University, China	http://www.lsp.nwsuaf.edu.cn/tcmsp.php	Contained 499 Chinese Parmacopoeia recorded TCMs and 29,384 compounds from these TCMs	[27]
Timtec	Timtec, Russia	http://www.timtec.net	Record more than 13,000 natural products and their derivatives structure information	[28]
TradiMed (Traditional Chinese medicine DB)	TradiMed, Korea	http://www.tradimed.com	Contains 11,810 prescriptions in 3199 Chinese and Korean traditional medicines and 20,012 chemical composition information	[29]
ZINC	University of California, USA	http://www.zinc.docking.org	Free compounds virtual screening database which included more than 35 million kinds of commercially available compounds 3D structure for docking	[30]

another set of system requirements for the oral administration of drugs that included the molecular flexibility, polar surface area (PSA) and number of hydrogen bonds, which were determined by a series of studies in rats: (1) no more than 10 rotatable bonds and (2) polar surface area no more than 140 Å^2 or no more than 12 hydrogen bonds and receptors [33]. However, there are still exceptions for special drug screening such as narcotic drug screening, which cannot rule out small molecular weight compounds, and those anti-tumour drugs cannot exclude metal organic compounds. Nowadays, several softwares can performing the drug-likeness prediction. Such as the Instant JChem from ChemAxon company which can calculate the RO5 properties, and the Discovery Studio software can both predict the Lipinski and Veber's rules [34].

ADME/T selection

When drug-likeness established from the analyses of the physiochemical properties and structural features of existing drug candidates, the ADME/T (absorption, distribution, metabolism, excretion and toxicity) properties play an important role in the drug filtering. So, we employed the ADME/T selection after other drug-likeness properties evaluated.

It is necessary to predict the situation and movement of a drug in the human body during the design of the drug molecule. During the early stages of drug design, the ADME/T properties of a drug are evaluated [35]. Absorption is the process of drug transport into the human circulatory system. Distribution is the penetration of the drug through the cell membrane barrier into the various tissues, organs or body fluids. As metabolism occurs, the initial (parent) compound is converted to new compounds called metabolites. The majority of small-molecule drug metabolism is carried out in the liver by redox enzymes, termed cytochrome P450 enzymes. Excretion is the removal of the initial form and metabolites of the drug from the human body. The toxicity of the drug also affects the human body. Several commercial software programs have equipped the ADME/T prediction module for drug molecules. For instance, the commercial software Discovery Studio provides an ADME/T descriptor module for candidate drug screening, which contains the following aspects: aqueous solubility, to predict the solubility of each compound in aqueous solvent; blood brain barrier penetration, to predict the ability of compounds to penetrate into the brain; and CYP2D6 enzyme binding capacity. The CYP2D6 enzyme is an important member of the CYP450 enzyme family and participates with the CYP3A4, CYP1A2, CYP2C9, and CYP2C19 enzymes in drug metabolism. The five major CYP enzymes are responsible for more than 95% of the drug metabolism in animals. The CYP2D6 enzyme normally accounts for approximately 2% of the CYP total but approximately 30% of the total drug metabolism. In clinical practice, the high CYP2D6 enzyme binding capacity of drug can reflect its excellent metabolism ability in the human body. The relevant criteria involve hepatotoxicity, the dose-dependent liver toxicity of the drug molecules; intestinal absorption, the absorption of drug molecules in the human body after oral administration; and plasma protein binding, the ability of the compound to bind to the carrier protein in the bloodstream.

Suitable pharmacokinetic properties and low toxicity during body absorption, distribution, metabolism and excretion are the key factors in successfully passing the clinical trials. Predicting the ADME/T properties of drug molecules prior to drug design and performing this screening can reduce the cost of drug development and improve the success rate of the whole procedure. For ADME/T properties rational predictive have been developed on mechanistic descriptions of the underlying biophysical processes. Some softwares can performing ADME/T such as Simulations Plus ADME/T predictor [36], PK-Map the Discovery Studio from Accerlary company [37].

Exclusion of false-positive compounds

Due to accidents or other reasons, some false-positive compounds are also included in the filtered sample library for the post-screening step. Most of these false-positive compounds are easily decomposed under hydrolytic conditions and react with proteins or biological nucleophiles (glutathione, dithiothreitol, etc.), which are easily detected by a positive result in an enzyme system or cell test. In fact, these false-positive compounds are mostly chemical reaction intermediates such as epoxides, aldehydes, haloalkanes, or compounds consisting of a conjugated system.

The concept and performance of virtual screening

The virtual screening of drugs can be defined as follows: based on the theories of drug design and new drug screening, with the aid of computer technology and professional software, selecting the theoretically active lead compounds from large quantities of compounds and then evaluating the activity experimentally. Virtual screening methods have three main theoretical foundations: molecular docking, pharmacophore theory, and small molecular shape similarity. According to the author's work experiences: these three methods have different applications and their own advantages and disadvantages (Table 2, Fig. 2).

Molecular docking relies on the characteristics of the receptor (drug target/protein/enzyme) itself and the interaction pattern with its small molecule ligand to

Table 2 Three virtual screening methods comparison

Methods	Molecular docking [38]	Pharmacophore model [39]	Small molecule shape similarity [40]
Theory basis	Molecular mechanics, quantum mechanics	Statistics	Graph theory and other mathematical methods
Overview	Obtain the receptor structure information and locate its binding site, mimic the interaction between the receptor and its ligands	Establish pharmacophore model, evaluate the matching degree between ligands 3D conformation and pharmacophore models	To investigate the structural similarity of unknown molecules by druggable molecules at known targets
Advantages	1. Algorithm is mature 2. A variety of optional softwares	1. High accuracy and efficiency 2. Several commercial pharmacophore databases	1. Fastest screening 2. Abundant data resources
Disadvantages	1. Relatively large amount of calculation 2. Huge data preparation workload 3. Results analysis takes a long time	1. Affected by the quality of pharmacophore model 2. Affected by the amount of protein crystals	1. Low accuracy and rough results 2. Require operator able to develop chemical software

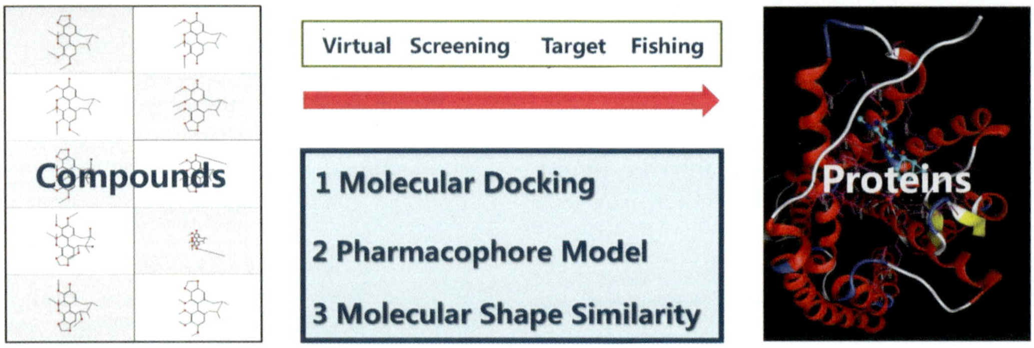

Fig. 2 Demonstration of virtual screening methods

perform drug design based on the ligand-receptor binding mode (the lock and key principle) [41]. The electrostatic interactions, hydrogen bonding, hydrophobic interaction and van der Waals forces are calculated to predict the ligand's binding mode and affinity. The pharmacophore is an abstract set of molecular features that are necessary for the molecular recognition of a ligand by a biological macromolecule [42]. The pharmacophore group refers to the spatial arrangement of the pharmacological characteristics of the small molecule in the drug, including the hydrogen bond donors, hydrogen bond acceptors, positive and negative charge centres, aromatic ring centre, hydrophobic groups, hydrophilic groups and geometric conformation. The biological activity of small molecules can be predicted by the summary of their pharmacological feature elements. Small molecule shape similarity can be defined as a database search technique based on the quantitative structure–activity relationships of compounds with the same mechanisms [43]. These three types of common screening software and their characteristics are listed in Table 3.

The focus of our research is to find the pharmacological basis of the effects of the constituents of medicinal plants. From this perspective, the pharmacophore model can be used to screen the large quantities of compounds from medicinal plants. In contrast, from the perspective of diseases and proteins, it is possible to use molecular docking to find the most likely active constituents.

Therefore, we design this core section methodology as follows: first, we perform batch screening based on the pharmacophore model theory to obtain the potential set of binding drugs. Subsequently, these results are verified by use of the small molecule shape similarity theory. Finally, when the target protein requires detailed study, molecular docking can be used to refine the active small molecules.

Virtual screening based on pharmacophore model

The geometrical matching and energy matching process between a drug molecule and its receptor are necessary features for the binding interaction. Different group structures exert different effects on the activity, while similar chemical characteristics have the same or similar pharmacological activities. The concept of the pharmacophore was first described by Paul Ehrlich in 1909 [63]. The pharmacophore refers to the molecular framework of

Table 3 Common virtual screening softwares overview

Softwares	Websites	Features	References
Molecular docking			
Affinity	http://www.accelrys.com/insight/affinity	Based on simulated annealing, molecular mechanics and molecular dynamics simulation of molecular pairs of procedures, the calculation is more accurate	[44]
AutoDock	http://www.scripps.edu/pub/olson-web/doc/autodock	Famous molecular docking program developed by the Scripps Institute. Which is one of the most widely used docking software	[44]
DOCK	http://www.dock.compbio.ucsf.edu	One of the most widely used molecular docking programs, free open access	[45]
DockVision	http://www.dockvision.com	A set of docking applets that support multiple algorithms	[46]
DockIt	http://www.metaphorics.com/dockit	Provide Energy, PLP and PMF evaluation methods	[47]
eHiTS	http://www.simbiosys.ca/ehits	eHiTS is an exhaustive flexible-docking method that systematically covers the part of the conformational and positional search space that avoids severe steric clashes, producing highly accurate docking poses at a speed practical for virtual high-throughput screening	[48]
FlexX	http://www.biosolveit.de/FlexX	The method can be used in the design process of specific protein ligands. It combines an appropriate model of the physico-chemical properties of the docked molecules with efficient methods for sampling the conformational space of the ligand	[49]
Glide	http://www.schrodinger.com/prods/glide	Glide approximates a complete systematic search of the conformational, orientational, and positional space of the docked ligand. In this search, an initial rough positioning and scoring phase that dramatically narrows the search space is followed by torsionally flexible energy optimization on an OPLS-AA nonbonded potential grid for a few hundred surviving candidate poses	[50]
GoldDock	http://www.ccdc.cam.ac.uk/prods/gold	GOLD is an automated ligand docking program that uses a genetic algorithm to explore the full range of ligand conformational flexibility with partial flexibility of the protein, and satisfies the fundamental requirement that the ligand must displace loosely bound water on binding. Numerous enhancements and modifications have been applied to the original technique resulting in a substantial increase in the reliability and the applicability of the algorithm	[51]
SystemsDock	http://www.systemsdock.unit.oist.jp	SystemsDock is a web server for network pharmacology-based prediction and analysis, which applies high-precision docking simulation and molecular pathway map to comprehensively characterize the ligand selectivity and to illustrate how a ligand acts on a complex molecular network	[52]
ZDOCK	http://www.zlab.bu.edu/rong/dock	Protein–Protein docking procedure based on geometric matching. With a goal of providing an accessible and intuitive interface, ZDOCK provide options for users to guide the scoring and the selection of output models, in addition to dynamic visualization of input structures and output docking models	[53]
Pharmacophore model			
Apex-3D	http://www.biosym.com/apex-3d	Activity prediction expert system with 3D-QSAR. pharmacophore identification based on logical structure analysis	[54]
DISCOtech	http://www.tripos.com/discotech	Distance comparison technique provide multi-drug group model for database search, auto recognize the priority	[55]
Discovery Studio	http://www.accelrys.com/	Powerful pharmacophore identification and database search software	[56]
GASP	http://www.tripos.com/gasp	Based on genetic algorithm to realize flexible stacking between drug molecules	[57]

Table 3 (continued)

Softwares	Websites	Features	References
SEAware	http://www.seachangepharma.com/store/academic/products	Chemically similar drugs often bind to biologically diverse targets, making it difficult to predict what off-target effects a drug might have by protein structure or sequence alone. The similarity ensemble approach (SEA) addresses this problem using a different strategy; it groups receptors according to the chemical similarity of their ligands, and can identify unknown relationships between ligands and receptors amenable to experimental testing	[58]
Small molecule shape similarity			
CerberuS		CerBeruS is a method developed for iterative screening. CerBeruS is based on Daylight fingerprints. CerBeruS proposes only highly similar molecules for testing. This strategy results in a high hit rate but is unlikely to identify new scaffolds or lead series	[59]
FlexS	http://www.biosolveit.de/FlexS/	FlexS is an incremental construction procedure. The molecules to be superimposed are partitioned into fragments. Starting with placements of a selected anchor fragment, computed by two alternative approaches, the remaining fragments are added iteratively. At each step, flexibility is considered by allowing the respective added fragment to adopt a discrete set of conformations. The mean computing time per test case is about 1:30 min on a common-day workstation	[60]
BRUTUS		BRUTUS aligns molecules using field information derived from charge distributions and van der Waals shapes of the compounds. Molecules can have similar biological properties if their charge distributions and shapes are similar, even though they have different chemical structures; that is, BRUTUS can identify compounds possessing similar properties, regardless of their structures	[61]
WEGA	http://www.rcdd.org.cn/home/program.html	(WEGA), is proposed to improve the accuracy of the first order approximation. The new approach significantly improves the accuracy of molecular volumes and reduces the error of shape similarity calculations by 37% using the hard-sphere model as the reference. The new algorithm also keeps the simplicity and efficiency of the FOGA (First Order Gaussian Approximation)	[62]

atoms with active and essential features that allow identification of their pharmacological activities. In 1977, Peter Gund further defined the pharmacophore as a group of molecular features that participate in a molecular biological activity. At present, the definition of the pharmacophore is pharmacodynamics elements and their spatial arrangement. These 'potency elements' can be specific atoms such as an oxygen atom or carbonyl group or abstract functional structures: hydrogen bond acceptor/donor, positive/negative ionizable charge, aromatic ring, hydrophilic group, the location and orientation of atoms, or the distance, tolerance and exclusion volume of atoms. The pharmacophore is a summary of a series of biologically active molecules that effectively describes the structural features that play the most important roles in activity. The pharmacophore is not representative of a single molecule or a specific functional group. It can represent a group of compounds and the important interaction information on the same receptor class or can be considered a large number of active compounds with common drug characteristics. The construction of a pharmacophore model can be used for the virtual screening of a small molecule library, searching for new skeletal active molecules, predicting the activity of compounds, and optimizing and modifying them. The pharmacophore can also qualitatively quantify the structure–activity relationships of compounds and elucidate the selectivity mechanism of the compounds [64]. During the process of virtual screening, the pharmacophore model can be used to characterize the active conformation of the ligand molecule by conformational search and molecular superposition, and the possible mode of action between the receptor and the ligand molecule can be deduced and explained accordingly.

In addition, a reverse search based on the pharmacophore can solve several common issues focused on the chemical constituents of the medicinal plants, such as its specific targets, therapeutic effect and how to find or construct a similar role among synthesized compounds. Currently, the active ingredients of the medicinal plans can be elucidated by utilizing different commercial software launched by many companies, which can afford virtual screening modules based on pharmacophore theory. We recommend The Discovery Studio developed by the Accelary Company, which equipped the PharmaDB and Hypo DB, these databases contained thousands of pharmacophore models from sc-PDB recorded information.

Validation based on ligand molecule shape similarity

Molecular shape similarity analysis is based on the similarity of small molecules as the index for the database mapping search. Similar to pharmacophore theory, molecular shape similarity analysis can effectively utilize the overall structural characteristics of those compounds. For now, molecular shape similarity analysis is specifically applied to scaffold hopping and shape discrimination [65].

Due to the rule that "molecules with similar structure may have similar or the same biological activity", during the drug design process, a pharmacist might choose the ligand shape similarity screening method. Generally, small molecule compounds with known activity and targets are used to search for the molecular structure of chemicals in the compound database according to the shape similarity of the potential sample compounds.

During the establishment of this methodology, since the molecular shape similarity screening approach involves a faster process but more challenging result limitations and peculiarities, this method is not suitable for use as the main approach in virtual screening but rather as a validation based on efficacy. At present, many commercial software programs can perform molecular shape similarity operations, including CerberuS, FlexS, and MIMIC. We suggest to choose the WEGA (weighted Gaussian algorithm), is a typical virtual screening method based on ligand shape similarity that was established by Professor Xu Jun's group from Sun Yat-sen University [56]. The WEGA already can performing in TianHe No. 2 supercomputing platform to ensure its efficiency. The accuracy of the results from another pathway can be evaluated by comparing the shape similarity between the small molecules of those ligands corresponding to the known drug targets and the small molecules yet to be tested.

Accurate verification based on molecular docking theory

The conceptual basis of molecular docking originated from the "lock and key principle model" proposed 100 years ago. The principle of molecular docking is to place a series of test compounds with known three-dimensional structures in turn at the active site of the biological target molecule [66]. The optimal binding conformation of the compound with the target molecule is found by continuously improving the conformation, position, dihedral angle of each rotatable bond, and amino acid residue side chain and backbone of the compound in space and predicting their combination patterns and affinities. The molecular docking method can use a variety of scoring standards to select the most natural conformation of the compound and optimize its affinity to the target according to theoretical analogue molecular interactions. Autodock, FlexX, ICM, GoldDocK, LigandFit and Glide can all perform molecular docking. Due to the accuracy, sensitivity and specificity of the molecular docking, we can use it to refine the results obtained from the pharmacophore model and shape similarity theory. The Autodock is the most used tool for molecular docking in recently years due to its fast and friendly interface. We also recommend LigandFit algorithm: A method employs a cavity detection algorithm for detecting invaginations in the protein as candidate active site regions. A shape comparison filter is combined with a Monte Carlo conformational search for generating ligand poses consistent with the active site shape. Candidate poses are minimized in the context of the active site using a grid-based method for evaluating protein–ligand interaction energies and due to its can comparing enormous poses of ligands, which is suitable for high-throughput screening.

Analysis of target sets

Analysis and annotation of target information

After obtaining the druggable targets by virtual screening, we need to analyse the relevant information on the targets: target type, protein structure, binding pocket shape, associated pathway and corresponding diseases. The targets are usually nominated according to their UniProt ID. UniProt is an abbreviation for the Universal Protein Database program, which consists of the Swiss-Prot, TrEMBL and PIR-PSD databases and is the largest database containing the most informative data resources and protein structures [67]. Using the UniProt ID, detailed information regarding the target protein can obtained at the UniProt website (http://www.uniprot.org/), including the protein name, gene name, organism, sequence information, taxonomy, family and domains, and related molecular functions and biological processes. This database can also link to other databases by searching based on the PDB ID, KEGG ID and other information. In addition to UniProt, many other databases and software programs can also analyse the category and function of these fished targets and their corresponding diseases. Table 4 summarizes the commonly used databases and analysis software.

Table 4 Common druggable targets/protein databases overview

Databases	Developers	Websites	Abstract	References
Binding DB	Skaggs School of Pharmacy & Pharmaceutical Sciences, USA	http://www.bindingdb.org/bind/index.jsp	BindingDB is a public, web-accessible database of measured binding affinities, focusing chiefly on the interactions of proteins considered to be candidate drug-targets with ligands that are small, drug-like molecules	[68]
BioGRID (Biological General Repository for Interaction Datasets)	BioGRID, Canada	http://www.thebiogrid.org	BioGRID is an interaction repository with data compiled through comprehensive curation efforts. Our current index is version 3.4.151 and searches 63,354 publications for 1,493,749 protein and genetic interactions, 27,785 chemical associations and 38,559 post translational modifications from major model organism species. All data are freely provided via our search index and available for download in standardized formats	[69]
DAVID (Database for Annotation, Visualization, and Integrated Discovery)	Laboratory of Human Retrovirology and Immunoinformatics, USA	http://www.david.ncifcrf.gov	The database for annotation, visualization and integrated discovery Able to perform: Identify enriched biological themes, discover enriched functional-related gene groups, list interacting proteins and other functions	[70]
DRUGBANK	Canadian Institutes of Health Research, Canada	http://www.drugbank.ca	The DrugBank database is a unique bioinformatics and cheminformatics resource that combines detailed drug data with comprehensive drug target information. The database contains 9591 drug entries including 2037 FDA-approved small molecule drugs, 241 FDA-approved biotech drugs, 96 nutraceuticals and over 6000 experimental drugs. Additionally, 4661 non-redundant protein (sequences are linked to these drug entries	[71]
GeneMANIA	University of Toronto, Canada	http://www.genemania.org	GeneMANIA finds other genes that are related to a set of input genes, using a very large set of functional association data. Association data include protein and genetic interactions, pathways, co-expression, co-localization and protein domain similarity. You can use GeneMANIA to find new members of a pathway or complex, find additional genes you may have missed in your screen or find new genes with a specific function, such as protein kinases. Your question is defined by the set of genes you input	[72]

Table 4 (continued)

Databases	Developers	Websites	Abstract	References
HPRD (Human Protein Reference Database)	Johns Hopkins University and the Institute of Bioinformatics, USA	http://www.hprd.org	HPRD is a database of curated proteomic information pertaining to human proteins. All the information in HPRD has been manually extracted from the literature by expert biologists who read, interpret and analyze the published data	[73]
IntAct	European Molecular Biology Laboratory	http://www.ebi.ac.uk/intact	IntAct is an open-source, open data molecular interaction database populated by data either curated from the literature or from direct data depositions	[74]
KEGG (Kyoto Encyclopedia of Genes and Genomes)	Kyoto University, Japan	http://www.kegg.jp	KEGG (Kyoto Encyclopedia of Genes and Genomes) is a database resource that integrates genomic, chemical and systemic functional information. In particular, gene catalogs from completely sequenced genomes are linked to higher-level systemic functions of the cell, the organism and the ecosystem. KEGG is widely used as a reference knowledge base for integration and interpretation of large-scale datasets generated by genome sequencing and other high-throughput experimental technologies. In addition to maintaining the aspects to support basic research, KEGG is being expanded towards more practical applications integrating human diseases, drugs and other health-related substances	[75]
MAS3.0	CapitalBio, China	http://www.bioinfo.capitalbio.com	MAS (Molecule Annotation System) is a whole data-mining and function annotation solution to extract and analyze biological molecules relationships from public knowledgebase of biological molecules and signification. MAS analysis platform is a web client program for interactive navigation in the knowledge base. MAS uses relational database of biological networks created from millions of individually modeled relationships between genes, proteins, diseases and tissues. MAS allow a view on your data, integrated in biological networks according to different biological context. This unique feature results from multiple lines of evidence which are integrated in MAS' database. MAS Help to understand relationship of gene expression data	[76]

Table 4 (continued)

Databases	Developers	Websites	Abstract	References
MINT (The Molecular INTeraction Database)	Department of Biology, University of Rome, Italy	http://www.mint.bio.uniroma2.it/	The MINT is a public repository for protein–protein interactions (PPI) reported in peer-reviewed journals. The database grows steadily over the years and at September 2011 contains approximately 235 000 binary interactions captured from over 4750 publications	[77]
PharmMapper Server	Shanghai Institute of Materia Medica, China	http://lilab.ecust.edu.cn/pharmmapper/index.php	PharmMapper Server is a freely accessed web-server designed to identify potential target candidates for the given probe small molecules (drugs, natural products, or other newly discovered compounds with binding targets unidentified) using pharmacophore mapping approach. Benefited from the highly efficient and robust mapping method, PharmMapper bears high throughput ability and can identify the potential target candidates from the database within a few hours	[78]
Potential Drug Target Database (PDTD)	Shanghai Institute of Materia Medica, China	http://www.dddc.ac.cn/pdtd/index.php	PDTD is a dual function database that associates an informatics database to a structural database of known and potential drug targets. PDTD is a comprehensive, web-accessible database of drug targets, and focuses on those drug targets with known 3D-structures. PDTD contains 1207 entries covering 841 known and potential drug targets with structures from the Protein Data Bank	[79]
RCSB PDB (Protein Data Bank)	Research Collaboratory for Structural Bioinformatics: Rutgers and UCSD/SDSC	http://www.rcsb.org/pdb/home	A global resource for the advancement of research and education in biology and medicine. Along with our Worldwide PDB collaborators, RCSB PDB curates, annotates, and makes publicly available the PDB data deposited by scientists around the globe. The RCSB PDB then provides a window to these data through a rich online resource with powerful searching, reporting, and visualization tools for researchers	[80]

Table 4 (continued)

Databases	Developers	Websites	Abstract	References
Reactome	European Bioinformatics Institute (EMBL-EBI)	http://www.reactome.org	The Reactome provides molecular details of signal transduction, transport, DNA replication, metabolism and other cellular processes as an ordered network of molecular transformations—an extended version of a classic metabolic map, in a single consistent data model	[81]
STITCH (search tool for interactions of chemicals)	European Molecular Biology Laboratory, Germany	http://www.stitch.embl.de	STITCH is a database of known and predicted interactions between chemicals and proteins. The interactions include direct (physical) and indirect (functional) associations; they stem from computational prediction, from knowledge transfer between organisms, and from interactions aggregated from other (primary) databases	[82]
STRING (Search Tool for the Retrieval of Interacting Genes/Proteins)	Swiss Institute of Bioinformatics, Switzerland	http://www.string-db.org	STRING is a database of known and predicted protein–protein interactions. The interactions include direct (physical) and indirect (functional) associations; they stem from computational prediction, from knowledge transfer between organisms, and from interactions aggregated from other (primary) databases	[83]
TTD (Therapeutic Target Database)	Department of Computational Science National University of Singapore, Singapore	http://www.bidd.nus.edu.sg/group/cjttd	Therapeutic target database (TTD) is a database to provide information about the known and explored therapeutic protein and nucleic acid targets, the targeted disease, pathway information and the corresponding drugs directed at each of these targets. Also included in this database are links to relevant databases containing information about target function, sequence, 3D structure, ligand binding properties, enzyme nomenclature and drug structure, therapeutic class, clinical development status. All information provided are fully referenced	[84]
Uniprot (Univeral Protein)	UniProt Consortium	http://www.uniprot.org	The Universal Protein Resource (UniProt) is a comprehensive resource for protein sequence and annotation data. The UniProt databases are the UniProt Knowledgebase (UniProtKB), the UniProt Reference Clusters (UniRef), and the UniProt Archive (UniParc)	[67]

Construction of network pharmacology

In contrast to the chemical drug action model, traditional medicinal herbs, TCMs or formulas all have a wide variety of ingredients, a broad range of drug targets and complex mechanistic characteristics, leading to challenges in elucidating their mechanisms and action models. Network pharmacology is based on the theory of systems biology. It treats each drug, target, gene, pathway and disease as a specific signal node and each action model as an edge to construct a topological network map of their complex relationships [85]. The multi-component, multi-target and multi-pathway mechanisms of medicinal plants can be elucidated by analysing the interrelationships in this topological network map, making traditional medicinal plants available for modern research and innovation. A variety of software programs and web databases can currently analyse the relevant information on target sets and their related pathways and diseases. Examples include the Ingenuity Pathway Analysis (IPA) software from QIAGEN Bioinformatics [86], the KEGG pathway database developed by Kyoto University [87] and MetaCore by Thomson Reuters [88]. The analyses of the principles and characteristics performed by each program also vary. The Causal Network Analysis and Upstream Regulator Analysis tools in IPA can predict the type of disease and associated signalling pathways that correspond to a list of genes and give separate weights for the resulting compound data set. MetaCore uses a massive collection of literature information to identify the small molecules and related proteins corresponding to the underlying disease pathways.

Through the above steps, we can obtain a large amount of information on a medicinal plant, compound, target, pathway, or disease and its interrelationships by analysing the results of the virtual screening and target analysis. Different network visualization tools can show the relationships between these related nodes. Commonly applied software programs and their features are summarized in Table 5. Among them, the open access software Cytoscape is currently the most widely used tool due to its powerful graphical effects and its extensive compatibility with other software programs and databases. The core function of Cytoscape is network construction, which can build a two-dimensional topological network map within each node by edges and then concisely and clearly analyse the pharmacological basis and mechanism of medicinal plants. Each type of node (protein, compound and disease) and their relationship strength can be edited and analysed separately. Cytoscape can also link directly to external public databases and currently offers a variety of plugins to satisfy diverse analysis requirements. Pajek means spider in Slovenian and is another software program for network analysis. Pajek has the ability to break a large and complex network into smaller networks to utilize more efficient methods for further processing. It can also supply powerful visualization tools to implement large-scale (subquadratic) network algorithm analysis.

Vine tea (VT) originates from the plant *Ampelopsis grossedentata*, which belongs to the family Vitaceae. VT is mainly distributed in the south of China, and pharmacological studies have shown that it has anti-inflammatory and anti-tumour functions and can decrease hypoglycaemia and protect liver function [96]. However, its specific activity components and their mechanism remain unclear. Using the methodology constructed previously, its mechanism can be adequately predicted.

Firstly, we collected 94 compounds from VT which were all reported, and all chemical structures were prepared in SD format. Molecular energy was minimized using the Energy Minimization module of Discovery Studio version 4.5 (DS 4.5; Accelrys Inc., San Diego, CA, USA) under the chemistry at Harvard Macromolecular Mechanics (CHARMM) force field and construction of the 3D multi-conformational VT compounds molecular structure database (VT-DB), which was generated by a Monte Carlo-based conformational analysis (FAST mode). After ADME/T selection in DS4.5 ADME/T property module, the pharmacophore-based target fishing was performed in DS4.5. All those fished protein targets were through the second refine by using WEGA validation. For each target, the protein name, gene name, and pathway information were collected from the PDB, KEGG, DRUNGBANK and TDD. The overall VT compound-target-pathway networks were generated using Cytoscape V3.2.

In Fig. 3, the topological analysis of the interaction network provides insights into its biologically relevant connectivity patterns. The pharmacological network of VT contains three types of nodes. The compounds extracted from VT form the external part of the network (pink octagon) and surround their fished target nodes (blue quadrangle). Each target is linked to at least one disease (green circle). A general overview of the global topological properties of the VT network can obtained from this figure. The figure clearly shows that the effects of the compounds in VT are usually "multiple to multiple", which reflects the material basis of the VT and its hypoglycaemic and lipid-lowering activities.

Conclusion and perspectives

In this paper, we have proposed a wide-ranging complete technical route that utilizes a series of in silico approaches to reveal the pharmacological basis of the effects of medicinal plants, first to determine the object of study and then to obtain its natural constituents and

Table 5 Common visualization tool overview

Tools	Websites	Features	References
CADLIVE	http://www.cadlive.jp	CADLIVE (Computer-Aided Design of LIVing systEms) is a comprehensive computational tool for constructing large-scale biological network maps, analyzing the topological features of them, and simulating their dynamics	[89]
Cytoscape	http://www.cytoscape.org	Cytoscape is an open source software platform for visualizing molecular interaction networks and biological pathways and integrating these networks with annotations, gene expression profiles and other state data	[90]
Graphviz	http://www.graphviz.org	Graphviz is open source graph visualization software. Graph visualization is a way of representing structural information as diagrams of abstract graphs and networks. It has important applications in networking, bioinformatics, software engineering, database and web design, machine learning, and in visual interfaces for other technical domains	[91]
Pajek	http://www.mrvar.fdv.unilj.si/pajek	Pajek is a program package for analysis and visualization of large networks (networks containing up to one billion of vertices, there is no limit-except the memory size-on the number of lines). It has been available for 20 years	[92]
VANTED	http://www.vanted.ipkgatersleben.de	VANTED is a tool for the visualization and analysis of networks with related experimental data. Data from large-scale biochemical experiments is uploaded into the software via a Microsoft Excel-based form. Then it can be mapped on a network that is either drawn with the tool itself, downloaded from the KEGG Pathway database, or imported using standard network exchange formats. Transcript, enzyme, and metabolite data can be presented in the context of their underlying networks	[93]
VisANT	http://www.visant.bu.edu/	VisANT is an application for integrating biomolecular interaction data into a cohesive, graphical interface. This software features a multi-tiered architecture for data flexibility, separating back-end modules for data retrieval from a front-end visualization and analysis package	[94]
YANAsquare	http://www.yana.bioapps.biozentrum.uni-wuerzburg.de	YANAsquare provides a software framework for rapid network assembly (flexible pathway browser with local or remote operation mode), network overview (visualization routine and YANAsquare editor) and network performance analysis (calculation of flux modes as well as target and robustness tests)	[95]

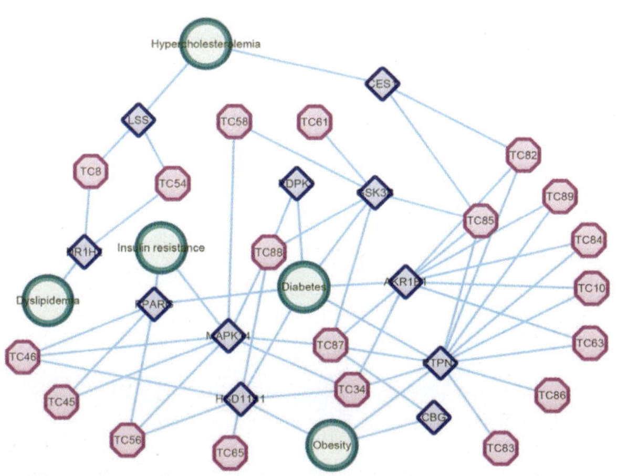

Fig. 3 The topological network relationships between compounds, targets and diseases associated with VT

construct the compound database. After pre-processing of the included compounds, a three-step virtual screening is performed. Finally, network pharmacology tools can be used to analyse the target set obtained from the screening; sketch out the network topological map of the medicinal plants, natural constituents, biological targets, associated pathways, related diseases and their interactions; and elaborate on the results.

The proposed joint methodology combines multiple in silico approaches and, through the full use of a series of virtual screening and network pharmacology tools, can clarify the substance basis and the mechanism of medicinal plants. The first half of this methodology uses software technology, including compound activity forecasting and virtual screening, all based on mass experimental data, to provide pinpoint accuracy. This methodology is superior to conventional screening because it requires only structural information on compounds and can perform multi-target screening of a vast number of compounds in a relatively short period of time, which can drastically reduce the cost and time of drug development. Moreover, combining this in silico methodology with pertinent pharmacological experiments could significantly enhance the efficiency of medicinal plant research and new drug discovery. The latter half of the methodology is guided by network pharmacology theory and uses multiple analysis tools and related databases to obtain relevant information from massive bio-information resources; build a network topological map of medicinal plants, chemical constituents, genes, proteins, pathways and diseases; and perform data mining and analysis.

This in silico methodology can resolve the status of medicinal plants that are difficult to study on a practical level and can predict and clarify the mechanisms of the active ingredients in medicinal plants.

Although computer-aided drug design and network pharmacology have been widely used and developed, there still have deficiencies and limitations: (1) The model maturity and computational accuracy of computer docking algorithms need to be further improved. (2) Due to the structure-based methodology, several compounds are not suitable for computer-aided design because of their special structure characteristics. (3) A large number of databases can improve different information for the obtained potential targets, the progress of the selection of these databases and their effective information annotation, still requires continuously practical activities to optimize. With the advancement of computer science, and the constant optimization of algorithms, including the maturity of the protein model. Through more practical researches and development examples to upgrade the entire process of in silico methodology, we believe that in the future, this methodological process will enable the discovery of new drugs more efficiently, accurately and quickly. This methodology will be more widely usable in future work on revealing and predicting the basis of medicinal materials.

Abbreviations

TCM: Traditional Chinese medicine; ADME/T: absorption, distribution, metabolism, excretion and toxicity; RO5: Lipinski's rule of five; WEGA: weighted Gaussian algorithm; VT: vine tea.

Authors' contributions

PGX and HBL designed the methodology. FY performed the experimental computing and data analysis, prepared the figures and wrote the paper. LL, LJX, YMD and HM collected the relevant information. All authors read and approved the final manuscript.

Author details

[1] Key Laboratory of Cosmetic, China National Light Industry, Beijing Technology and Business University, No. 11/33, Fucheng Road, Haidian District, Beijing 100048, People's Republic of China. [2] Beijing Key Laboratory of Plant Resources Research and Development, Beijing Technology and Business University, No. 11/33, Fucheng Road, Haidian District, Beijing 100048, People's Republic of China. [3] Institute of Medicinal Plant Development, Chinese Academy of Medical Sciences, Peking Union Medical College, Beijing, 151 Malianwa North Road, Haidian District, Beijing 100193, People's Republic of China.

Acknowledgements

We very grateful to Pr. Jun Xu (Research Centerfor Drug Discovery, School of Pharmaceutical Sciences, Sun Yat-sen University, Guangzhou) for his valuable suggestions.

Competing interests

The authors declare that they have no competing interests.

Funding

This study was supported by the Beijing Technology and Business University Youth Scholars Fund: PXM2018_014213_000033; and the Key Laboratory of Cosmetic, China National Light Industry, Beijing Technology and Business University Innovation Fund ID: KLC-2017-YB3.

References

1. Schippmann U, Cunningham AB, Leaman DJ. Impact of cultivation and gathering of medicinal plants on biodiversity: global trends and issues. Rome: FAO; 2002. p. 142–67.
2. Koutsoukas A, et al. From in silico target prediction to multi-target drug design: current databases, methods and applications. J Proteom. 2011;74(12):2554–74.
3. Zhang X, et al. Danshen-Chuanxiong-Honghua Ameliorates cerebral impairment and improves spatial cognitive deficits after transient focal ischemia and identification of active compounds. Front Pharmacol. 2017;8:452.
4. Yi F, et al. In silico approach for anti-thrombosis drug discovery: P2Y1R structure-based TCMs screening. Front Pharmacol. 2016;7:531.
5. Yi F, et al. In silico profiling for secondary metabolites from Lepidium meyenii (maca) by the pharmacophore and ligand-shape-based joint approach. Chin Med. 2016;11(1):42.
6. Tu Y. The discovery of artemisinin (qinghaosu) and gifts from Chinese medicine. Nat Med. 2011;17(10):1217–20.
7. Zaman MA, Oparil S, Calhoun DA. Drugs targeting the renin-angiotensin-aldosterone system. Nat Rev Drug Discov. 2002;1(8):621–36.
8. Ghosh AK, Gemma S. Structure-based design of drugs and other bioactive molecules. Hoboken: John Wiley & Sons; 2015. p. 397–409.
9. Rubio-Perez C, et al. In silico prescription of anticancer drugs to cohorts of 28 tumor types reveals targeting opportunities. Cancer Cell. 2015;27(3):382–96.
10. Zhang Y, et al. Pathway of PPAR-gamma coactivators in thermogenesis: a pivotal traditional Chinese medicine-associated target for individualized treatment of rheumatoid arthritis. Oncotarget. 2016;7(13):15885–900.
11. Ehrman TM, Barlow† DJ, Hylands‡ PJ. Phytochemical informatics of Traditional Chinese medicine and therapeutic relevance. J Chem Inf Model. 2007;47(6):2316–34.
12. Liu C, et al. Uncovering pharmacological mechanisms of Wu-tou decoction acting on rheumatoid arthritis through systems approaches: drug-target prediction, network analysis and experimental validation. Scientific Rep. 2015;5:9463.
13. Gao B, et al. Platelet P2Y12 receptors are involved in the haemostatic effect of notoginsenoside Ft1, a saponin isolated from Panax notoginseng. Br J Pharmacol. 2014;171(1):214.
14. Ji W, et al. Water-compatible molecularly imprinted polymers for selective solid phase extraction of dencichine from the aqueous extract of Panax notoginseng. J Chromatogr B. 2016;1008:225.
15. Esparza E, et al. Bioactive maca (Lepidium meyenii) alkamides are a result of traditional Andean postharvest drying practices. Phytochemistry. 2015;116:138–48.
16. Li Z, et al. Antioxidant and anti-inflammatory activities of berberine in the treatment of diabetes mellitus. Evid Based Complement Altern Med eCAM. 2014;2014(33):289264.
17. Liu H-K. Artemisinin, GABA signaling and cell reprogramming: when an old drug meets modern medicine. Sci Bull. 2017;62(6):386–7.
18. Boonen J, et al. Alkamid database: chemistry, occurrence and functionality of plant N-alkylamides. J Ethnopharmacol. 2012;142(3):563–90.
19. Umashankar V, Nandhitha S, Kalabharath P. InPACdb—Indian plant anticancer compounds database. Bioinformation. 2009;4(2):71–4.
20. Kim S-K, et al. TM-MC: a database of medicinal materials and chemical compounds in Northeast Asian traditional medicine. BMC Complement Altern Med. 2015;15(1):218.
21. Fang X, et al. CHMIS-C: a comprehensive herbal medicine information system for cancer. J Med Chem. 2005;48(5):1481–8.
22. Chen L, et al. Identification of compound–protein interactions through the analysis of gene ontology, KEGG enrichment for pro-

teins and molecular fragments of compounds. Mol Genet Genomics. 2016;291(6):2065–79.
23. Loub WD, et al. NAPRALERT: computer handling of natural product research data. J Chem Inf Comput Sci. 1985;25(2):99–103.
24. Ihlenfeldt WD, et al. Enhanced CACTVS browser of the open NCI database. J Chem Inf Comput Sci. 2002;42(1):46.
25. Chen CY-C. TCM Database@ Taiwan: the world's largest traditional Chinese medicine database for drug screening in silico. PLoS ONE. 2011;6(1):e15939.
26. Xue R, et al. TCMID: Traditional Chinese medicine integrative database for herb molecular mechanism analysis. Nucleic Acids Res. 2013;41(Database issue):D1089.
27. Ru J, et al. TCMSP: a database of systems pharmacology for drug discovery from herbal medicines. J Cheminform. 2014;6(1):13.
28. Luo M, Reid T-E, Simon Wang X. Discovery of natural product-derived 5-HT1A receptor binders by cheminfomatics modeling of known binders, high throughput screening and experimental validation. Comb Chem High Throughput Screen. 2015;18(7):685–92.
29. Yi Y-D, Chang I-M. An overview of traditional Chinese herbal formulae and a proposal of a new code system for expressing the formula titles. Evid Based Complement Altern Med. 2004;1(2):125–32.
30. Irwin JJ, et al. ZINC: a free tool to discover chemistry for biology. J Chem Inf Model. 2012;52(7):1757–68.
31. Kerns EH, Li D. Drug-like properties: concepts, structure design and methods. Oxford: Elsevier LTD; 2008. p. 125–6.
32. Lipinski CA, et al. Experimental and computational approaches to estimate solubility and permeability in drug discovery and development settings1. Adv Drug Deliv Rev. 2001;46(1–3):3–26.
33. Veber DF, et al. Molecular properties that influence the oral bioavailability of drug candidates. J Med Chem. 2002;45(12):2615–23.
34. Eldehna WM, et al. Synthesis and cytotoxic activity of biphenylurea derivatives containing indolin-2-one moieties. Molecules. 2016;21(6):762.
35. Van De Waterbeemd H, Gifford E. ADMET in silico modelling: towards prediction paradise? Nature reviews. Drug Discov. 2003;2(3):192.
36. Dhiman V, et al. Characterization of stress degradation products of amodiaquine dihydrochloride by liquid chromatography with high-resolution mass spectrometry and prediction of their properties by using ADMET predictor. J Sep Sci. 2017;40(23):4530–40.
37. Willmann S, Lippert J, Schmitt W. From physicochemistry to absorption and distribution: predictive mechanistic modelling and computational tools. Expert Opin Drug Metab Toxicol. 2005;1(1):159–68.
38. Morris GM, Limwilby M. Molecular docking. New York: Humana Press; 2008. p. 365–82.
39. Sun H. Pharmacophore-based virtual screening. Curr Med Chem. 2008;15(10):1018–24.
40. Najmanovich RJ, et al. Analysis of binding site similarity, small-molecule similarity and experimental binding profiles in the human cytosolic sulfotransferase family. Bioinformatics. 2007;23(2):e104.
41. Ewing TJA, et al. DOCK 4.0: search strategies for automated molecular docking of flexible molecule databases. J Comput Aided Mol Des. 2001;15(5):411–28.
42. Yang H, et al. X-ray crystallographic structure of a teixobactin analogue reveals key interactions of the teixobactin pharmacophore. Chem Commun. 2017;53(18):2772–5.
43. Chen YC, et al. Prediction of protein pairs sharing common active ligands using protein sequence, structure, and ligand similarity. J Chem Inf Model. 2016;56(9):1734–45.
44. Cosconati S, et al. Virtual screening with AutoDock: theory and practice. Expert Opin Drug Discov. 2010;5(6):597–607.
45. Allen WJ, et al. DOCK 6: impact of new features and current docking performance. J Comput Chem. 2015;36(15):1132–56.
46. Hart TN, Ness SR, Read RJ. Critical evaluation of the research docking program for the CASP2 challenge. Proteins. 1997;29(Suppl 1):205–9.
47. Sullivan DC, Martin EJ. Exploiting structure-activity relationships in docking. J Chem Inf Model. 2008;48(4):817–30.
48. Zsoldos Z, et al. eHiTS: a new fast, exhaustive flexible ligand docking system. J Mol Graph Model. 2007;26(1):198–212.
49. Rarey M, et al. A fast flexible docking method using an incremental construction algorithm. J Mol Biol. 1996;261(3):470–89.
50. Friesner RA, et al. Glide: a new approach for rapid, accurate docking and scoring. 1. Method and assessment of docking accuracy. J Med Chem. 2004;47(7):1739–49.
51. Jones G, et al. Development and validation of a genetic algorithm for flexible docking. J Mol Biol. 1997;267(3):727–48.
52. Hsin KY, et al. systemsDock: a web server for network pharmacology-based prediction and analysis. Nucleic Acids Res. 2016;44(W1):W507–13.
53. Pierce BG, et al. ZDOCK server: interactive docking prediction of protein-protein complexes and symmetric multimers. Bioinformatics. 2014;30(12):1771–3.
54. Arockia Babu M, et al. Development of 3D-QSAR models for 5-lipoxygenase antagonists: chalcones. Bioorg Med Chem. 2002;10(12):4035–41.
55. Liu GY, et al. 3D-QSAR studies of insecticidal anthranilic diamides as ryanodine receptor activators using CoMFA, CoMSIA and DISCOtech. Chemosphere. 2010;78(3):300–6.
56. Vora J, et al. Molecular docking, QSAR and ADMET based mining of natural compounds against prime targets of HIV. J Biomol Struct Dyn. 2018. https://doi.org/10.1080/07391102.2017.1420489.
57. Patel Y, et al. A comparison of the pharmacophore identification programs: catalyst, DISCO and GASP. J Comput Aided Mol Des. 2002;16(8–9):653–81.
58. Irwin JJ, et al. Predicted biological activity of purchasable chemical space. J Chem Inf Model. 2017. https://doi.org/10.1021/acs.jcim.7b00316.
59. Engels MF, et al. CerBeruS: a system supporting the sequential screening process. J Chem Inf Comput Sci. 2000;40(2):241–5.
60. Lemmen C, Lengauer T, Klebe G. FLEXS: a method for fast flexible ligand superposition. J Med Chem. 1998;41(23):4502–20.
61. Tervo AJ, et al. BRUTUS: optimization of a grid-based similarity function for rigid-body molecular superposition. 1. Alignment and virtual screening applications. J Med Chem. 2005;48(12):4076–86.
62. Yan X, et al. Enhancing molecular shape comparison by weighted Gaussian functions. J Chem Inf Model. 2013;53(8):1967–78.
63. Wermuth CG. Pharmacophores: historical perspective and viewpoint from a medicinal chemist. Methods Princ Med Chem. 2006;32:3.
64. Zuo Z, MacMillan DW. Decarboxylative arylation of α-amino acids via photoredox catalysis: a one-step conversion of biomass to drug pharmacophore. J Am Chem Soc. 2014;136(14):5257–60.
65. Cereto-Massagué A, et al. Molecular fingerprint similarity search in virtual screening. Methods. 2015;71:58–63.
66. Ferreira LG, et al. Molecular docking and structure-based drug design strategies. Molecules. 2015;20(7):13384–421.
67. Consortium, U. UniProt: the universal protein knowledgebase. Nucleic Acids Res. 2017;45(D1):D158–69.
68. Liu T, et al. BindingDB: a web-accessible database of experimentally determined protein-ligand binding affinities. Nucleic Acids Res. 2007;35(Database issue):D198–201.
69. Chatr-aryamontri A, et al. The BioGRID interaction database: 2017 update. Nucleic Acids Res. 2017;45(D1):D369–79.
70. Dennis G, et al. DAVID: database for annotation, visualization, and integrated discovery. Genome Biol. 2003;4(9):R60.
71. Wishart DS, et al. DrugBank: a comprehensive resource for in silico drug discovery and exploration. Nucleic Acids Res. 2006;34(suppl_1):D668–72.
72. Mostafavi S, et al. GeneMANIA: a real-time multiple association network integration algorithm for predicting gene function. Genome Biol. 2008;9(1):S4.
73. Keshava Prasad TS, et al. Human protein reference database-2009 update. Nucleic Acids Res. 2009;37(Database issue):D767–72.
74. Orchard S, et al. The MIntAct project—IntAct as a common curation platform for 11 molecular interaction databases. Nucleic Acids Res. 2014;42(D1):D358–63.
75. Kanehisa M, et al. KEGG: new perspectives on genomes, pathways, diseases and drugs. Nucleic Acids Res. 2017;45(D1):D353–61.
76. Deng L, et al. MTA1 modulated by miR-30e contributes to epithelial-to-mesenchymal transition in hepatocellular carcinoma through an ErbB2-dependent pathway. Oncogene. 2017;36(28):3976–85.
77. Licata L, et al. MINT, the molecular interaction database: 2012 update. Nucleic Acids Res. 2012;40(1):D857–61.
78. Wang X, et al. PharmMapper 2017 update: a web server for potential drug target identification with a comprehensive target pharmacophore database. Nucleic Acids Res. 2017. https://doi.org/10.1093/nar/gkx374

79. Gao Z, et al. PDTD: a web-accessible protein database for drug target identification. BMC Bioinform. 2008;9:104.
80. Goodsell DS. The protein data bank, in atomic evidence. Berlin: Springer; 2016. p. 1–4.
81. Croft D, et al. The reactome pathway knowledgebase. Nucleic Acids Res. 2014;42(Database issue):D472.
82. Kuhn M, et al. STITCH: interaction networks of chemicals and proteins. Nucleic Acids Res. 2007;36(suppl_1):D684–8.
83. Szklarczyk D, et al. STRING v10: protein–protein interaction networks, integrated over the tree of life. Nucleic Acids Res. 2014;43(D1):D447–52.
84. Zhu F, et al. Therapeutic target database update 2012: a resource for facilitating target-oriented drug discovery. Nucleic Acids Res. 2011;40(D1):D1128–36.
85. Li S. Mapping ancient remedies: applying a network approach to traditional Chinese medicine. Science. 2015;350(6262):S72–4.
86. Krämer A, et al. Causal analysis approaches in ingenuity pathway analysis. Bioinformatics. 2013;30(4):523–30.
87. Du J, et al. KEGG-PATH: Kyoto encyclopedia of genes and genomes-based pathway analysis using a path analysis model. Mol BioSyst. 2014;10(9):2441–7.
88. Ekins S, et al. Algorithms for network analysis in systems-ADME/Tox using the MetaCore and MetaDrug platforms. Xenobiotica. 2006;36(10–11):877–901.
89. Kurata H, et al. Extended CADLIVE: a novel graphical notation for design of biochemical network maps and computational pathway analysis. Nucleic Acids Res. 2007;35(20):e134–e134.
90. Shannon P, et al. Cytoscape: a software environment for integrated models of biomolecular interaction networks. Genome Res. 2003;13(11):2498–504.
91. Fitts B, et al. dot-app: a Graphviz-Cytoscape conversion plug-in. F1000Research. 2016;5:2543.
92. De Nooy W, Mrvar A, Batagelj V. Exploratory social network analysis with Pajek, vol. 27. Cambridge: Cambridge University Press; 2011.
93. Junker BH, Klukas C, Schreiber F. VANTED: a system for advanced data analysis and visualization in the context of biological networks. BMC Bioinform. 2006;7(1):109.
94. Hu Z, et al. VisANT: data-integrating visual framework for biological networks and modules. Nucleic Acids Res. 2005;33(suppl_2):W352–7.
95. Schwarz R, et al. Integrated network reconstruction, visualization and analysis using YANAsquare. BMC Bioinform. 2007;8(1):313.
96. Wan W, et al. Metabolomics reveals that vine tea (Ampelopsis grossedentata) prevents high-fat-diet-induced metabolism disorder by improving glucose homeostasis in rats. PLoS ONE. 2017;12(8):e0182830.

3

Chemical characterization of wound ointment (WO) and its effects on fracture repair: a rabbit model

Zhixue Ou[1†], Qi Cheng[2†], Yueping Chen[1], Tao Chen[1], Xiangbin Rong[1], Feipan Long[1], Xiaoyun Zhang[1], Qinghua Liang[1] and Zhe Feng[1*]

Abstract

Background: Wound ointment (WO), a kind of Chinese medicine, can significantly promote fracture healing. The study aimed at analyzing the chemical composition and the effects of WO on fracture of rabbits and tried to explore the corresponding molecular mechanism in cytokine.

Methods: The qualitative and quantitative analysis of WO was conducted by liquid chromatography-mass spectrometry (LC–MS). Fifty-four Zealand mature male rabbits were randomly divided into 3 groups: Control group, Yunnan Baiyao (YB) group and WO group. All the rabbits suffered a fracture of right radius and were then stabilized with an external fixator. Treated with different methods, fracture healing was observed. The bone specimens were subjected to radiograph, immunohistochemistry (IHC) analysis, hematoxylin–eosin staining (HE), western blot and enzyme linked immunosorbent assay (ELISA).

Results: A total of 12 active compositions were detected by LC–MS. Radiographs showed a considerably better bone healing and remodeling of the fracture in WO group. HE experiments showed that a large number of osteoclasts appeared in the early stage when treated with WO. In immunohistochemistry (IHC), western blot and ELISA test, significant increases in vascular endothelial growth factor (VEGF) expression were observed in WO group compared with other two groups.

Conclusions: Wound ointment contained active compositions which efficiently promoted fracture healing through increasing the expression of VEGF.

Keywords: Animals, Osteoclasts, Fracture healing, Wound ointment (WO), Radius fracture, VEGF

Background

Bone fracture is a very common disease, which is usually caused by high force, stress, or a minimal trauma injury. An average fracture incidence of 1.17% in males and 1.07% in females has been reported in UK and over 6 million cases occurred in the United States per year [1–4]. Fracture healing is a complicated process, including granulation tissue formation, cartilage callus formation, lamellar bone deposition and remodeling to original bone contour. Surgical management is the most common treatment for fractures, while there is still a risk of morbidity and mortality among the elderly population [5]. Thus, finding a safer and more efficient treatment for fracture is essential. Vascular endothelial growth factor (VEGF) is a sub-family member of growth factors which are important to both vasculogenesis and angiogenesis process. In addition, it has been widely accepted that VEGF played a vital role in bone regeneration through accelerating the process of angiogenesis, which has been confirmed through several animal models as well [6, 7].

*Correspondence: chizf0618@163.com
†Zhixue Ou and Qi Cheng contributed equally to this work
[1] Department of Traumatic Orthopedics and Hand Surgery, Ruikang Hospital Affiliated to Guangxi University of Chinese Medicine, Block B, No 10 Huadong Road, Nanning 530011, Guangxi, China
Full list of author information is available at the end of the article

There are sufficient evidences supporting that the high expression of VEGF protein can accelerate the healing of femoral fractures in mice and remedy radius segmental defects in rabbits [8, 9].

Yunnan Baiyao (YNBY) is one of the most popular prescriptions of Chinese herbal medicine which possesses haemostatic functions of both open and closed wounds. It is deemed as "a must for first aid" therapy in China of both internal and external hemorrhage as well as open and closed wounds due to its renowned haemostatic functions. It was also reported that YNBY can effectively reduce the severity of murine experimental colitis by both immune-suppressing and wound-healing mechanisms [10–12].

Wound ointment (WO) is made from Chinese medicinal herbs, containing panax, notoginseng, drynaria fortunei and rhubarb etc. Those herbal remedies have active compositions with synergism to relieve pain, prevent infection, and promote healing with less side effects. Antibacterial constituents and analgesic were added in several WOs to bitterly treat wounds and prevent infection. Some uncommon ointments enriching vitamins, including vitamin E, vitamin A and vitamin D can promote skin healing from scrapes, cuts and burns.

The main usage of WOs is to treat soft tissue injury, accelerate blood circulation and relieve congestion, swelling and pain. WO also has anti-inflammatory and antibacterial effects with non-stimulation to skin, heart, liver, kidney and other organs. After traditional disinfection, WO may be dressed directly, or painted onto gauze. It was first applied for fracture regeneration by Chinese medicine doctors [13, 14]. With a clinical application for 30 years, WO has its positive effects on the union of bone confirmed, and exerted a certain influence in China and Southeast Asia [15, 16]. However, there was no relative animal experiment or clinical study to evaluate its efficacy on fracture healing systematically, and its functional mechanism remains unknown to the public due to a lack of researches. These factors mentioned above have largely limited the wide application of WO in clinic. Thus, in this research, we utilized rabbits for radius fracture model to investigate the effects of WO on fracture healing and illustrate the potential mechanisms of WO.

Methods

Preparation of sample solutions

A total of 4.0 g WO sample was extracted with 40 mL methanol using Soxhlet extractor for 12 h until the complete extraction. Afterwards, the solution was filtered and evaporated. The crude remnants were uniformly mixed with 5 mL methanol for further analysis.

Analysis of liquid chromatography-mass spectrometry (LC–MS)

LC–MS was performed using Waters Acquity UPLC system (Waters, Milford, MA, USA) coupled with TOF mass spectrometer (Bruker, Bremen, Germany). The results were acquired using Hystar software (Bruker). Acquity UPLC BEH C18 column (2.1 mm × 100 mm, 1.7 μm) served as the stationary phase, 0.1% formic acid in pure water (A) and 0.1% formic acid in acetonitrile (B) with a flow rate of 0.4 mL/min were utilized as the mobile phase. The conditions were as follows: 0–1 min, 5% B; 1–4 min, 20% B; 4–6 min, 25% B; 6–10 min, 40% B; 10–12 min, 60% B; 12–15 min, 100% B; 15–16 min, 40% B; 16–20 min, 5% B. The column temperature was maintained at 40 °C, and the injection volume of each sample was 2 μL.

The mass spectrometer was operated in the negative mode, the scanning range of m/z from 100 to 3000. The mass conditions were as follows: gas (N2) flow rate was 8 L/min and the temperature was 180 °C; the capillary voltage was 4500 V.

Animal model and fracture surgery

Fifty-Four New Zealand white male rabbits (provided by Animal Center of Guangxi University of Chinese Medicine, Guangxi, China), which were 10 months old with body weight ranging from 2.0 to 2.5 kg, were involved in this study. All rabbits were kept singly and fed with a standard laboratory diet and tap water under climate-controlled conditions (25 °C; 55% humidity; 12 h of light alternating with 12 h of darkness). A small patch of skin dermis was excised from the back and the right forelimb of each rabbit. After the injection of anesthetic (30 mg/mL, sodium pentobarbital sodium solution, Sigma-Aldrich, MO, USA) into the vein of the rabbit ear, all the following procedures were performed in disinfection area with rabbits in supine position. A 1.5 cm longitudinal incision was made to expose the middle part of radius. The periosteum was cut and peeled off, and then the radial shaft was exposed. A fracture model was established by bone sheared with peripheral vessel, muscle and cartilage tissue preserved, keeping the ulna integrate. The research was approved by the ethical committee of Ruikang Hospital Affiliated to Guangxi University of Chinese Medicine. The Minimum Standards of Reporting Checklist contained details of the experimental design, statistics and resources used in this study (Additional file 1).

Grouping and treatment

The rabbits were categorized into three groups (n = 18 each group). Rabbits received normal saline only were in control group, those treated with Yunnan Baiyao (YB, Yunnan Baiyao group Co., Ltd., Yunnan, China) were regarded as YB group, and WO group consisted of rabbits treated with WO (Ruikang Hospital Affiliated to Guangxi University of Chinese Medicine, Guangxi, China). Five milligram/kilogram of YB and WO were externally applied on the fracture three times a day with bandage being put on and dressings were changed every 3 days. The fracture parts of control group were bandaged without any drug applied.

Preparation and treatment of specimens

The rabbits were killed at different time point (3, 7, 14, 21, 28, 35 days after operation) by being injected 10–15 mL air into the syringes. After the skin of the fracture was cut immediately, the surrounding muscles, tendons and other soft tissues were stripped. Hyperplastic soft tissue, fibrous and bones callus were halved. One part was fixed in 10% neutral formalin solution and prepared for the following HE stain and IHC analysis; other part was wrapped by tin foil and stored at − 80 °C for western blot. The sacrifice of rabbits and the preservation of the specimens were completed within 10 min to prevent protein degradation and cell autolysis rupture.

Radiography analysis

The procedure of X-ray and micro-CT observation was similar to the previous studies [17, 18]. Briefly, fracture morphology was detected by digital X-ray equipment (Siemens, Chicago, USA). Three-dimensional (3D) images were rendered. A laboratory micro-CT scanner (Scanco Medical AG, Brüttisellen, Switzerland) and the VGStudio MAX software (Dürr, Bietigheim-Bissingen, Germany) were used for the micro-CT examination. The proportion about total void area of all area in transverse section image was calculated, and the fraction of mineralized callus was quantified.

Alkaline phosphatase (ALP) assay

At each time point, 4 mL ear margin venous blood stewed in the bio-tube for 30 min was centrifugalized at the speed of 2500 r/min. Then, the upper layer of the serum was removed and ALP activity of the lower layer was detected with ALP assay kit (Sigma-Aldrich, St. Louis, MO, USA). The measurement was performed using Beckman LX 20 Analyzer (Beckman Coulter, Inc., CA, USA).

Hematoxylin–eosin (HE) staining

The bone specimens were fixed in 10% formaldehyde solution for 48 h and decalcified in 15% ethylene diamine tetraacetic acid (EDTA) for 3 weeks. Then, the decalcified samples were embedded in paraffin, cut into 4 mm-thick sections and dehydrated with gradient ethanol. After that, the sections were stained with HE and assessed with the optical microscope.

Immunohistochemistry

The bone specimen sections, which were dewaxed and rehydrated with xylene solution and gradient ethanol, were then hot fixed with 0.01 M Citrate repair solution (pH 6.0) for 2 min in hyperbaric condition. 100 μL anti-VEGF receptor 1 (rabbit, 1: 800, ABcam, US) was added and incubated overnight. Then the sections were incubated with horseradish enzyme labeled goat anti-rabbit IgG (Beijing Zhong Jin Jinqiao company, Biological Technology Co., Ltd., Beijing, China) for 40 min. Afterwards, the sections were treated with 3,3′-diaminobenzidine (DAB) coloring agent for 20 s, hematoxylin re-infection for 1 min and dehydrated. The figures were analyzed with the MIQAS medical image quantitative analysis system (Motic China Group Co., Ltd., Guangdong, China), 5 fields of vision were selected randomly with about 100 cells in each field. In each field, mean optical density, the positive reaction area and total area of cells were measured (cells area was 0.15 mm^2). Subsequently, the average rate of positive area was calculated.

Western blot

The harvested bone specimens were cut into pieces, weighed and grinded into powder in liquid nitrogen with radio-immunoprecipitation assay (RIPA) buffer. The total proteins were extracted using protein extraction kit (Millipore, Billerica, MA, USA). Equal weight of proteins were loaded and separated by sodium dodecyl sulfate-polyacrylamide gel electrophoresis (SDS-PAGE), transferred to polyvinylidene fluoride (PVDF) membranes and then blocked with 5% skim milk at room temperature for 1 h. Primary antibody anti-rabbit F-box protein 32 (FBXO32) diluted with Tris buffered saline solution (TBST, 1: 2500) was added to the membranes and incubated at 4 °C overnight. The membranes were then incubated with goat monoclonal anti-rabbit, the secondary antibody marked with horseradish peroxidase (HRP, 1: 2000), for 2 h at room temperature. Glyceraldehyde-3-phosphate dehydrogenase (GAPDH) served as the internal control. Signal detection was performed using Chemiluminescence reagent kit (Amersham, IL, USA). The antibodies mentioned above were all bought from Beijing Zhong Shan Jinqiao Biological Technology Co., Ltd. (Beijing, China).

Enzyme linked immunosorbent assay (ELISA)

The bone specimens were cut off and rinsed with pre-cooled phosphate buffered solution (PBS) (0.01 M, pH = 7.4) to remove residual blood and weighted. The specific volume of PBS (1:9 w/w) was added to a glass homogenizer and sufficiently grinded on ice. After 5000*g* homogenate were ultrasonically broken and thawed, it was centrifuged for 10 min and the supernatant was collected. Rabbit VEGF specific enzyme-linked immunoassay kit (TWp027731, TongWei, Shanghai, China) was used to detect the VEGF expression level. Manufacturer's protocol was strictly followed and the optical density (OD) was measured at 450 nm.

Statistical analysis

All statistical analyses were performed by SPSS 19.0 software (SPSS, IL, USA). The significant differences in numerical data (mean ± SD) were estimated with the analysis of variance (ANOVA). Differences between two groups were analyzed by unpaired *t* tests. *P* value less than 0.05 was defined as statistical significance.

Results

12 compositions were detected in WO

As shown in Table 1, a total of 12 compositions were detected in WO. The structures of the active compounds were shown in Additional file 2: Figure S1. Most of compositions have the property of antioxidant, anti-inflammatory and antibacterial. Some compositions have been verified to play a crucial role in the fracture healing, especially asperosaponin VI, which could accelerate the proliferation of the bone marrow mesenchymal stem cells and their differentiation toward osteoblasts [19].

Fracture healing was the fastest in WO group

The control group showed the common process of fracture healing (Fig. 1), where the fracture line was still clearly observed 21 days after the operation. At the 35th day, the fracture line became blurry, and the bone callus formed. While in YB group, the speed of fracture healing was much faster than that of control group. At the 21st day, the fracture line was fuzzy with massive callus appeared at the fracture end. At the last observation in day 35, the fracture line was almost disappeared, but fracture ghosting still existed. In WO group, the recovery rate of fractured bone was faster than that of other two groups. At the 21st day, the obscure space was very narrow with massive bone callus proliferated. At the 35th day, the fracture line disappeared and the fractured limbed was almost repaired. As shown in Fig. 2, micro-CT results further verified the healing progress and presented more distinct fracture healing condition. The YB group and WO group were much superior to that of control group. In the WO group, the fracture was almost recovered at the 35th day. As bone volume shown in Table 2, the volume of YB and WO group had significant difference compared with that of control group. WO group also showed larger volume in YB group in the 21st day. The results showed that WO and YB could promote the fracture healing in a short time, and the WO had the better effect during the interim period.

Table 1 Comprehensive analysis of WO by LC–MS

Retention time (min)	*m/z*	Mol. wt	Formula	Compounds
2.23	137	154.12	$C_7H_5O_3$	Protocatechuic acid
2.81	289	308.28	$C_{15}H_{14}O_6$	Catechin
2.86	137	138.12	$C_7H_6O_3$	p-Hydroxybenzoic acid
4.55	595	596.53	$C_{27}H_{32}O_{15}$	Neoeriocitrin
5.27	579	580.53	$C_{27}H_{32}O_{14}$	Naringin
7.98	269	270.23	$C_{15}H_{10}O_5$	Emodin
9.36	928	929.1	$C_{47}H_{76}O_{18}$	Asperosaponin VI
10.02	266	283.21	$C_{15}H_7O_6$	Rhein
10.32	271	272.25	$C_{15}H_{12}O_5$	Naringenin
11.4	285	286.23	$C_{15}H_{10}O_6$	Kaempferol
12.63	283	284.27	$C_{16}H_{12}O_5$	Physcion
13.29	861	862.75	$C_{42}H_{38}O_{20}$	Sennoside A

Tissues grew fastest in WO group

As shown in Fig. 3, at the 7th day, tissue necrosis and reactive periosteum hyperplasia occurred in control group, with inflammatory cell gathered and capillary proliferated. At the 14th day, little fibrocyte formed with slight reaction while at the 21st day, the proliferation became active and at the 35th day, the bone callus joint with no woven bone molded. As in YB group, there was periosteal reaction and proliferation, and fibroblast gathered obviously at the 7th day. The chondrocyte appeared the 14th day and proliferated at the 21st day with primary callus formed, when subperiosteum ossification, endochondral ossification and primitive trabecula bone could be observed at the fracture end. At the 28th day, fracture was connected with a great deal of woven bones formed. At the last observation, primary marrow cavity appeared, but there was no connection between the upper and lower cavum ossis. Meanwhile, the bone recovery process in WO group was similar to that in YB group during the first 14 days. However, massive bone callus appeared and connected at the 21st day, primary marrow cavity formed at the 28th day and both ends of bone medullary cavity were connected in the last examination. In summary, the WO group showed the best bone healing effect.

ALP concentration was the highest in WO group

ALP activity is an indicator that measures the self-repaired ability. Osteon recovery is strongly associated with the increase of ALP. As shown in Fig. 4, the value of ALP in serum showed an upward tendency in three groups. ALP value in WO group increased significantly compared with the control group ($P < 0.01$) at the 28th

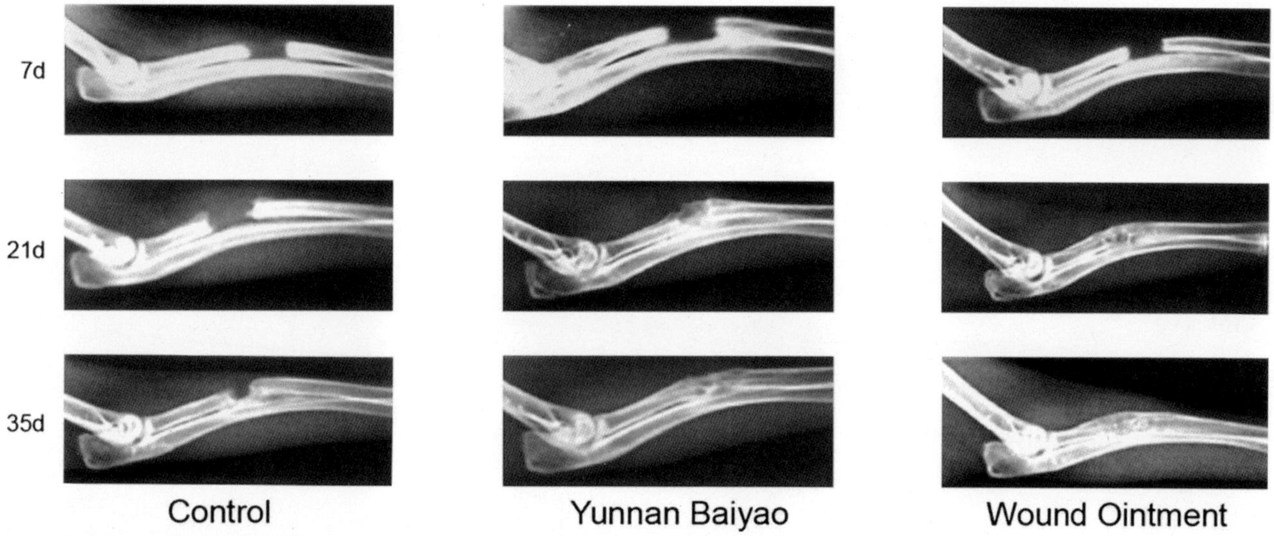

Fig. 1 Fracture healing was the fastest in WO group detected by X-ray. X-ray observation of fracture healing conditions at 7, 21 and 35 days after fracture in the control group, Yunnan Baiyao (YB) group and Wound Ointment (WO) group. WO group turned out to be the fastest recovery of fracture

day, the relevant phenomena was the surprising speed of bone formation. 35 day after the operation, the ALP level in the YB group and WO group both showed the significant increase compared with the control group ($P < 0.01$).

WO accelerated fracture healing by promoting the release of VEGF

The positive substance was located in cytoplasm, in other words, the claybank cytoplasm showed a positive signal (Fig. 5). At the 7th day, in NC group, VEGF expressed high in dense fibrous connective tissue and expressed low in few hyperplastic chondrocytes. The expression of VEGF in YB was stronger than that in control group, and more chondrocytes showed positive VEGF signal. WO group showed the higher expression of VEGF in both the dense connective tissue and the chondrocytes compared with other two groups. In the 14th day, the proliferation of cartilage was active and VEGF was significantly increased while the hypertrophic chondrocytes were less and the contained VEGF was negative. In YB group, the new bone was arranged into trabeculae which was consisted of cartilage and fibrous bones and covered with osteoblasts. These osteoblasts showed positive expression of VEGF signal. Compared with YB group, WO group showed the similar results, while the number of osteoblasts was more and the positive VEGF signal was also stronger. At the 21st day, the typical trabeculae was found and covered a large number of osteoblasts containing VEGF. The number of osteoblasts significantly decreased, however, the size of callus increased in YB and WO group and there was no significant difference between them. After 28 days, there were more callus in control group showed negative expression of VEGF and the number of osteoblasts decreased. In YB and WO group, primary bone marrow cavity appeared and showed slightly positive expression of VGEF, and the expression level was higher in WO than in YB group. At the 35th day, the NC group was in the primary bone marrow cavity stage, YB group and WO group has developed more secondary bone marrow cavity which was relatively more in the WO group and showed higher positive expression of VEGF. The expressions of VEGF in YB group and WO group were much higher than that in control group at each time point ($P < 0.01$), and both reached the peak at the 28th days while the control group increased gradually during the monitoring time. In conclusion, we might speculate that WO promoted the release of VEGF in a short time.

VEGF was highly expressed in WO group

Results of western blot further confirmed the regular expression of VEGF protein in the fracture of rabbits during fracture healing in control group, YB group and

Table 2 The bone volume of uCT in 7, 21 and 35 days

	Control	YB	WO
7 days	0.479 ± 0.026	0.627 ± 0.047**	0.855 ± 0.057***
21 days	0.684 ± 0.043	0.942 ± 0.061***	1.197 ± 0.066***###
35 days	0.875 ± 0.056	1.225 ± 0.073***	1.301 ± 0.105***

** $P < 0.01$, *** $P < 0.001$. There was significant difference between the control group and two treatment group; ### $P < 0.001$. There was significant difference between the YB group and WO group

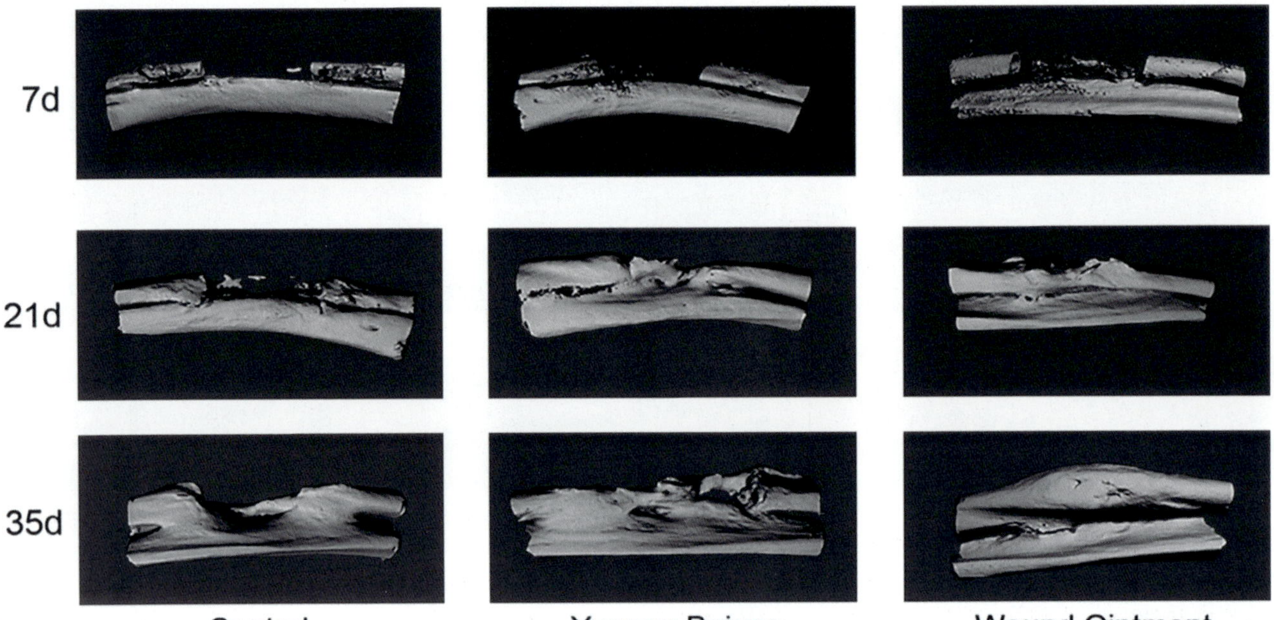

Fig. 2 Fracture healing was the fastest in WO group detected by Micro-CT. Micro-CT observation of fracture healing conditions at 7, 21 and 35 days after fracture in the control group, Yunnan Baiyao (YB) group and Wound Ointment (WO) group. Recovery of WO group was the best among all the three groups

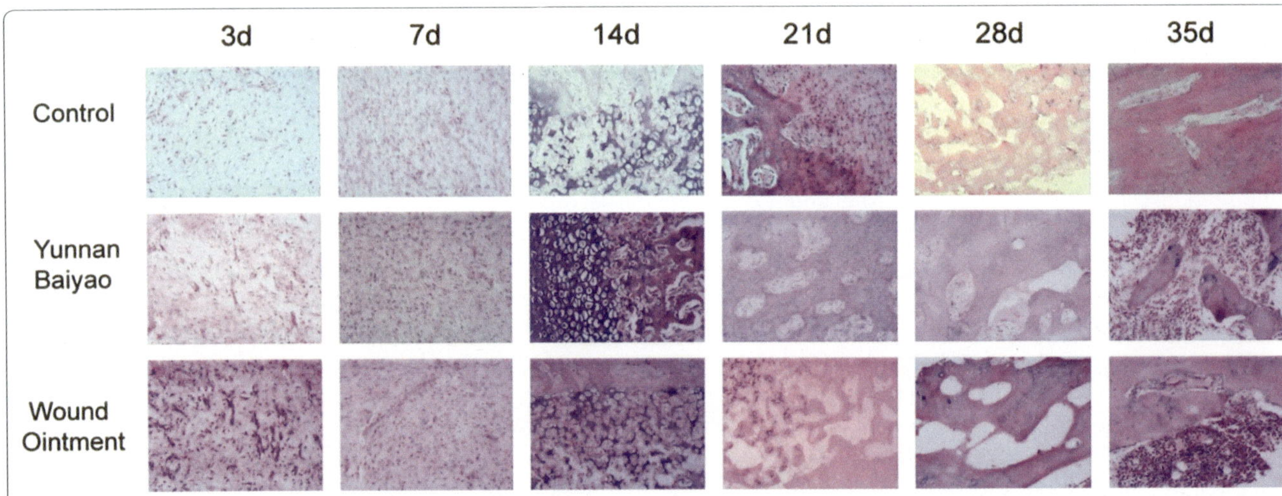

Fig. 3 Tissues and VEGF grew fastest in WO group. HE staining of positive signal of vascular endothelial growth factor (VEGF) within the fracture end at each time point (3, 7, 14, 21, 28 and 35 days) in the control group, Yunnan Baiyao (YB) group and Wound Ointment (WO) group. WO group showed the best bone healing effect. *HE* hematoxylin eosin

WO group (Fig. 6a). In the process of fracture healing, the expression level of VEGF in control group was the lowest but increased gradually. After 14 days, the growth was accelerated distinctly. In both YB group and WO group, the expressions of VEGF were augmented dramatically and peaked at the 28th day, and then dropped slightly. Overall, the VEGF expressions in YB and WO group were significantly higher than that in control group ($P < 0.01$). The results were consistent with the IHC analysis.

Results of ELISA confirmed that secretion of VEGF protein in control group, YB group and WO group

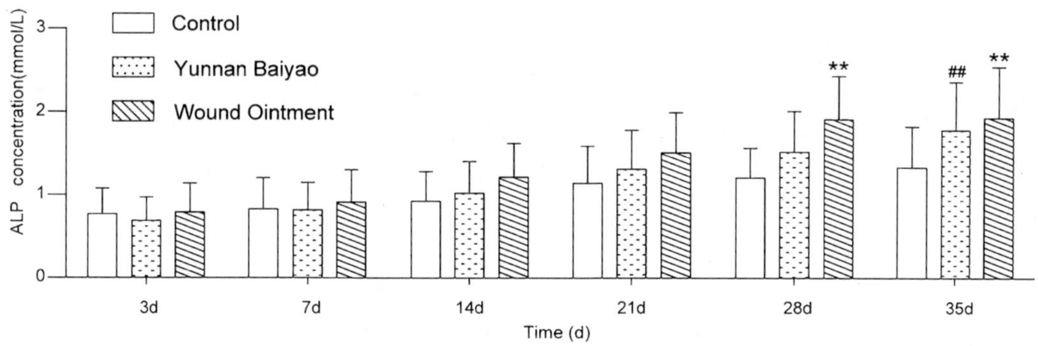

Fig. 4 ALP concentration was the highest in WO group. ALP assay detected the value of ALP in fracture tissue at each time point (3, 7, 14, 21, 28 and 35 days) in the control group, Yunnan Baiyao (YB) group and Wound Ointment (WO) group. WO group increased the fastest, suggesting a surprising speed of bone formation. ##$P < 0.01$, YB group versus control group; **$P < 0.01$, WO group versus control group. *ALP* alkaline phosphatase

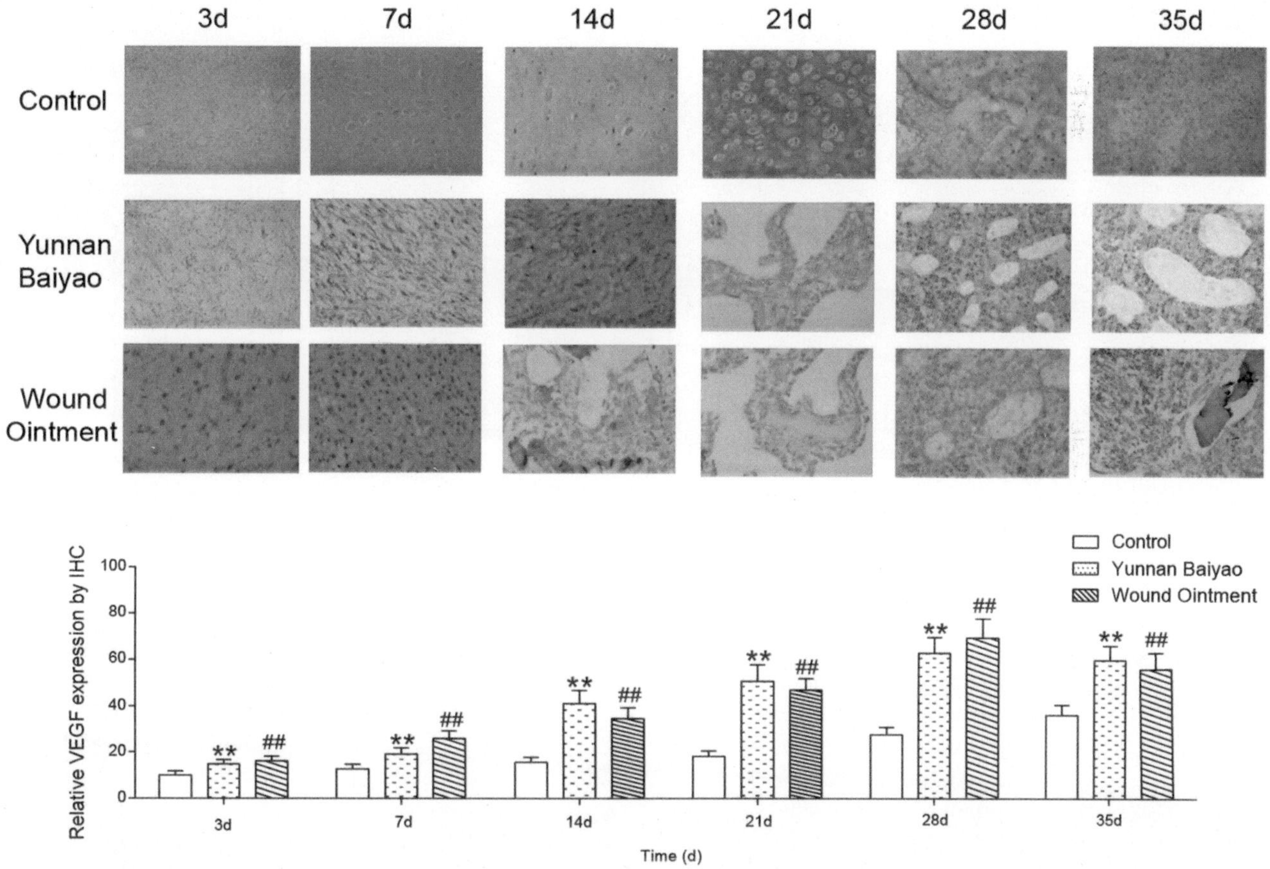

Fig. 5 WO accelerated fracture healing by promoting the release of VEGF. Immunohistochemistry of positive signal of vascular endothelial growth factor (VEGF) within the fracture end at each time point (3, 7, 14, 21, 28 and 35 days) in the control group, Yunnan Baiyao (YB) group and Wound Ointment (WO) group. **$P < 0.01$, YB group versus control group; ##$P < 0.01$, WO group versus control group

(Fig. 6b). The trend in the three groups in 35 days was coordinated with that of western blot. The expression of VEGF was higher in the WO group especially in the 28th day, nearly 3000 pg/mL.

Discussion

A series of physiological processes are involved in bone fracture healing, each of which has fundamental roles in contributing to the healing process [20]. As one of the

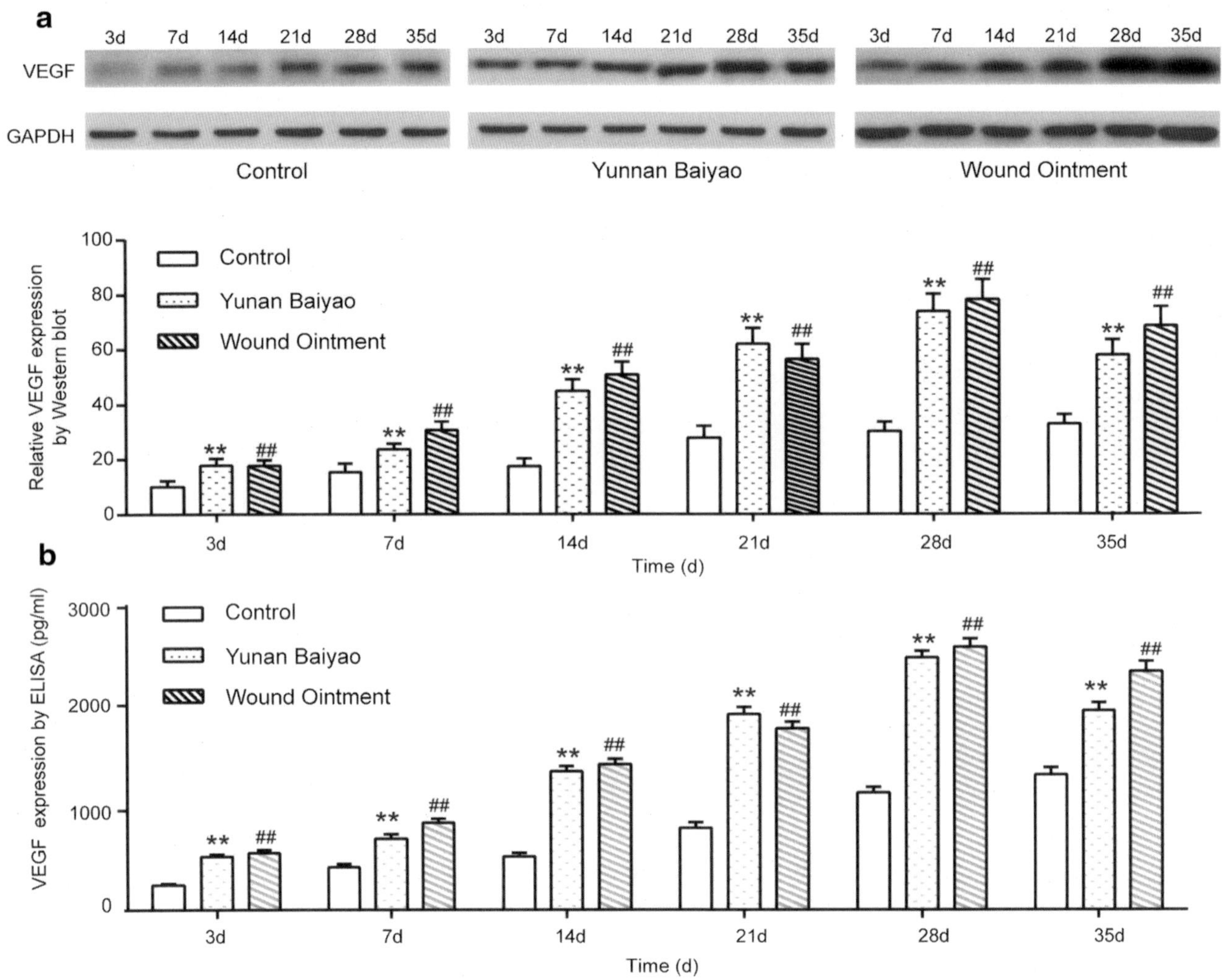

Fig. 6 VEGF was higher expressed in WO group. Western blot analysis (**a**) and ELISA (**b**) of VEGF expression within the fracture end at each point (3, 7, 14, 21, 28 and 35 days) in the control group, Yunnan Baiyao (YB) group and Wound Ointment (WO) group. GAPDH was used as loading control. $^{**}P < 0.01$, YB group versus control group; $^{\#\#}P < 0.01$, WO group versus control group. *VEGF* vascular endothelial growth factor

most important factors in influencing fracture healing, VEGF can stimulate local vascular regeneration in the fracture [21]. There are many studies showing that the application of VEGF can work effectively on angiogenesis and speed the process of bone repair [22–24]. Meanwhile, establishment of animal fracture model will be of great value in the understanding of fracture repair process [25]. The purpose of this research is to investigate whether WO could facilitate the expression of VEGF and accelerate fracture union. Our research was mainly based on a rabbit model of radius fracture. After treatment of Yunnan Baiyao or WO, the healing situation was assessed and compared with the control group. The experimental data showed that WO behaved well in promote neovascularization and callus regeneration via up-regulating the expression of VEGF, which contributed to accelerating fracture healing.

X-ray and micro-CT were logically applied to evaluate the fracture degree, bone strength, as well as fracture healing degree, because of their functions in quantitatively analyzing the microarchitecture of bones [26, 27]. Our observations of X-ray and micro-CT in different time points revealed that in terms of the degree of callus formation and mineralization in fracture healing, WO group came out to be the best-performing one, followed by the YB group, and the control group was the worst.

Results of histomorphometric analysis in the three groups (control, YB and WO group) showed a similar bone formation process. The first change observed by light microscope was the regeneration of chondroblasts and the formation of hyaline cartilage. Loose connective tissue reverted to dense connective tissue gradually and developed into fibrous callus. With the proliferation, differentiation and growth of osteoblasts, fracture callus gradually replaced fibrous callus. At the last stage, osteoclasts became active. Fracture healing was in the phase of remodeling original bone contour. In WO group, the granulation tissue formation, chondroblasts and osteoblasts proliferation, fibrous callus and fracture callus remodeling process occurred at 3 or 7 days after fracture, which was faster than other groups. Significant cartilaginous osteogenesis and faster new bone growth were seen in WO group. These evidences indicated that WO could accelerate new bone growth through promoting cartilaginous osteogenesis. IHC analysis, Western blot and ELISA assay demonstrated that YB and WO played the same role in influencing VEGF expression, while VEGF showed a stronger expression in WO group than in YB group. When compared with control group, both WO and YB groups could improve the expression of VEGF at different stages of fracture repair, which was consistent to the results of HE analysis.

In this research, we investigated the effect of WO on the expression of VEGF during fracture healing in rabbit radius fracture model for the first time. The conclusion conformed to the results of clinical practices. However, there were still some limitations. First, although the positive control of this study, YB is widely utilized to promote fracture healing in China, but it's unacquainted for other researchers. The mechanisms concerning how YB accelerated fracture healing were also not widely reported. Second, there are some other proteins such as bone morphogenetic protein 2, osteocalcin and type I collagen that also contributing to fracture healing which were not studied in the present research. Whether WO or YB affects expressions of those factors during the treatment still needs other evidences. Moreover, the real conditions of fracture were different from the experimental condition. The causes for bone fractures are very complex and there are great individual differences among patients. Fractures are associated with different complications such as soft tissue damage, massive bleeding, severe pain, infection, visceral injury and even shock. Thus, experiments in animals are not enough and the mechanism of WO on the treatment of fracture needs more studies.

Conclusions

In conclusion, we had detected the composition of WO and confirmed that its effect on increasing the VEGF expression in the process of bone regeneration was good for neovascularization and callus regeneration, as well as acceleration of fracture healing. This research will deepen our understanding of the function of WO, and will be of value in the development and application of WO.

Abbreviations

ALP: alkaline phosphatase; DAB: diaminobenzidine; EDTA: ethylene diamine tetraacetic acid; FBXO32: F-box protein 32; GAPDH: glyceraldehyde-3-phosphate dehydrogenase; HE: hematoxylin–eosin staining; PVDF: polyvinylidene fluoride; RIPA: radio-immunoprecipitation assay; SDS-PAGE: sodium dodecyl sulfate-polyacrylamide gel electrophoresis; VEGF: vascular endothelial growth factor; WO: wound ointment; YB: Yunnan Baiyao; YNBY: Yunnan Baiyao; LC–MS: liquid chromatograph-mass spectrometer; ELISA: enzyme linked immunosorbent assay.

Authors' contributions

Study design and conception: ZO, QC; data collection: ZO, QC, YC, TC; data analysis: ZO, QC, XR, FL, XZ, QL; data interpretation: ZO, QC, FL, XZ, QL; manuscript drafting: ZO, QC; critical revising the manuscript: ZF. All authors read and approved the final manuscript.

Author details

Department of Traumatic Orthopedics and Hand Surgery, Ruikang Hospital Affiliated to Guangxi University of Chinese Medicine, Block B, No 10 Huadong Road, Nanning 530011, Guangxi, China. [2] Department of Traumatic Orthopedics, Daye Hospital of Traditional Chinese Medicine, Daye 435100, Hubei, China.

Acknowledgements

Not applicable.

The work was done in Department of Traumatic Orthopedics and Hand Surgery, Ruikang Hospital Affiliated to Guangxi University of Chinese Medicine, Nanning, 530011, Guangxi, China.

Competing interests

The authors declare that they have no competing interests.

Consent for publication

Not applicable.

Funding

This study was supported by Guangxi Zhuang Autonomous Region Science and Technology Agency Research Project (No. 0816004-37).

References

1. Dombrowski S, Jacob L, Hadji P, Kostev K. Oral contraceptive use and fracture risk-a retrospective study of 12,970 women in the UK. Osteoporos Int. 2017;28(8):2349–55.
2. Cunningham TD, Martin BC, DeShields SC, Romero CC. The impact of osteoporotic fractures compared with other health conditions in older adults living in Virginia, United States. Osteoporos Int. 2016;27:2979–88.
3. Benetou V, Orfanos P, Feskanich D, Michaelsson K, Pettersson-Kymmer U, Eriksson S, et al. Fruit and vegetable intake and hip fracture incidence in older men and women: the CHANCES project. J Bone Miner Res. 2016;31:1743–52.
4. Ogilvie CM, Lu C, Marcucio R, Lee M, Thompson Z, Hu D, et al. Vascular endothelial growth factor improves bone repair in a murine nonunion model. Iowa Orthop J. 2012;32:90–4.
5. Karres J, Heesakkers NA, Ultee JM, Vrouenraets BC. Predicting 30-day mortality following hip fracture surgery: evaluation of six risk prediction models. Injury. 2015;46:371–7.
6. Du B, Liu W, Deng Y, Li S, Liu X, Gao Y, et al. Angiogenesis and bone regeneration of porous nano-hydroxyapatite/coralline blocks coated with rhVEGF165 in critical-size alveolar bone defects in vivo. Int J Nanomed. 2015;10:2555–65.
7. Grassmann JP, Schneppendahl J, Sager M, Hakimi AR, Herten M, Loegters TT, et al. The effect of bone marrow concentrate and hyperbaric oxygen therapy on bone repair. J Mater Sci Mater Med. 2015;26:5331.

8. Katagiri W, Kawai T, Osugi M, Sugimura-Wakayama Y, Sakaguchi K, Kojima T, et al. Angiogenesis in newly regenerated bone by secretomes of human mesenchymal stem cells. Maxillofac Plast Reconstr Surg. 2017;39:8.
9. Sukul M, Nguyen TB, Min YK, Lee SY, Lee BT. Effect of local sustainable release of BMP2-VEGF from nano-cellulose loaded in sponge biphasic calcium phosphate on bone regeneration. Tissue Eng Part A. 2015;21:1822–36.
10. Frederick J, Boysen S, Wagg C, Chalhoub S. The effects of oral administration of Yunnan Baiyao on blood coagulation in beagle dogs as measured by kaolin-activated thromboelastography and buccal mucosal bleeding times. Can J Vet Res. 2017;81:41–5.
11. Murphy LA, Panek CM, Bianco D, Nakamura RK. Use of Yunnan Baiyao and epsilon aminocaproic acid in dogs with right atrial masses and pericardial effusion. J Vet Emerg Crit Care (San Antonio). 2017;27:121–6.
12. Li R, Alex P, Ye M, Zhang T, Liu L, Li X. An old herbal medicine with a potentially new therapeutic application in inflammatory bowel disease. Int J Clin Exp Med. 2011;4:309–19.
13. Zhou J, Ni M, Liu X, Ren Z, Zheng Z. Curcumol promotes vascular endothelial growth factor (VEGF)-mediated diabetic wound healing in streptozotocin-induced hyperglycemic rats. Med Sci Monit. 2017;23:555–62.
14. Tang QL, Han SS, Feng J, Di JQ, Qin WX, Fu J, et al. Moist exposed burn ointment promotes cutaneous excisional wound healing in rats involving VEGF and bFGF. Mol Med Rep. 2014;9:1277–82.
15. Ho TJ, Jiang SJ, Lin GH, Li TS, Yiin LM, Yang JS, et al. The in vitro and in vivo wound healing properties of the Chinese herbal medicine "Jinchuang Ointment". Evid Based Complement Alternat Med. 2016;2016:1654056.
16. Arti H, Khorami M, Ebrahimi-Nejad V. Comparison of negative pressure wound therapy (NPWT) & conventional wound dressings in the open fracture wounds. Pak J Med Sci. 2016;32:65–9.
17. Yang GE, Duan X, Lin D, Li T, Luo D, Wang L, et al. Rapamycin-induced autophagy activity promotes bone fracture healing in rats. Exp Ther Med. 2015;10:1327–33.
18. Murphy CM, Schindeler A, Cantrill LC, Mikulec K, Peacock L, Little DG. PTH(1-34) treatment increases bisphosphonate turnover in fracture repair in rats. J Bone Miner Res. 2015;30:1022–9.
19. Ke K, Li Q, Yang X, Xie Z, Wang Y, Shi J, et al. Asperosaponin VI promotes bone marrow stromal cell osteogenic differentiation through the PI3K/AKT signaling pathway in an osteoporosis model. Sci Rep. 2016;6:35233.
20. Berendsen AD, Pinnow EL, Maeda A, Brown AC, McCartney-Francis N, Kram V, et al. Biglycan modulates angiogenesis and bone formation during fracture healing. Matrix Biol. 2014;35:223–31.
21. Ozturk BY, Inci I, Egri S, Ozturk AM, Yetkin H, Goktas G, et al. The treatment of segmental bone defects in rabbit tibiae with vascular endothelial growth factor (VEGF)-loaded gelatin/hydroxyapatite "cryogel" scaffold. Eur J Orthop Surg Traumatol. 2013;23:767–74.
22. Song N, Zhao Z, Ma X, Sun X, Ma J, Li F, et al. Naringin promotes fracture healing through stimulation of angiogenesis by regulating the VEGF/VEGFR-2 signaling pathway in osteoporotic rats. Chem Biol Interact. 2017;261:11–7.
23. Hu K, Olsen BR. Osteoblast-derived VEGF regulates osteoblast differentiation and bone formation during bone repair. J Clin Invest. 2016;126:509–26.
24. Stegen S, van Gastel N, Carmeliet G. Bringing new life to damaged bone: the importance of angiogenesis in bone repair and regeneration. Bone. 2015;70:19–27.
25. Issa JP, Ingraci de Lucia C, Dos Santos Kotake BG, Goncalves Gonzaga M, Tocchini de Figueiredo FA, Mizusaki Iyomasa D, et al. The effect of simvastatin treatment on bone repair of femoral fracture in animal model. Growth Factors. 2015;33:139–48.
26. Lee JY, Son SJ, Son JS, Kang SS, Choi SH. Bone-healing capacity of PCL/PLGA/Duck beak scaffold in critical bone defects in a rabbit model. Biomed Res Int. 2016;2016:2136215.
27. De Kock T, Boone MA, De Schryver T, Van Stappen J, Derluyn H, Masschaele B, et al. A pore-scale study of fracture dynamics in rock using X-ray micro-CT under ambient freeze-thaw cycling. Environ Sci Technol. 2015;49:2867–74.

4

Wenyang Huazhuo Tongluo formula inhibits fibrosis via suppressing Wnt/β-catenin signaling pathway in a Bleomycin-induced systemic sclerosis mouse model

Qian Wang[1,2], Wenhua Zang[1,2], Li Han[1,2], Lei Yang[1,2], Songshan Ye[1,2], Jingfeng Ouyang[3], Chaoyun Zhang[1], Yuefeng Bi[4], Cuiyue Zhang[1] and Hua Bian[1,2*]

Abstract

Background: Systemic sclerosis (SSc) is an autoimmune disease characterized by fibrosis of the skin and internal organs. So far, no Western medicine treatment can completely inhibit or reverse the progress of SSc, while at the same time, our previous series of studies have shown that the treatment of SSc by the Wenyang Huazhuo Tongluo formula (WYHZTL), a Chinese herbal decoction, shows a delightful prospect. The aim of this study is to further investigate the mechanism of anti-fibrosis of WYHZTL formula in SSc mouse model.

Methods: The Bleomycin-induced SSc mouse model was treated with saline (BLM), high-dosage of WYHZTL formula (WYHZTL-H), medium-dosage of WYHZTL formula (WYHZTL-M), low-dosage of WYHZTL formula (WYHZTL-L) and XAV-939, a small molecule inhibitor of Wnt/β-catenin signaling pathway, by the intragastric administration and intraperitoneal injection, respectively. The mRNA and protein levels of Wnt/β-catenin signaling pathway associated genes, fibrosis markers and histopathology were detected by reverse transcription-quantitative polymerase chain reaction, Western blotting and hematoxylin/eosin-staining. The levels of Wnt1, CTGF and DKK1 protein in serum were detected by enzyme-linked immunosorbent assay.

Results: Compared with BLM group, the WYHZTL formula and XAV-939 could significantly inhibit the thickness of the skin tissue of the SSc mouse model. The mRNA expression levels of GSK3β and DKK1 in the WYHZTL formula and XAV-939-treated group were significantly higher than those in the BLM group, while Wnt1, β-catenin, TCF4, cyclin D1, survivin, VEGF, CTGF, FN1, collagen I/III were decreased. Compared with BLM group, the protein expression levels of GSK3β and DKK1 in the WYHZTL formula and XAV-939-treated group were upregulated, while Wnt1, β-catenin, cyclin D1, survivin, CTGF, FN1, collagen I/III were downregulated. WYHZTL formula and XAV-939 could inhibit expression of Wnt1 and CTGF, but promoted DKK1 in serum. Furthermore, WYHZTL-H seemed more effective than WYHZTL-M and/or XAV-939 on regulating Wnt1, β-catenin, TCF4, GSK3β, DKK1, cyclin D1, survivin, VEGF, CTGF, FN1 and collagen I/III.

Conclusion: This present study demonstrates that WYHZTL formula has anti-fibrosis effect in Bleomycin-induced SSc mouse model in a dosage-dependent manner, and the molecular mechanism may be related to the inhibition of Wnt/β-catenin signaling pathway.

Keywords: Wenyang Huazhuo Tongluo formula, SSc mouse model, Anti-fibrosis, Wnt/β-catenin signaling pathway

Background

Systemic sclerosis (SSc) is an autoimmune disease characterized by fibrosis of the skin and internal organs. Fibrosis is a typical pathological feature of SSc, which is closely related to its prognosis and mortality [1, 2]. So far,

*Correspondence: biancrown@163.com
[1] Zhang Zhongjing College of Chinese Medicine, Nanyang Institute of Technology, Changjiang Road 80, Nanyang 473004, Henan, China
Full list of author information is available at the end of the article

there is no drug that can completely inhibit or reverse the progress of SSc, neither the plasma exchange treatment indicating by clinical score [3]. Encouragingly, hematopoietic stem cell transplantation shows a certain effect on the treatment of SSc, but needs a long way for clinical applications [4].

Studies have shown that the occurrence, development and prognosis of SSc fibrosis depends on the "net effect" of the synthesis and degradation processes of extracellular matrix (ECM). Fibrosis occurs when collagen fibers are excessively synthesized and relatively less degraded [5, 6]. Wnt signal pathway plays an important role in regulating the adhesion, migration, epithelial transformation and growth of cells, and maintaining the stability of tissues and organs [7, 8]. When the Wnt/β-catenin signaling pathway, the classical Wnt signaling pathway, is inactive, Axin, APC, GSK3β and CK1 in the cytoplasm form a degraded complex that binds to β-catenin, leading β-catenin degraded by proteasomes. On the other hand, when the Wnt protein binds to the receptors of Frizzled family on the cell membrane, the Wnt/β-catenin signaling pathway is activated, causing the accumulation of β-catenin in the cytoplasm to promote the translocation of β-catenin to the nucleus to form transcriptional activation complex with TCF/LEF family proteins, followed by the upregulation of a series of target genes, such as c-myc and cyclin D1 and so on [9, 10].

Previous studies showed that Wnt/β-catenin signaling pathway was closely related to fibrosis in skin, lung, liver and kidney [11–15], which played an important role in the pathogenesis of SSc fibrosis. In the process of SSc fibrosis, Wnt/β-catenin signaling pathway was overactive, and the expression level of target genes, such as cyclinD1, VEGF, CTGF and ET-1 are abnormal [16, 17]. Compared with normal subjects, the accumulation of β-catenin in the SSc skin fibroblasts was increased, which resulted in higher transcription level of the target genes. At the same time, the expression levels of Wnt-1 and Wnt-10b were increased in the fibrotic skin and lung tissue [18]. In the Bleomycin-induced fibrosis model or Tsk mice, Wnt/β-catenin signaling pathway was also overactivated [18–20]. Similarly, Liu et al. [21] found that the expression level of cyclin D1 and TGF-β in pulmonary fibrosis were elevated in the Bleomycin-induced animal model. On the contrary, Dkk1 inhibited Wnt/β-catenin signaling pathway by binding to LRP5 and LRP6, the Wnt receptor complex [22]. Akhmetshina et al. [23, 24] found that DKK1 expression was absent in SSc dermal fibroblasts and also significantly reduced in pulmonary fibrosis. The animal experiments showed that DKK1 overexpression inhibited Bleomycin-induced fibrosis [18]. By injecting DKK siRNA into mouse ears, scientists found that expression level of DKK was decreased, and dermal was thickening, which accompanied by increased fibroblast growth and β-catenin expression [25]. All the results showed that DKK1 deletion was one of the causes of Wnt/β-catenin signaling pathway overactivation and played an important role in the pathogenesis of SSc.

The current western medicine treatment of SSc is not satisfactory, so it is essential to explore another treatment option. In the traditional Chinese medicine treatment of SSc, Wenyangchubi formula and Yiqihuoxue formula were representative examples. Studies have shown that Wenyangchubi formula could reduce the expression of connective tissue growth factor (CTGF) and collagen I, improve the skin fibrosis of SSc mouse model [26]. And Yiqihuoxue formula could inhibit the expression of collagen in SSc dermal fibroblasts and TGF-β1-induced NIH/3T3 fibroblasts by regulating TGF-β/smad3 signaling pathway [27]. In 2000, our team invented Wenyang Huazhuo Tongluo formula (WYHZTL formula, Patent No. CN201310351880.2), and applied to the treatment of SSc. Our previous studies have shown that WYHZTL formula could effectively improve the skin score of SSc patients, Renault phenomenon and nail fold microcirculation, reduce plasma endothelin, FVC, DLco and other indicators [28]. In vitro, WYHZTL formula could inhibit the expression of cyclin D1, survivin, TGF-β1 and collagen I/III in skin fibroblasts of SSc patients [29, 30]. WYHZTL formula promoted MMP-9 secretion, inhibited TIMP-1 production, regulated MMP-9/TIMP-1 imbalance, and reduced the serum PIIINP levels while upregulated ICTP levels in SSc patients, thereby reducing fibrosis [31]. However, the mechanism of WYHZTL formula in the treatment of SSc fibrosis based on Wnt/β-catenin signaling pathway has not been reported.

The aim of this study was to further explore the molecular mechanism of anti-SSc fibrosis of WYHZTL formula, and investigate the effect of WYHZTL formula on Wnt/β-catenin signaling pathway in SSc mouse model.

Methods

The Minimum Standards of Reporting Checklist contains details of the experimental design, and resources used in this study (Additional file 1).

Composition and preparation of Wenyang Huazhuo Tongluo formula

WYHZTL formula contains Herba Epimedii, Radix Astragali membranacei, Herba Glechomae longitubae, Ramulus Cinnamomi cassiae, Radix Dioscoreae oppositae, Semen Sinapis lbae, Radix Codonopsitis pilosulae, Fasciculus vascularis Luffae, Radix Rehmanniae praeparata and Capparis zeylanica Linn. The preparation procedure of WYHZTL was performed as our previous protocol [29]. The ingredients of WYHZTL formula were

purchased from the First Affiliated Hospital of Nanyang Institute of Technology.

The establishment of Bleomycin-induced systemic sclerosis mouse model

Specific pathogen-free (SPF) C57BL/6 mice were purchased from Beijing Vital River Laboratory Animal Technology Co., Ltd. (Beijing, China). By local injection of Bleomycin in 7-week-old female mice for 3 weeks, the skin fibrosis was induced. Briefly, Bleomycin dissolved in sterile saline to a concentration of 200 μg/ml, and subcutaneous injection of 100 μl of Bleomycin to the restricted area of the upper back each day [27]. 100 μl of phosphate buffer saline (PBS) was subcutaneously injected as controls. All the animal protocols were approved by Zhang Zhongjing College of Chinese Medicine, Nanyang Institute of Technology, China.

The experimental group and drug treatment regimens

Eight mice on a C57BL/6 background were randomly selected as normal groups. Then, the Bleomycin-induced SSc mouse models were randomly divided into five groups, and each group has eight mice. The five groups were named as Bleomycin group (BLM), WYHZTL formula low-dosage group (BLM + WHHZTL-L), WYHZTL formula medium-dosage group (BLM + WYHZTL-M), WYHZTL formula high-dosage group (BLM + WYHZTL-H), and XAV-939 group (BLM + XAV-939), respectively. The PBS group (PBS) received PBS administered daily by subcutaneous injection into defined areas of upper back of normal C57BL/6 mouse, while the normal group (Normal) didn't receive any administration. Normal, PBS, and BLM group received saline (1 ml/day) administered daily by intragastric administration, while BLM + WYHZTL-L group, BLM + WYHZTL-M group, BLM + WYHZTL-H group received low-dosage of WYHZTL formula (11.75 g/kg/d), medium-dosage of WYHZTL formula (23.50 g/kg/day), high-dosage of WYHZTL formula (47.00 g/kg/day) administered daily by intragastric administration of Bleomycin-induced SSc mouse models, respectively. BLM + XAV-939 group received XAV-939 (10 mg/kg/day) administered daily by intraperitoneal injection of Bleomycin-induced SSc mouse models. All the treatments lasted for 4 weeks, then the mice of each group were anaesthetized and then euthanized, and skin tissues were harvested, stored at − 80 °C, to analyze expression levels of target genes and proteins.

Morphometric dermal measurements

The measurement of skin thickness, skinfold (pinch) thickness and breaking strength of skin were performed as previously described protocol [32]. Briefly, skin thickness was measured using a skin caliper on 12-mm punch biopsy samples obtained from the upper back, away from previous sites of drug injection. A skin caliper was used to measure skinfold (pinch) thickness at the same area of the upper back of the mouse. The measurement of breaking strength of skin was performed by a tensiometer, with a forceps clamped to one side of the 12-mm skin tissue sample and coupled to another forceps clamped to the furthermost extreme of the tissue sample. The value of maximal stress was recorded before tearing of the tissue sample [33]. All measurements were undertaken in a blinded manner.

Histopathological analysis

Skin tissue samples were fixed with 4% paraformaldehyde, and embedded in paraffin, then cutted into 3 μm-thick sample sections for hematoxylin/eosin staining [34]. For hematoxylin/eosin stained tissue samples, a SCN400 Digital Slide Scanner (Leica Microsystems, Wetzlar, Germany) was used to examine and acquire images to identify histopathological changes. The diagnosis was performed by two independent examiners in a blinded manner.

Western blotting analysis

The effects of the WYHZTL formula on Wnt/β-catenin signaling pathway was analyzed by Western blotting as previously described protocol [35]. Briefly, 1 day after WYHZTL formula and XAV-939 administration, the mice were killed to obtain skin tissues. Then the skin tissues were emulsified by ultrasound in RIPA lysis buffer (Beyotime Biotechnology, China). The protein concentrations were detected by BCA assay (Beyotime Biotechnology, China). 40 μg of protein was electrophoresed via sodium dodecyl sulphate polyacrylamide gel electrophoresis (SDS-PAGE), and transferred onto polyvinylidene fluoride (PVDF) membranes (Millipore, USA). Then the membranes were blocked using 5% skimmed milk powder at room temperature for 1 h. After blocking, membranes were incubated with specific antibodies against Wnt1 (1:500 dilution; abcam, UK), β-catenin, TCF4, DKK1, GSK3β, cyclin D1, survivin, CTGF, VEGF, Fibronectin, Collagen I, Collagen III (1:1000 dilution; Proteintech, USA), and GAPDH (1:5000 dilution; Proteintech, USA) overnight. After washing membranes with TBST buffer, membranes were incubated with corresponding horseradish peroxidase (HRP)-conjugated secondary antibody at a 1:5000 dilution for 1 h at 37 °C. Finally, the membranes were washed with TBST three times and developed using an BeyoECL Plus Kit by automated chemiluminescence system (Tanon, China) according to the manufacturer's instructions. The optical density of immunoreactive bands was measured with a computer-assisted imaging analysis system (Tanon, China) and the relative protein expression levels were normalized to optical density of GAPDH.

RT-qPCR analysis

Total RNA of each skin tissue samples was extracted using TRIzol reagent (Invitrogen, USA). All handling procedures perform under a laminar flow hood and RNAse-free conditions. The extracted RNA was dissolved in 30 μl RNase-free water and quantified by Nanodrop 2000 ultraviolet spectrophotometer (Thermo Fisher Scientific, Inc.), then stored at − 80 °C until used. RNA (2 μg) was reverse transcribed into complementary DNA (cDNA) using M-MLV Reverse Transcriptase (Thermo Fisher Scientific, Inc.) according to the manufacturer's instructions. RT-qPCR analysis was performed using ABI Power SYBR Green PCR Master Mix Kit on an ABI Step One Plus instrument (Thermo Fisher Scientific, Inc.). The reaction condition follows denaturation for 2 min at 95 °C, 40 cycles including 95 °C for 15 s, 60 °C for 20 s and 72 °C for 30 s. Each experiment was performed 3 times independently. PCR products were mixed with 6× loading buffer (TaKaRa Biotechnology, Dalian, China) and then electrophoresed in 1.5% agarose gels containing ethidium bromide. The images were captured using a 4600SF Gel Image System (Tanon, China). The relative expression level of target gene was normalized to GAPDH and calculated with $2^{-\Delta\Delta Ct}$ method [36]. The primers for mRNA analysis for RT-qPCR were listed in the Table 1.

Table 1 Sequences of oligonucleotide primers and products size of RT-qPCR

mRNA	Primers (5′→ 3′) F: Forward R: Reverse	Product size (bp)
Wnt1	F: TGTTGACGGATTCCAAGAGT R: GAAGTAGACGAGGTCGTGAG	235
β-catenin	F: GGCAACCCTGAGGAAGAAGA R: AGCGTCAAACTGCGTGGAT	192
DKK1	F: ATCAATTCCAACGCGATCAA R: GGTCAGAGGGCATGCATATT	325
GSK3β	F: CCTGGTGCTGGACTATGT R: CAAGAGGTTCTGTGGTTTAA	214
TCF4	F: ACCACATGACTAGCAGGGATCT R: GGAGGAACTTTTCGGACTTTCT	298
VEGF	F: TTACTGCTGTACCTCCACC R: ACAGGACGGCTTGAAGATG	189
cyclin D1	F: GAGAAGTTGTGCATCTACAC R: GAAGGGCTTCAACTGTTCC	375
Survivin	F: GCTCTATGTAAGATCGCTTC R: CGTGAATCGCCATAATTATCC	389
CTGF	F: GTGTGTGACGAGCCCAAGGA R: AGTTGGGTCTGGGCCAAATGT	112
Fn1	F: ACCATACCTGCCGAATGTAG R: CTCCTCTCCAATGGCGTAAT	439
Collagen I	F: TGTTCGTGGTTCTCAGGGTAG R: TTGTCGTAGCAGGGTTCTTTC	245
Collagen III	F: TGCCCACAGCCTTCTACACCT R: CAGCCATTCCTCCCACTCCAG	254
GAPDH	F: TGGGTGTGAACCACGAGAA R: GGCATGGACTGTGGTCATGA	143

Enzyme-linked immunosorbent assay (ELISA) analysis

One day after WYHZTL formula and XAV-939 administration, the animals were sacrificed. Collecting blood sample and standing to clot for 2 h at room temperature. Then centrifugation at 1000×*g* for 10 min, and obtain upper serum carefully to assay immediately. ELISA analysis was performed using enzyme-linked immunosorbent assay kit (Cusabio Technology, China) on a SpectraMax iD3 microplate reader instrument (Molecular Devices, USA). Reagents, and samples or standards were prepared, and experiments were performed according to the manufacturer's instructions. Briefly, standard or sample were added to each well separately, and incubated at 37 °C for 2 h. Then standards or samples were removed without washing. Add Biotin-antibody to each well, and incubate at 37 °C for 1 h. Remove liquid of each well and wash. Add HRP-avidin to each well, and incubate at 37 °C for 1 h. Remove liquid of each well and wash. Add TMB Substrate to each well, and incubate at 37 °C for 20 min. Add Stop Solution to each well, and immediately detect the optical density of each well by a SpectraMax iD3 microplate reader instrument set to 450 nm. At last, the concentration of target protein was calculated according to standard curve. Each experiment was performed three times independently.

Statistical analysis

Results were represented as mean ± SD. Data were analyzed by one-way analysis of variance, as appropriate, followed by Bonferroni post hoc test if F achieved $P < 0.05$ and there was no significant variance in homogeneity. All statistical analyses were performed with Graphpad Prism 6.0 Software. $P < 0.05$ was considered to indicate a statistically significant difference. All data and statistical analysis complied with the recommendations on experimental design and analysis in pathology.

Results

WYHZTL formula could ameliorate skin fibrosis in Bleomycin-induced SSc mouse model

To confirm whether the Bleomycin-induced SSc mouse model was successfully constructed in this study, and detected the effect of WYHZTL formula and XAV-939 on skin fibrosis in mouse models, the skin of each mouse model group was dissected using paraffin sections, and the skin pathological changes of the mouse model were observed by hematoxylin and eosin stained (HE) staining. The results of HE staining showed that there was excessive accumulation of collagen and other extracellular matrix components in BLM group, which was attenuated with WYHZTL formula or XAV-939 treatment (Fig. 1a). The skin tissue of BLM group was significantly thicker than that of the PBS group. Compared with the BLM group, BLM+WYHZTL-L, BLM+WYHZTL-M, BLM+WYHZTL-H and BLM+XAV-939 groups displayed significantly reduced skin thickness ($P<0.05$, $P<0.01$, $P<0.01$, $P<0.01$, respectively) (Fig. 1b) and skinfold thickness ($P<0.05$, $P<0.01$, $P<0.001$, $P<0.01$, respectively) (Fig. 1c). These results were consistent with the higher dermal tensile strength, measured as breaking tension ($P<0.05$, $P<0.05$, $P<0.01$, $P<0.01$, respectively) (Fig. 1d). In addition, for skin thickness, skinfold thickness, and breaking tension, BLM+WYHZTL-H group showed more reduction than BLM+WYHZTL-L, BLM+WYHZTL-M, and BLM+XAV-939 groups ($P<0.05$) (Fig. 1b–d). These results confirmed that WYHZTL formula or XAV-939 could significantly improve the thickening degree of the skin tissue, in addition, more importantly, the effect of WYHZTL formula was in a dosage-dependent manner, and WYHZTL-H had more advantage than XAV-939.

Effect of WYHZTL formula on Wnt/β-catenin signal pathway in SSc mouse model

In order to determine whether the therapeutic effect of WYHZTL formula on SSc mouse model was related to Wnt/β-catenin signaling pathway, we collected the skin tissues of mice in each group, and detected the components of Wnt/β-catenin signal pathway using RT-qPCR and Western blotting.

The results of RT-qPCR showed that the mRNA expression level of GSK3β in BLM+WYHZTL-H, and BLM+XAV-939 group were significantly higher than that in BLM group ($P<0.01$), while BLM+WYHZTL-L, BLM+WYHZTL-M groups had no significant changes ($P>0.05$) (Fig. 2d). And the expression level of GSK3β in BLM+WYHZTL-H group was higher than BLM+WYHZTL-M, and BLM+XAV-939 group ($P<0.01$, $P<0.05$, respectively) (Fig. 2d). The expression level of DKK1 mRNA in BLM+WYHZTL-L, BLM+WYHZTL-M, BLM+WYHZTL-H, and BLM+XAV-939 group were significantly higher than that in BLM group ($P<0.01$, $P<0.05$, $P<0.01$, $P<0.01$, respectively) (Fig. 2e). And the expression level of DKK1 mRNA was higher than BLM+WYHZTL-L, BLM+WYHZTL-M group ($P<0.05$, $P<0.01$, respectively), rather than BLM+XAV-939 group ($P>0.05$)

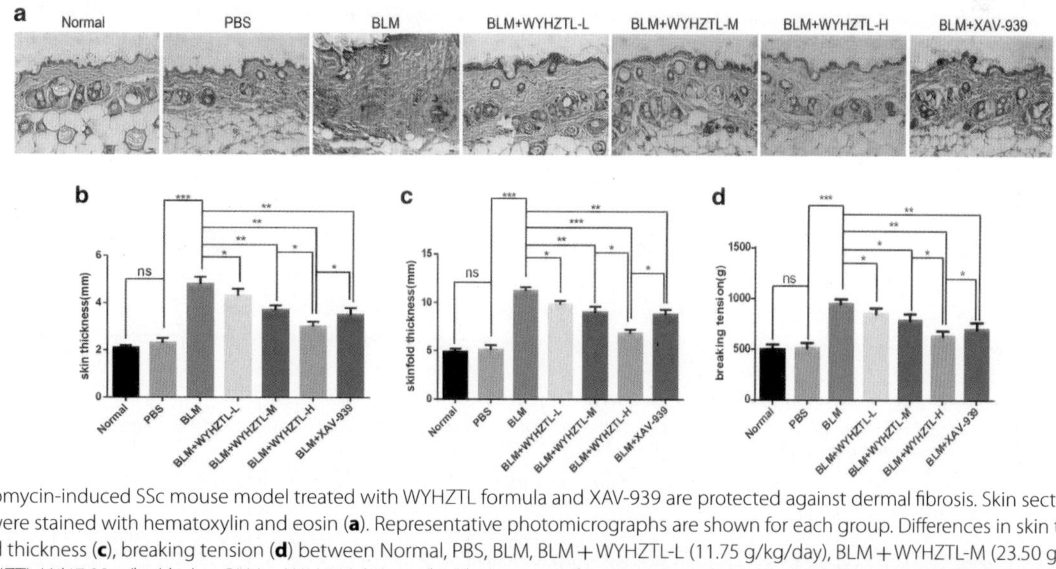

Fig. 1 Bleomycin-induced SSc mouse model treated with WYHZTL formula and XAV-939 are protected against dermal fibrosis. Skin sections for histology were stained with hematoxylin and eosin (**a**). Representative photomicrographs are shown for each group. Differences in skin thickness (**b**), skinfold thickness (**c**), breaking tension (**d**) between Normal, PBS, BLM, BLM+WYHZTL-L (11.75 g/kg/day), BLM+WYHZTL-M (23.50 g/kg/day), BLM+WYHZTL-H (47.00 g/kg/day) or BLM+XAV-939 (10 mg/kg/day) groups after injections of Bleomycin (BLM) or phosphate buffered saline (PBS) for 3 weeks. The mean values ± SD (n = 8 per group) was shown for each bar. *(P < 0.05) or **(P < 0.01) or ***(P < 0.001) represents significance. Original magnification: ×20 (**a**). BLM: Bleomycin, WYHZTL: Wenyang Huazhuo Tongluo formula, WYHZTL-L: low-dosage of WYHZTL formula, WYHZTL-M: medium-dosage of WYHZTL formula, WYHZTL-H: high-dosage of WYHZTL formula

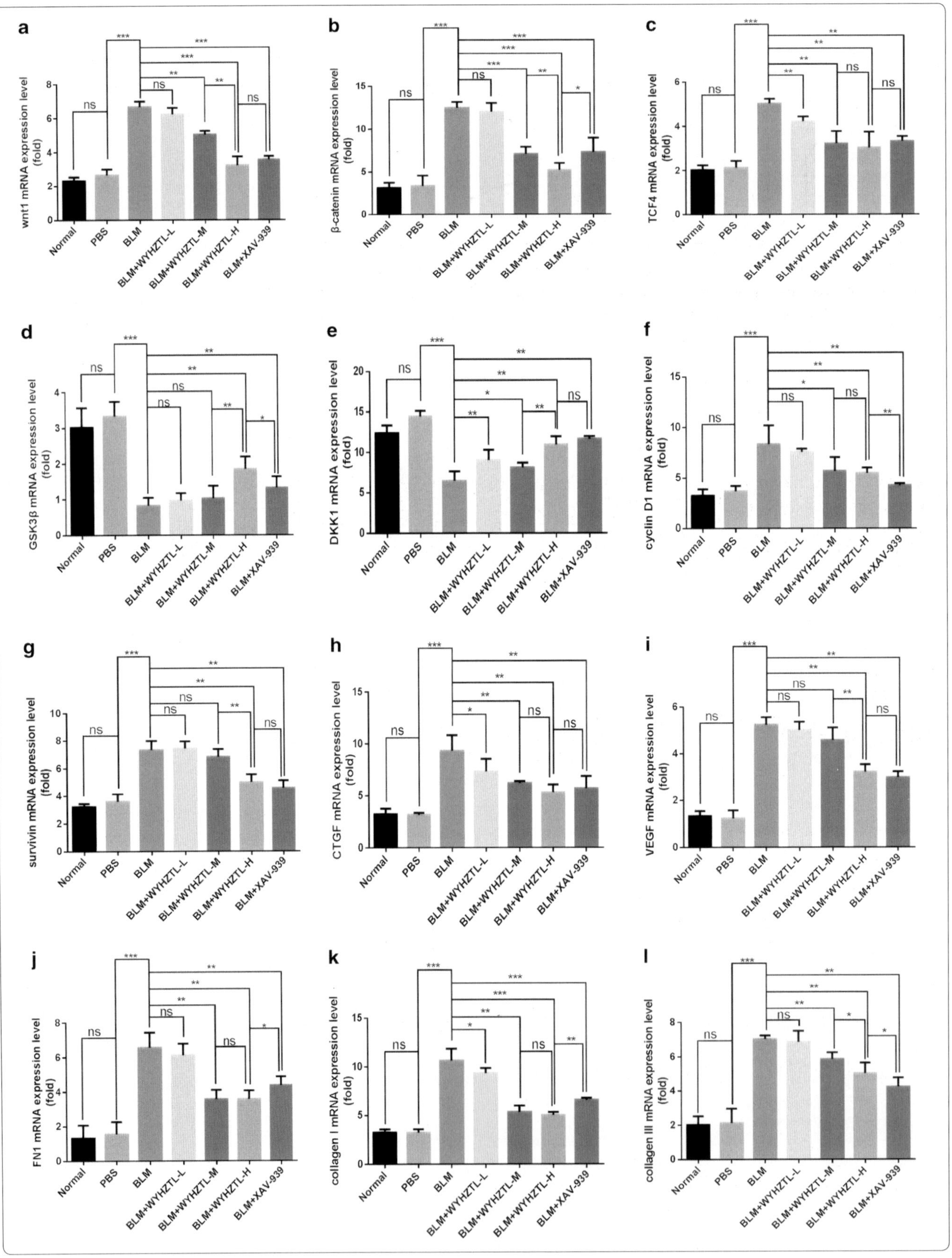
a
wnt1 mRNA expression level (fold)
b
β-catenin mRNA expression level (fold)
c
TCF4 mRNA expression level (fold)
d
GSK3β mRNA expression level (fold)
e
DKK1 mRNA expression level (fold)
f
cyclin D1 mRNA expression level (fold)
g
survivin mRNA expression level (fold)
h
CTGF mRNA expression level (fold)
i
VEGF mRNA expression level (fold)
j
FN1 mRNA expression level (fold)
k
collagen I mRNA expression level (fold)
l
collagen III mRNA expression level (fold)
Normal
PBS
BLM
BLM+WYHZTL-L
BLM+WYHZTL-M
BLM+WYHZTL-H
BLM+XAV-939
ns
*
**
***

(See figure on previous page)

Fig. 2 The ratios of the mRNA expression level of Wnt1, β-catenin, TCF4, GSK3β, DKK1, cyclin D1, survivin, CTGF, VEGF, FN1, Collagen I and Collagen III relative to that of GAPDH. The mRNA expression level ratios of Wnt1 (**a**), β-catenin (**b**), TCF4 (**c**), GSK3β (**d**), DKK1 (**e**), cyclin D1 (**f**), survivin (**g**), CTGF (**h**), VEGF (**i**), FN1 (**j**), Collagen I (**k**) and Collagen III (**l**) relative to GAPDH were calculated by RT-qPCR. The mean values ± SD (n = 8 per group) was shown for each bar. *(P < 0.05) or **(P < 0.01) or ***(P < 0.001) represents significance, ns represents no significance. BLM: Bleomycin, WYHZTL: Wenyang Huazhuo Tongluo formula, WYHZTL-L: low-dosage of WYHZTL formula, WYHZTL-M: medium-dosage of WYHZTL formula, WYHZTL-H: high-dosage of WYHZTL formula. RT-qPCR: Reverse transcription-quantitative polymerase chain reaction

(Fig. 2e). Compared to BLM group, the expression level of Wnt1 and β-catenin in BLM + WYHZTL-M, BLM + WYHZTL-H and BLM + XAV-939 group was significantly decreased ($P<0.01$, $P<0.001$, $P<0.001$; all $P<0.001$, respectively), while BLM + WYHZTL-L group had no significant changes ($P>0.05$) (Fig. 2a, b). And the expression level of β-catenin in BLM + WYHZTL-H was lower than BLM + WYHZTL-M ($P<0.01$) and BLM + XAV-939 ($P<0.05$) group while the expression level of Wnt1 in BLM + WYHZTL-H were lower than BLM + WYHZTL-M ($P<0.01$), other than BLM + XAV-939 group ($P>0.05$) (Fig. 2a, b). Compared to BLM group, the expression level of TCF4 in BLM + WYHZTL-L, BLM + WYHZTL-M, BLM + WYHZTL-H and BLM + XAV-939 group was significantly decreased ($P<0.01$) (Fig. 2c).

As shown in Fig. 3a, b, the result of Western blotting showed that compared with the BLM group, the

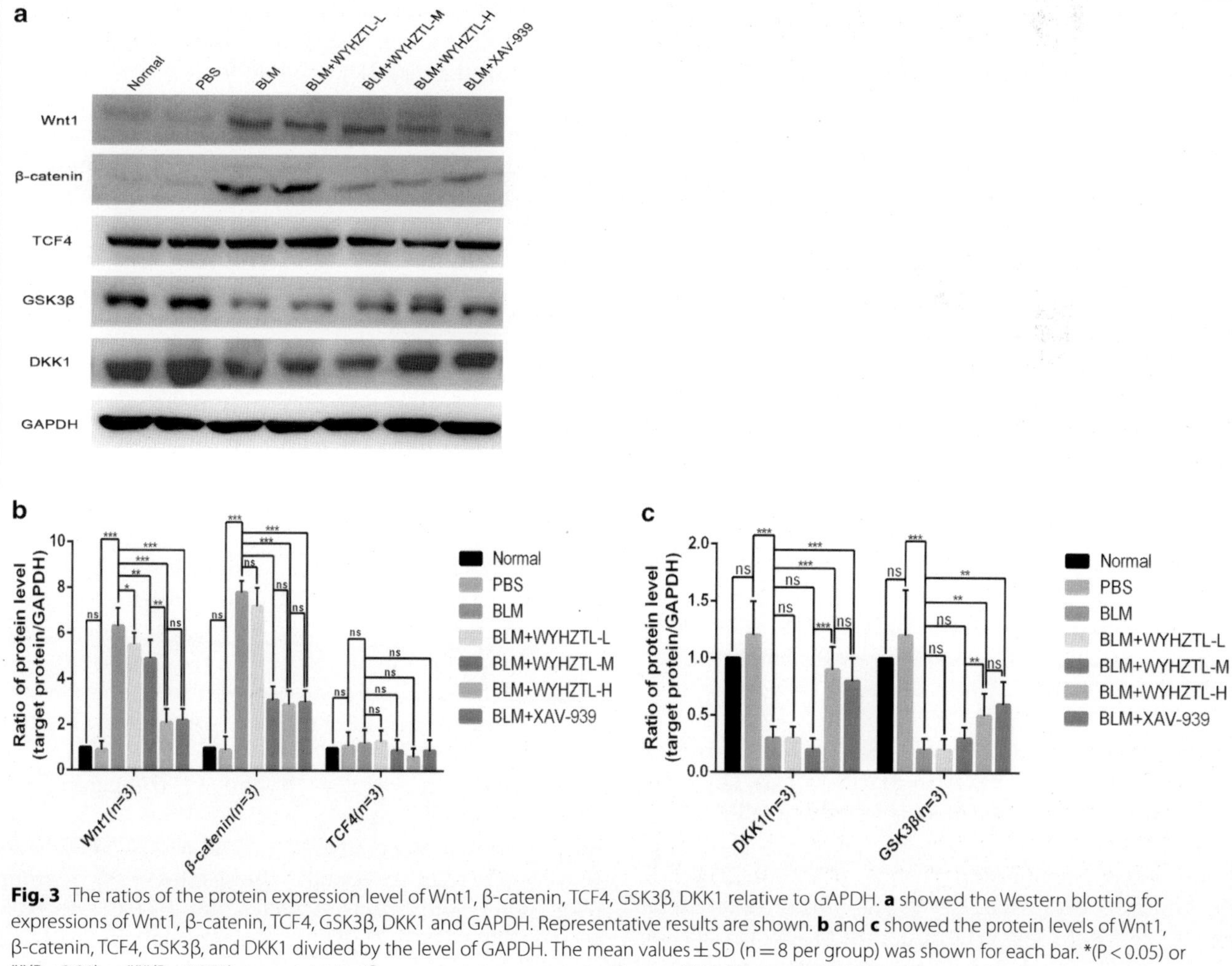

Fig. 3 The ratios of the protein expression level of Wnt1, β-catenin, TCF4, GSK3β, DKK1 relative to GAPDH. **a** showed the Western blotting for expressions of Wnt1, β-catenin, TCF4, GSK3β, DKK1 and GAPDH. Representative results are shown. **b** and **c** showed the protein levels of Wnt1, β-catenin, TCF4, GSK3β, and DKK1 divided by the level of GAPDH. The mean values ± SD (n = 8 per group) was shown for each bar. *(P < 0.05) or **(P < 0.01) or ***(P < 0.001) represents significance, ns represents no significance. BLM: Bleomycin, WYHZTL: Wenyang Huazhuo Tongluo formula, WYHZTL-L: low-dosage of WYHZTL formula, WYHZTL-M: medium-dosage of WYHZTL formula, WYHZTL-H: high-dosage of WYHZTL formula

expression level of Wnt1 protein in BLM + WYHZTL-L, BLM + WYHZTL-M, BLM + WYHZTL-H, and BLM + XAV-939 group were significantly decreased, while BLM + WYHZTL-H was even lower than BLM + WYHZTL-M group, other than BLM + XAV-939 group. Compared with the BLM group, the expression level of β-catenin protein in BLM + WYHZTL-M, BLM + WYHZTL-H, and BLM + XAV-939 group were significantly decreased, while BLM + WYHZTL-L had no significant changes ($P > 0.05$), and among BLM + WYHZTL-M, BLM + WYHZTL-H, and BLM + XAV-939 group, there were no significant difference ($P > 0.05$). However, in this study, we didn't detect any significant difference among Normal group, PBS group and BLM group. And WYHZTL formula or XAV-939 also had no effect on the expression level of TCF4 protein.

As shown in Fig. 3a, c, the expression level of DKK1 and GSK3β protein in BLM + WYHZTL-H and BLM + XAV-939 group were significantly higher than that in BLM group ($P < 0.001$, $P < 0.01$, respectively), while BLM + WYHZTL-L and BLM + WYHZTL-M group didn't have significant difference with BLM group ($P > 0.05$). And the expression level of DKK1 and GSK3β protein in BLM + WYHZTL-H were all higher than BLM + WYHZTL-M group ($P < 0.001$, $P < 0.01$, respectively), but not BLM + XAV-939 group ($P > 0.05$).

The effect of WYHZTL formula on target genes of Wnt/β-catenin signaling pathway and fibrosis marker

In order to further study on regulating SSc fibrosis by WYHZTL formula via Wnt/β-catenin signaling pathway, we investigated the expression level of target genes of Wnt/β-catenin signaling pathway and fibrosis markers in the skin tissues of each mouse model by RT-qPCR and Western blotting.

The results of RT-qPCR showed that compared with the BLM group, the mRNA expression levels of cyclin D1, FN1 and collagen III in BLM + WYHZTL-M, BLM + WYHZTL-H and BLM + XAV-939 group were downregulated ($P < 0.05$, $P < 0.01$, $P < 0.01$; all $P < 0.01$; all $P < 0.01$, respectively), while BLM + WYHZTL-L group didn't significantly change ($P > 0.05$) (Fig. 2f, j and l). Compared with the BLM group, the mRNA expression levels of survivin and VEGF in BLM + WYHZTL-H and BLM + XAV-939 group were downregulated (all $P < 0.01$), while BLM + WYHZTL-L and BLM + WYHZTL-M group didn't significantly change ($P > 0.05$) (Fig. 2i). The mRNA expression levels of CTGF and collagen I in BLM + WYHZTL-L, BLM + WYHZTL-M, BLM + WYHZTL-H and BLM + XAV-939 group were all lower than BLM group ($P < 0.05$, $P < 0.01$, $P < 0.01$, $P < 0.01$; $P < 0.05$, $P < 0.01$, $P < 0.001$, $P < 0.001$, respectively) (Fig. 2h, k).

In addition, the mRNA expression levels of survivin, VEGF and collagen III in BLM + WYHZTL-H group were even lower than BLM + WYHZTL-M group ($P < 0.01$, $P < 0.01$, $P < 0.05$, respectively), while the mRNA expression levels of FN1, collagen I in BLM + WYHZTL-H group were even lower than BLM + XAV-939 group ($P < 0.05$, $P < 0.01$, respectively) (Fig. 2g, i–l). Besides that, the mRNA expression levels of cyclin D1 and collagen III in BLM + XAV-939 group were lower than BLM + WYHZTL-H group ($P < 0.01$, $P < 0.05$, respectively) (Fig. 2f, l).

As shown in Fig. 4a, b and c, the results of Western blotting showed that compared with the BLM group, the protein expression levels of cyclin D1, survivin, FN1 and collagen I/III in BLM + WYHZTL-L, BLM + WYHZTL-M, BLM + WYHZTL-H and BLM + XAV-939 group were all downregulated ($P < 0.01$, $P < 0.001$, $P < 0.001$, $P < 0.001$; all $P < 0.001$; all $P < 0.001$; all $P < 0.001$, respectively), while CTGF in BLM + WYHZTL-M, BLM + WYHZTL-H and BLM + XAV-939 group was decreased (all $P < 0.001$). In addition, the protein expression levels of cyclin D1, CTGF, FN1 in BLM + WYHZTL-H group were even lower than BLM + WYHZTL-M group (all $P < 0.001$), while the protein expression levels of collagen I in BLM + WYHZTL-H group was lower than BLM + XAV-939 group ($P < 0.01$). Besides that, the protein expression levels of CTGF in BLM + XAV-939 group was even lower than BLM + WYHZTL-H group ($P < 0.01$).

Furthermore, compared to Normal and PBS group, we found that VEGF was upregulated in BLM group ($P < 0.001$), but there was no significant difference among BLM, BLM + WYHZTL-L, BLM + WYHZTL-M, BLM + WYHZTL-H and BLM + XAV-939 group ($P > 0.05$).

Effect of WYHZTL formula on the protein level of Wnt-1, DKK1 and CTGF in serum of SSc mouse model

In order to further identify the regulation of Wnt/β-catenin signaling pathway by WYHZTL formula, we collected the serum of each group of mouse model and detected the protein level of Wnt1, DKK1 and CTGF in serum by ELISA.

As shown in Fig. 5a, b and c, compared with BLM group, the protein level of Wnt1 and CTGF in BLM + WYHZTL-L, BLM + WYHZTL-M, BLM + WYHZTL-H and BLM + XAV-939 group were significantly downregulated (all $P < 0.01$; $P < 0.05$, $P < 0.001$, $P < 0.001$, $P < 0.001$, respectively), while DKK1 was upregulated ($P < 0.05$, $P < 0.01$, $P < 0.01$, $P < 0.01$, respectively), in which WYHZTL-H became more

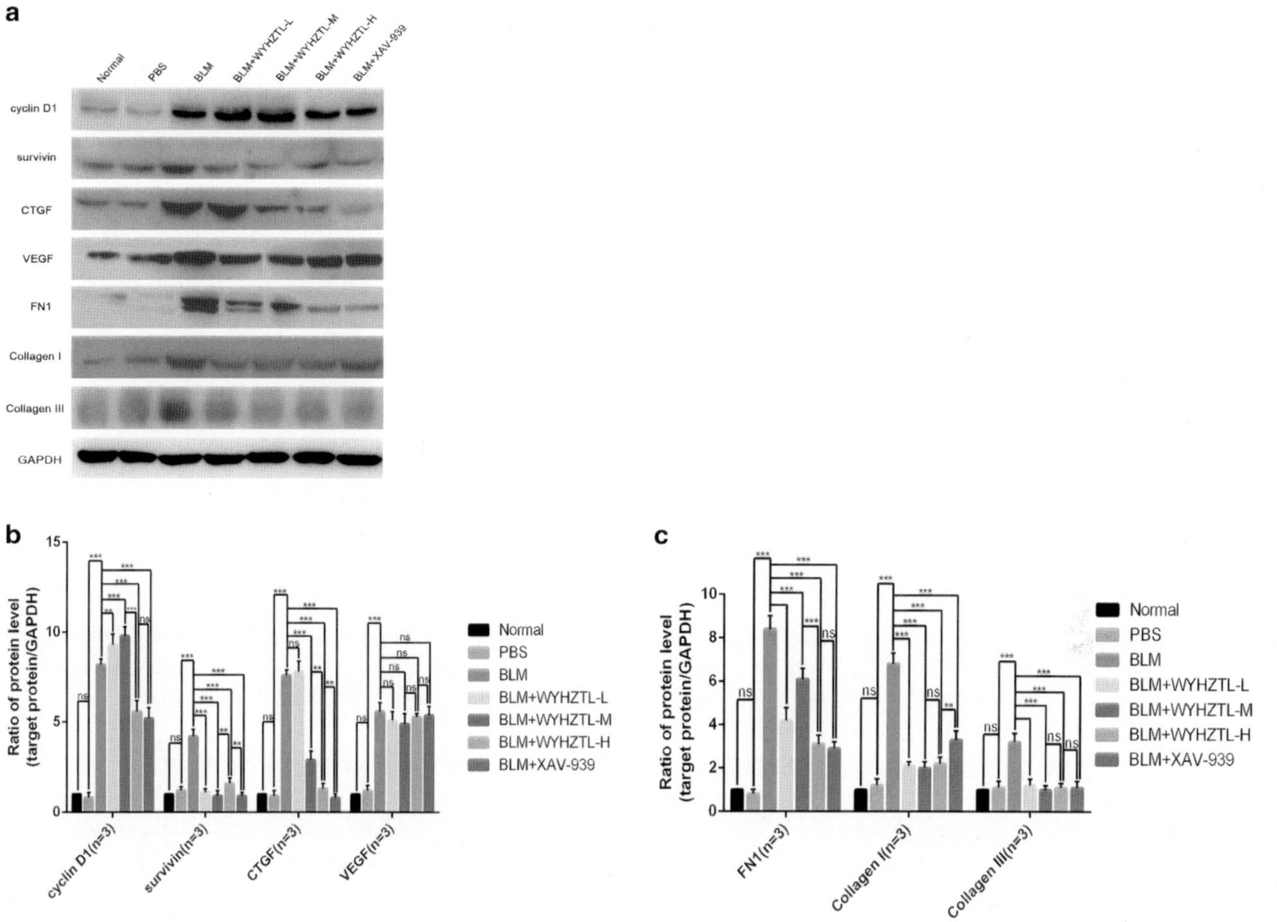

Fig. 4 The ratios of the protein expression level of cyclin D1, survivin, CTGF, VEGF, FN1, Collagen I and Collagen III relative to GAPDH. **a** showed the Western blotting for expressions of cyclin D1, survivin, CTGF, VEGF, FN1, Collagen I, Collagen III and GAPDH. Representative results are shown. **b** and **c** showed the protein levels of cyclin D1, survivin, CTGF, VEGF, FN1, Collagen I, Collagen III divided by the level of GAPDH. The mean values ± SD (n = 8 per group) was shown for each bar. ***(P < 0.001) represents significance, ns represents no significance. BLM: Bleomycin, WYHZTL: Wenyang Huazhuo Tongluo formula, WYHZTL-L: low-dosage of WYHZTL formula, WYHZTL-M: medium-dosage of WYHZTL formula, WYHZTL-H: high-dosage of WYHZTL formula

effective on promoting DKK1 ($P < 0.001$), while inhibiting Wnt1 and CTGF (all $P < 0.001$) than WYHZTL-M. Furthermore, compared with BLM + XAV-939 group, WYHZTL-H was more effective in downregulating Wnt1, and upregulating DKK1 (all $P < 0.001$).

Discussion

Wnt/β-catenin signaling pathway could induce fibrosis. Wnt1 and human skin fibroblasts were co-incubated to significantly stimulate the expression of α-SMA and type II collagen, which meant that Wnt1 could induce the transformation of resting fibroblasts to myofibroblasts, and stimulate collagen release [18, 37]. Previous works exhibited that Wnt signal overactivates in SSc patients which played an important role in myofibroblast differentiation and fibroblast proliferation, and also inducing adipose precursor cells transform to fibroblasts by DNA chip analysis and immunohistochemistry technology [38, 39]. At the same time, overexpressing Wnt-10b in normal fibroblasts could upregulate the expression level of fibrosis-related genes [19, 40]. In vivo experiments had also shown that Wnt-10b transgenic mice appear skin fibrosis, progressive subcutaneous fat loss, collagen accumulation, fibroblast activation, myofibroblast aggregation and other phenomena, while Wnt/β-catenin signaling pathway was overactivated in skin fibroblasts [19, 41], which further confirmed that activation of Wnt/β-catenin signaling pathway could induce fibrosis. In the present study, we also found that Wnt/β-catenin signaling pathway was overactivated in the

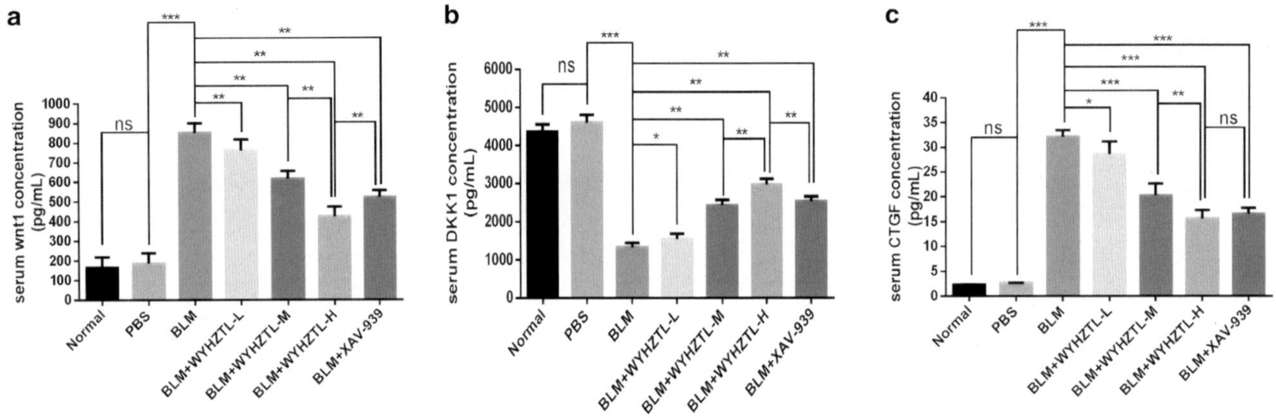

Fig. 5 The protein expression level of Wnt1, DKK1 and CTGF in serum. The protein concentrations of Wnt1 (**a**), DKK1 (**b**) and CTGF (**c**) were detected by ELISA. The mean values ± SD (n = 8 per group) was shown for each bar. *(P < 0.05) or **(P < 0.01) or ***(P < 0.001) represents significance, ns represents no significance. BLM: Bleomycin, WYHZTL: Wenyang Huazhuo Tongluo formula, WYHZTL-L: low-dosage of WYHZTL formula, WYHZTL-M: medium-dosage of WYHZTL formula, WYHZTL-H: high-dosage of WYHZTL formula. *ELISA* enzyme-linked immunosorbent assay

BLM-induced SSc mouse model, suggesting that Wnt/β-catenin signaling pathway indeed played an important role in the pathogenesis of SSc. More importantly, WYHZTL formula could significantly improve skin fibrosis in SSc mouse model. Further study found that WYHZTL formula could inhibit the Wnt/β-catenin signaling pathway. These results suggested that WYHZTL formula may exert anti-SSc fibrosis effect by inhibiting Wnt/β-catenin signaling pathway.

Fibrosis, atrophy and vascular occlusive vasculitis of connective tissue were basic pathological changes of SSc [6]. Fibrosis may involve multiple visceral systems, such as the gastrointestinal tract, lung, kidney, heart, blood vessels, skeletal muscle system, causing dysfunction of corresponding organs [42]. Among them, the skin tissue fibrosis and dermal thickening were the most important and common pathological features of SSc. Yamamoto and colleagues [43] used the Bleomycin (BLM) treatment to establish a new mouse model of SSc: subcutaneous injection of BLM can induce dermal and pulmonary fibrosis, autoantibody production and skin inflammatory infiltration, which was one of the best animal models for studying on systemic sclerosis. In this study, we used Bleomycin-induced mice on a C57BL/6 background to construct systemic sclerosis model. We identified Bleomycin-induced mouse skin tissue by HE staining, showing that fibrosis, dermal thickening, inflammatory cell infiltration and other pathological changes, suggesting that Bleomycin-induced systemic sclerosis mouse model was successfully constructed. Then we treated the SSc mouse model with WYHZTL formula and XAV-939, respectively. The result of HE staining showed that compared with the model group, the thickening degree of skin of the SSc mouse model was significantly thinner in WYHZTL formula and XAV-939 group, moreover, we found that the effect of WYHZTL formula was more significant than XAV-939.

The overexpression of target genes of Wnt/β-catenin signaling pathway were closely related to SSc fibrosis. The target genes include c-myc, cyclin D1, survivin, vascular endothelial growth factor (VEGF), transforming growth factor-β (TGF-β), connective tissue growth factor (CTGF), endothelin-1 (ET-1), and extracellular matrix components, such as fibronectin (FN) [44]. Therefore, Wnt/β-catenin signaling pathway may be acted as an important target for the treatment of SSc fibrosis. It may be one of effective ways to treat SSc fibrosis by regulating Wnt/β-catenin signaling pathway and its target genes [24]. In our previous study, we had found WYHZTL formula could inhibit the expression of cyclin D1 and survivin in skin fibroblasts of SSc patients [29]. The results of this study showed that WYHZTL formula could upregulate the mRNA expression of GSK3β and DKK1, while downregulated Wnt1, β-catenin, TCF4, cyclin D1, survivin, VEGF, CTGF, FN1, Type I/III collagen. More importantly, after treatment of WYHZTL formula, the protein expression level of DKK1 was increased, while the protein expression levels of Wnt1, β-catenin, cyclin D1, survivin, CTGF, FN1, collagen I/III were decreased. In addition, it was interesting that we also found that the regulation of Wnt/β-catenin signaling pathway and fibrotic-related protein by WYHZTL formula was in a dosage-dependent manner, which was to say, high-dosage of WYHZTL formula seemed more effective than low-dosage or medium-dosage. This discovery prompted us to consider the impact of dosage when we applied

WYHZTL formula to the SSc treatment. These results suggested that WYHZTL formula could inhibit fibrosis in SSc by regulating Wnt/β-catenin signaling pathway, which was consistent with our previous findings in SSc fibroblasts [29].

In addition, considering that Wnt1, DKK1 and CTGF are secreted proteins, we detected the protein expression levels of Wnt1, DKK1 and CTGF in serum of mice by ELISA. We found that WYHZTL formula and XAV-939 could significantly reduce the protein level of Wnt1 and CTGF, while increase the protein level of DKK1 in serum, which was consistent with the results in the study of skin tissue, suggesting that WYHZTL formula could indeed inhibit the development of fibrosis by regulating Wnt/β-catenin signal pathway.

XAV-939 was widely used as an inhibitor of Wnt/β-catenin signaling pathway [45]. Our previous studies [29] also demonstrated that XAV-939 inhibit expression of cyclin D1 and survivin, target genes of Wnt/β-catenin signaling pathway, in SSc fibroblasts. In this study, we firstly applied XAV-939 to the SSc mouse model. The results showed that XAV-939 could significantly inhibit

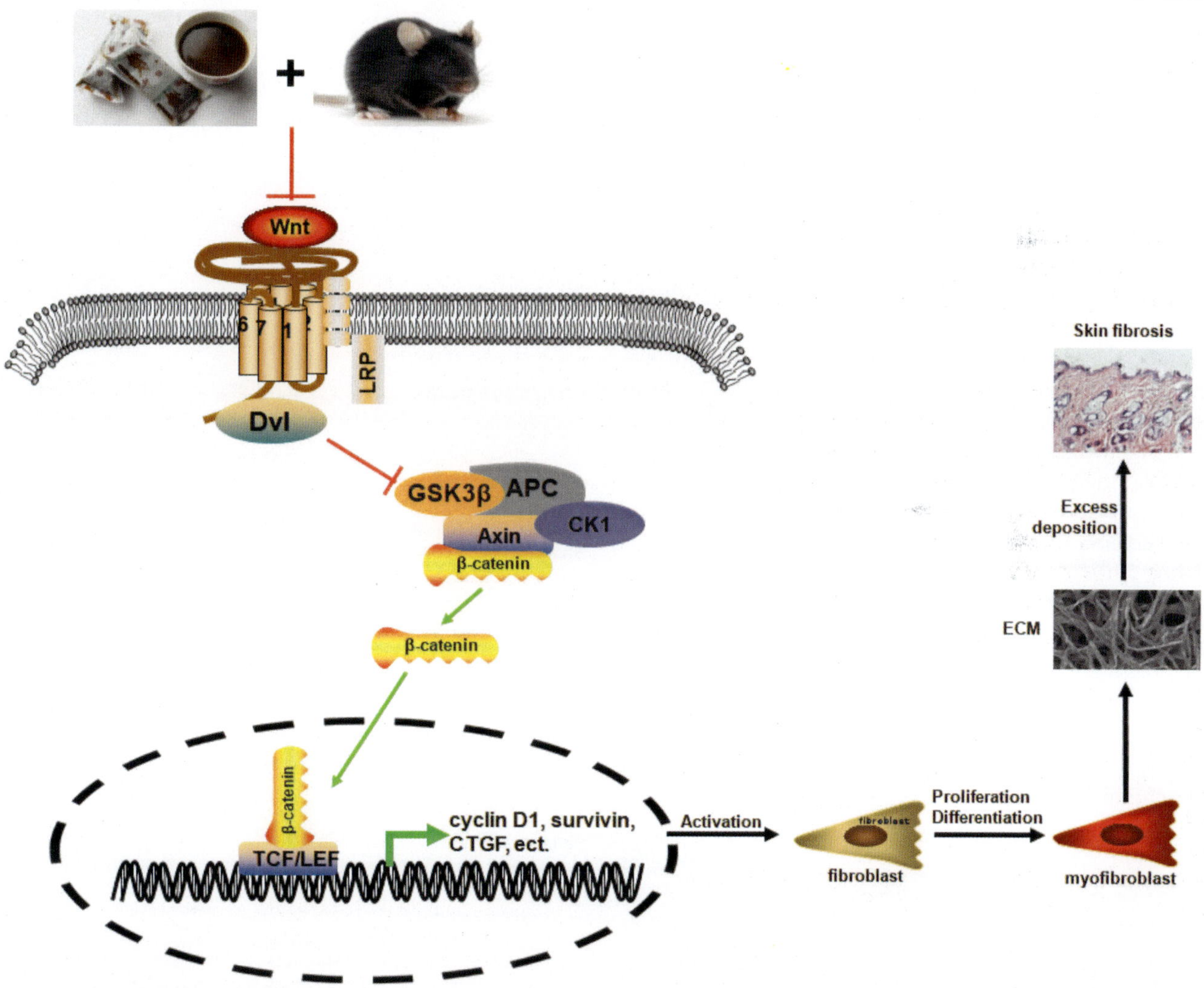

Fig. 6 A schematic diagram illustrating the mechanism of WYHZTL formula in regulating Wnt/β-catenin signaling pathway. When Wnt protein binds to the transmembrane frizzled receptor (Frizzled family member, Frz) and co-receptor LRP on the cell membrane, cytoplasmic disheveled (Dsh) inhibits activity of the Glycogen synthase kinase 3β (GSK3β) which causes the depolymerization of β-catenin destruction complex-Axin/APC/casein kinase Iα (CKIα)/GSK3β. The degradation of β-catenin is inhibited, then enriched in the cytoplasm and entered into the nucleus, which interacts with transcription factor T cell factor/lymphoid enhancer (TCF/LEF) to form a transcription complex that initiates downstream target genes expression. The target genes include cyclin D1, survivin, connective tissue growth factor (CTGF), which results in activation and transformation of fibroblast to myofibroblast. At last, the excess deposition of extracellular matrix (ECM) leads to the occurrence of skin fibrosis. In our present study, we reveal a mechanism of WYHZTL formula in inhibiting Wnt/β-catenin signaling pathway which can ameliorate skin fibrosis in Bleomycin-induced SSc mouse model

Wnt/β-catenin signaling pathway and fibrotic-related protein in vivo. More importantly, our results suggested that WYHZTL formula was more effective than XAV-939, that was to say, WYHZTL formula could inhibit Wnt/β-catenin signal pathway as XAV-939 worked in treatment of SSc mouse model, but WYHZTL formula may have another mechanism of anti-fibrosis except Wnt/β-catenin signal pathway. As was known to all, in addition to the Wnt/β-catenin signaling pathway, there was another signaling pathway that also played an important role in the pathogenesis of SSc, such as the TGF-β/smad signaling pathway [46]. In our previous study, we had found that WYHZTL formula could inhibit TGF-β/smad signaling pathway, thereby inhibiting collagen expression in SSc skin fibroblasts and exerting anti-fibrosis effect [30]. So this may explain that in our study, although the effect of low-dosage of WYHZTL formula on Wnt/β-catenin signaling pathway was not obvious, it may exert anti-SSc fibrosis through other mechanisms, such as TGF-β/smad signaling pathway. In addition, autoimmune abnormality was also an important marker of SSc and play a key role in the development of SSc [47]. The level of IL-17A expression was positively correlated with skin and lung inflammation scores and skin fibrosis in BLM-induced mice model. IL-17A could significantly enhance the proliferation of lung fibroblasts in vitro [48]. And Th17 cells in peripheral blood, skin and lung tissue of SSc mouse model were significantly increased, and were closely related to the inflammation and fibrosis of skin and lung tissue [49]. In our previous study, we had found WYHZTL formula could achieve its therapeutic effect on SSc patients by regulating Th17/Treg imbalance and inhibit the expression of IL-17 [31]. All of these results showed that WYHZTL formula worked by many mechanisms, except for regulating Wnt/β-catenin signaling pathway, suggesting that the effect of WYHZTL formula in SSc treatment should be multi-mechanism and multi-level.

Conclusions

In conclusion, our results validated the function of anti-fibrosis in SSc treatment for WYHZTL formula, and also proposed a new molecular mechanism of anti-fibrosis by inhibiting Wnt/β-catenin signaling pathway in Bleomycin-induced SSc mouse model (Fig. 6). At present, WYHZTL formula is widely used in the treatment of SSc, and our results provides a scientific explanation for its treatment mechanism.

Abbreviations

SSc: systemic sclerosis; WYHZTL: Wenyang Huazhuo Tongluo formula; DKK1: Dickkopf 1; CTGF: connective tissue growth factor; GSK3β: glycogen synthase kinase 3β; TCF4: T cell factor 4; VEGF: vascular endothelial growth factor; FN: fibronectin; APC: adenomatous polyposis coli; CK1: casein kinase 1; ET-1: endothelin-1; MMP-9: matrix metalloproteinase-9; GAPDH: glyceraldehyde-3-phosphate dehydrogenase; TIMP-1: tissue inhibitor of metalloproteinases-1; PIIINP: procollagen III N-terminal peptide; ICTP: I-collagen carboxyl terminal telopeptide; ECM: excessive accumulation of extracellular matrix; FVC: forced vital capacity; DLco: carbon monoxide diffusing capacity; ELISA: enzyme-linked immunosorbent assay; Ct: cycle threshold; RT-qPCR: reverse transcription-quantitative polymerase chain reaction.

Authors' contributions

QW and WZ carried out the molecular biology assay and drafted the manuscript. HB provided the WYHZTL formula, designed the study and helped to draft the manuscript. CZ (Chaoyun Zhang) and JO performed the statistical analysis, YB participated in the study design, LY and LH constructed mouse model, SY and CZ (Cuiyue Zhang) helped the in vivo study. All authors read and approved the final manuscript.

Author details

[1] Zhang Zhongjing College of Chinese Medicine, Nanyang Institute of Technology, Changjiang Road 80, Nanyang 473004, Henan, China. [2] Henan Key Laboratory of Zhang Zhongjing Formulae and Herbs for Immunoregulation, Nanyang Institute of Technology, Nanyang, Henan, China. [3] Experimental Research Center, China Academy of Chinese Medical Sciences, Beijing, China. [4] School of Pharmaceutical Sciences, Zhengzhou University, Zhengzhou, Henan, China.

Acknowledgements

Not applicable.

Competing interests

The authors declare no potential conflict of interest. Dr. Hua Bian holds a patent on the tested WYHZTL formula (No. CN201310351880.2).

Consent for publication

Not applicable.

Funding

The present study was supported by the National Natural Science Foundation of China (Grant Nos. 81373627, 81774300), the science and technology research project of Henan province (Grant No. 182102310595), and the Open Project Fund of Henan Key Laboratory of Zhang Zhongjing Formulae and Herbs for Immunoregulation (Grant No. kfkt201703).

References

1. Manetti M. Emerging biomarkers in systemic sclerosis. Curr Opin Rheumatol. 2016;28(6):606–12.
2. Gabrielli A, Avvedimento EV, Krieg T. Scleroderma. N Engl J Med. 2009;360(19):1989–2003.
3. Cozzi F, Marson P. Plasma-exchange in the treatment of systemic rheumatic diseases: past and present experience. Reumatismo. 2009;61(3):161–4.
4. Burt RK, Shah SJ, Dill K, Grant T, Gheorghiade M, Schroeder J, Craig R, Hirano I, Marshall K, Ruderman E, et al. Autologous non-myeloablative haemopoietic stem-cell transplantation compared with pulse cyclophosphamide once per month for systemic sclerosis (ASSIST): an open-label, randomised phase 2 trial. Lancet. 2011;378(9790):498–506.
5. Adigun R, Bhimji S: Systemic sclerosis (CREST syndrome). In: StatPearls, edn. Treasure Island (FL); 2017.
6. Katsumoto TR, Whitfield ML, Connolly MK. The pathogenesis of systemic sclerosis. Ann Rev Pathol. 2011;6:509–37.

7. van Amerongen R, Nusse R. Towards an integrated view of Wnt signaling in development. Development. 2009;136(19):3205–14.
8. Kahn M. Can we safely target the WNT pathway? Nat Rev Drug Discovery. 2014;13(7):513–32.
9. MacDonald BT, Tamai K, He X. Wnt/beta-catenin signaling: components, mechanisms, and diseases. Dev Cell. 2009;17(1):9–26.
10. Nusse R, Clevers H. Wnt/beta-catenin signaling, disease, and emerging therapeutic modalities. Cell. 2017;169(6):985–99.
11. Guo Y, Xiao L, Sun L, Liu F. Wnt/beta-catenin signaling: a promising new target for fibrosis diseases. Physiol Res. 2012;61(4):337–46.
12. Blyszczuk P, Muller-Edenborn B, Valenta T, Osto E, Stellato M, Behnke S, Glatz K, Basler K, Luscher TF, Distler O, et al. Transforming growth factor-beta-dependent Wnt secretion controls myofibroblast formation and myocardial fibrosis progression in experimental autoimmune myocarditis. Eur Heart J. 2017;38(18):1413–25.
13. Lam AP, Herazo-Maya JD, Sennello JA, Flozak AS, Russell S, Mutlu GM, Budinger GR, DasGupta R, Varga J, Kaminski N, et al. Wnt coreceptor Lrp5 is a driver of idiopathic pulmonary fibrosis. Am J Respir Crit Care Med. 2014;190(2):185–95.
14. Arellanes-Robledo J, Reyes-Gordillo K, Shah R, Dominguez-Rosales JA, Hernandez-Nazara ZH, Ramirez F, Rojkind M, Lakshman MR. Fibrogenic actions of acetaldehyde are beta-catenin dependent but Wingless independent: a critical role of nucleoredoxin and reactive oxygen species in human hepatic stellate cells. Free Radic Biol Med. 2013;65:1487–96.
15. Li Z, Zhou L, Wang Y, Miao J, Hong X, Hou FF, Liu Y. (Pro)renin receptor is an amplifier of Wnt/beta-catenin signaling in kidney injury and fibrosis. J Am Soc Nephrol. 2017;28:2393–408.
16. Serrati S, Chilla A, Laurenzana A, Margheri F, Giannoni E, Magnelli L, Chiarugi P, Dotor J, Feijoo E, Bazzichi L, et al. Systemic sclerosis endothelial cells recruit and activate dermal fibroblasts by induction of a connective tissue growth factor (CCN2)/transforming growth factor beta-dependent mesenchymal-to-mesenchymal transition. Arthritis Rheum. 2013;65(1):258–69.
17. Riccieri V, Stefanantoni K, Vasile M, Macri V, Sciarra I, Iannace N, Alessandri C, Valesini G. Abnormal plasma levels of different angiogenic molecules are associated with different clinical manifestations in patients with systemic sclerosis. Clin Exp Rheumatol. 2011;29(2 Suppl 65):S46–52.
18. Akhmetshina A, Palumbo K, Dees C, Bergmann C, Venalis P, Zerr P, Horn A, Kireva T, Beyer C, Zwerina J, et al. Activation of canonical Wnt signalling is required for TGF-beta-mediated fibrosis. Nat Commun. 2012;3:735.
19. Wei J, Melichian D, Komura K, Hinchcliff M, Lam AP, Lafyatis R, Gottardi CJ, MacDougald OA, Varga J. Canonical Wnt signaling induces skin fibrosis and subcutaneous lipoatrophy: a novel mouse model for scleroderma? Arthritis Rheum. 2011;63(6):1707–17.
20. Bayle J, Fitch J, Jacobsen K, Kumar R, Lafyatis R, Lemaire R. Increased expression of Wnt2 and SFRP4 in Tsk mouse skin: role of Wnt signaling in altered dermal fibrillin deposition and systemic sclerosis. J Invest Dermatol. 2008;128(4):871–81.
21. Liu L, Carron B, Yee HT, Yie TA, Hajjou M, Rom W. Wnt pathway in pulmonary fibrosis in the bleomycin mouse model. J Environ Pathol Toxicol Oncol. 2009;28(2):99–108.
22. Bilic J, Huang YL, Davidson G, Zimmermann T, Cruciat CM, Bienz M, Niehrs C. Wnt induces LRP6 signalosomes and promotes dishevelled-dependent LRP6 phosphorylation. Science. 2007;316(5831):1619–22.
23. Dees C, Schlottmann I, Funke R, Distler A, Palumbo-Zerr K, Zerr P, Lin NY, Beyer C, Distler O, Schett G, et al. The Wnt antagonists DKK1 and SFRP1 are downregulated by promoter hypermethylation in systemic sclerosis. Ann Rheum Dis. 2014;73(6):1232–9.
24. Daoussis D, Tsamandas A, Antonopoulos I, Filippopoulou A, Papachristou DJ, Papachristou NI, Andonopoulos AP, Liossis SN. B cell depletion therapy upregulates Dkk-1 skin expression in patients with systemic sclerosis: association with enhanced resolution of skin fibrosis. Arthritis Res Ther. 2016;18(1):118.
25. Kabashima K, Sakabe J, Yoshiki R, Tabata Y, Kohno K, Tokura Y. Involvement of Wnt signaling in dermal fibroblasts. Am J Pathol. 2010;176(2):721–32.
26. Yan XN, Feng J, Li WB, Cui R, Shi BJ. Effects of Wenyang Chubi Decoction on connective tissue growth factor and collagen-I in a mouse model of scleroderma. Zhong Xi Yi Jie He Xue Bao. 2007;5(5):526–30.
27. Wu T, Chu H, Tu W, Song M, Chen D, Yuan J, Yu L, Ma Y, Liu Q, Jin L, et al. Dissection of the mechanism of traditional Chinese medical prescription-Yiqihuoxue formula as an effective anti-fibrotic treatment for systemic sclerosis. BMC complement Altern Med. 2014;14:224.
28. Bian H, Fan YS, Lou LH, Mao BY, Shi JY. Effect of Wenyang Huazhuo Tongluo recipe contained serum on proliferation and cell cycle of systemic sclerosis skin fibroblasts. Zhong Yao Cai. 2009;32(6):936–9.
29. Han L, Bian H, Ouyang J, Bi Y, Yang L, Ye S. Wenyang Huazhuo Tongluo formula, a Chinese herbal decoction, improves skin fibrosis by promoting apoptosis and inhibiting proliferation through down-regulation of survivin and cyclin D1 in systemic sclerosis. BMC complement Altern Med. 2016;16:69.
30. Bian H, Lv Q, Huang XZ, Hu JL, Yang L, Mao BY. Effects of Wenyang Huazhuo Tongluo recipe containing serum on transforming growth factor beta1/Smad signaling pathway of skin fibroblasts in systemic sclerosis. Zhongguo Zhong Xi Yi Jie He Za Zhi. 2015;35(9):1054–9.
31. Bian H, Yuan M, Gao ZM, Bi XD, Han L, Hu JL, Mao BY. Effect of Wenyang Huazhuo Tongluo recipe on peripheral blood Thl7/Treg cell balance in systemic sclerosis patients. Zhongguo Zhong Xi Yi Jie He Za Zhi. 2015;35(8):975–80.
32. Zhang J, Corciulo C, Liu H, Wilder T, Ito M, Cronstein B. Adenosine A2a receptor blockade diminishes Wnt/beta-catenin signaling in a murine model of bleomycin-induced dermal fibrosis. Am J Pathol. 2017;187(9):1935–44.
33. Chan ES, Fernandez P, Merchant AA, Montesinos MC, Trzaska S, Desai A, Tung CF, Khoa DN, Pillinger MH, Reiss AB, et al. Adenosine A2A receptors in diffuse dermal fibrosis: pathogenic role in human dermal fibroblasts and in a murine model of scleroderma. Arthritis Rheum. 2006;54(8):2632–42.
34. Heap BJ, Kiernan JA. Mast cells and gastric secretion in the rat. Q J Exp Physiol Cogn Med Sci. 1975;60(4):307–13.
35. Tan SQ, Geng X, Liu JH, Pan WH, Wang LX, Liu HK, Hu L, Chao HM. Xue-fu-Zhu-Yu decoction protects rats against retinal ischemia by down-regulation of HIF-1alpha and VEGF via inhibition of RBP2 and PKM2. BMC complement Altern Med. 2017;17(1):365.
36. Yang W, Bancroft L, Nicholas C, Lozonschi I, Augenlicht LH. Targeted inactivation of p27kip1 is sufficient for large and small intestinal tumorigenesis in the mouse, which can be augmented by a Western-style high-risk diet. Cancer Res. 2003;63(16):4990–6.
37. Wei J, Fang F, Lam AP, Sargent JL, Hamburg E, Hinchcliff ME, Gottardi CJ, Atit R, Whitfield ML, Varga J. Wnt/beta-catenin signaling is hyperactivated in systemic sclerosis and induces Smad-dependent fibrotic responses in mesenchymal cells. Arthritis Rheum. 2012;64(8):2734–45.
38. Lam AP, Flozak AS, Russell S, Wei J, Jain M, Mutlu GM, Budinger GR, Feghali-Bostwick CA, Varga J, Gottardi CJ. Nuclear beta-catenin is increased in systemic sclerosis pulmonary fibrosis and promotes lung fibroblast migration and proliferation. Am J Respir Cell Mol Biol. 2011;45(5):915–22.
39. Wei J, Bhattacharyya S, Tourtellotte WG, Varga J. Fibrosis in systemic sclerosis: emerging concepts and implications for targeted therapy. Autoimmun Rev. 2011;10(5):267–75.
40. Bergmann C, Akhmetshina A, Dees C, Palumbo K, Zerr P, Beyer C, Zwerina J, Distler O, Schett G, Distler JH. Inhibition of glycogen synthase kinase 3beta induces dermal fibrosis by activation of the canonical Wnt pathway. Ann Rheum Dis. 2011;70(12):2191–8.
41. Paik DT, Rai M, Ryzhov S, Sanders LN, Aisagbonhi O, Funke MJ, Feoktistov I, Hatzopoulos AK. Wnt10b gain-of-function improves cardiac repair by arteriole formation and attenuation of fibrosis. Circ Res. 2015;117(9):804–16.
42. Miller LS, Liu JB, Klenn PJ, Holahan MP, Varga J, Feld RI, Troshinsky M, Jimenez SA, Castell DO, Goldberg BB. Endoluminal ultrasonography of the distal esophagus in systemic sclerosis. Gastroenterology. 1993;105(1):31–9.
43. Wu MH, Yokozeki H, Takagawa S, Yamamoto T, Satoh T, Kaneda Y, Katayama I, Nishioka K. Hepatocyte growth factor both prevents and ameliorates the symptoms of dermal sclerosis in a mouse model of scleroderma. Gene Ther. 2004;11(2):170–80.
44. Chen S, McLean S, Carter DE, Leask A. The gene expression profile induced by Wnt 3a in NIH 3T3 fibroblasts. J Cell Commun Signal. 2007;1(3–4):175–83.
45. Esfandiari F, Fathi A, Gourabi H, Kiani S, Nemati S, Baharvand H. Glycogen synthase kinase-3 inhibition promotes proliferation and neuronal

differentiation of human-induced pluripotent stem cell-derived neural progenitors. Stem Cells Dev. 2012;21(17):3233–43.

46. Viswanath V, Phiske MM, Gopalani VV. Systemic sclerosis: current concepts in pathogenesis and therapeutic aspects of dermatological manifestations. Indian J Dermatol. 2013;58(4):255–68.
47. Dijkstra KK, Hoeks SB, Prakken BJ, de Roock S. TH17 differentiation capacity develops within the first 3 months of life. J Allergy Clin Immunol. 2014;133(3):891 e895–894 e895.
48. Okamoto Y, Hasegawa M, Matsushita T, Hamaguchi Y, Huu DL, Iwakura Y, Fujimoto M, Takehara K. Potential roles of interleukin-17A in the development of skin fibrosis in mice. Arthritis Rheum. 2012;64(11):3726–35.
49. Lei L, Zhong XN, Zhao C, Mi CD, Li JQ, Zeng JJ. Expression and significance of Th17 cells and related cytokines in a murine model of systemic sclerosis. Beijing Da Xue Xue Bao Yi Xue Ban. 2012;44(2):259–64.

5

Comparative study of the polyphenol content-related anti-inflammatory and antioxidant activities of two *Urera aurantiaca* specimens from different geographical areas

Carla Marrassini*, Ignacio Peralta and Claudia Anesini

Abstract

Background: *Urera aurantiaca* is an Argentinean species that has been traditionally used to treat symptoms of inflammation. The aim of this study was to determine and compare the anti-inflammatory and antioxidant effects of two specimens of *Urera aurantiaca* obtained in the provinces of Salta and Misiones, which are two different geographical areas of Argentina.

Methods: The anti-inflammatory activity of the extracts was tested in LPS-stimulated macrophages through the DPPH radical scavenging activity, the SOD-like activity, the reducing power and the inhibition of lipid peroxidation. The anti-inflammatory activity was also evaluated by the inhibition of albumin denaturation and proteinase inhibitory action tests. The total polyphenols, flavonoids and tannins content were quantified.

Results: Both extracts were able to reduce the augmented NO release in LPS-activated macrophages and showed antioxidant and in vitro anti-inflammatory activities. The polyphenols content was higher in the extract obtained from the specimen from Salta than in that obtained in Misiones. This finding accounts for the higher anti-inflammatory and antioxidant properties obtained with the former.

Conclusion: The differences in chemical composition and the biological activities observed between the extracts are probably related to the different environmental conditions found in both provinces.

Keywords: *Urera aurantiaca*, Inflammation, Antioxidant activity, Macrophages, Polyphenols

Background

Inflammation is a defence mechanism against tissue damage caused by either mechanical, chemical, or microbial stimuli. The main cells involved in the inflammatory response are monocytes/macrophages, polymorphonuclear leucocytes, and endothelial cells. When these cells become activated, they aggregate and infiltrate tissues where the respiratory burst is triggered to increase the oxygen consumption and the production of cytokines and reactive oxygen species (ROS), as well as other inflammation mediators [1]. The ROS that are produced during the inflammatory response facilitating it; however, when produced for prolonged periods, these mediators can promote oxidative stress and chronic inflammation-associated disorders. It is known that inflammation and oxidative stress are interrelated processes [2].

In living organisms, the energy production is achieved through oxidation processes. Thus, the aerobic metabolism entails the generation of different ROS, such as singlet oxygen, superoxide, peroxyl and hydroxyl

*Correspondence: cmarra@ffyb.uba.ar
Facultad de Farmacia y Bioquímica, Instituto de la Química y Metabolismo del Fármaco (IQUIMEFA), Consejo Nacional de Investigaciones Científicas y Técnicas, Universidad de Buenos Aires, Buenos Aires, Argentina

radicals, and reactive nitrogen species (RNS), including peroxynitrite and nitric oxide (NO). Apart from their physiological activity, ROS and RNS oxidise membrane lipids, proteins and DNA, leading to diseases, such as cancer, cardiovascular diseases, cataracts, asthma, hepatitis, liver injury and immunodeficiency diseases [3].

During inflammation, ROS and RNS are largely produced by macrophages, which play a central role in both innate and adaptive immunity. Macrophages are known to perform several functions such as killing foreign organisms, presenting antigens, phagocytising foreign invaders, and producing chemical mediators, such as cytokines and those of oxidative stress. These cells interact with T and B cells, natural killer and dendritic cells, neutrophils, and fibroblasts.

The lipopolysaccharide (LPS), which is a component of cell walls and the major virulence factor of Gram-negative bacteria, can induce oxidative stress in macrophages [4].

Nowadays, there is an increasing interest in the use of plant antioxidants for dietary, pharmaceutical and cosmetic purposes. This is mainly due to their strong biological activity, exceeding those of many carcinogenic synthetic antioxidants. Many plants contain antioxidant compounds and these compounds protect cells against the damaging effects of ROS. Epidemiological studies have indicated the beneficial effects of plant antioxidants in patients with chronic diseases [5]. Thus, the antioxidant activity of plant-derived compounds is currently being studied, as regards the free radical quenching ability, mainly of polyphenol compounds.

Urera aurantiaca Wedd. (Urticaceae), commonly known as "ortiga colorada", "pino guasú", and "pica pica", is an Argentinean native herb also growing in Paraguay, Uruguay, Bolivia, and Brazil. *U. aurantiaca* is used in folk medicine to treat rheumatic pain, varicose veins, furuncles, bruises, inflammation, tooth pain, dermal diseases, and trauma [6].

In a previous work, the in vivo anti-inflammatory and antinociceptive effects of a methanolic extract of *U. aurantiaca* from Paraguay have been reported [7]. Its modulatory effect on immune and tumoral cells during inflammation has also been demonstrated [8].

Species of the Urticaceae family have been used in traditional Chinese medicine. For example, *Laportea bulbifera* (Siebold & Zucc.) Wedd. (Urticaceae) is used for the treatment and management of urinary stones [9]; *Gonostegia hirta* (Blume) Miq. (Urticaceae) is used to treat many types of injuries [10]; *Pilea microphylla* (L.) Liebm. (Urticaceae) is used for the treatment of osteoarthritis [11]; *Pellionia repens* (Lour.) Merr. (Urticaceae) is used for the treatment of skin injuries [12]; *Boehmeria nivea* (L.) Gaudich. (Urticaceae) is employed as a pro-coagulant, to reduce swelling and as detoxifying [13].

Urera aurantiaca is distributed in different phytogeographic zones in Argentina. It is known that specimens of the same species growing under different environmental conditions differ in the production levels of primary and secondary metabolites. This phenomenon is due to the different metabolic requirements to accomplish long term acclimation or local adaptation, seasonal differences related to phenology or environmental changes of both biotic and abiotic factors, geographical differences involving different populations (genetic differences within a plant species), etc. [14, 15].

Considering the popular medicinal use of *U. aurantiaca* and the biological activities previously reported for this species, the objectives of this work were to analyse and compare the antioxidant effect of two species of *U. aurantiaca* obtained in the provinces of Salta and Misiones, which are two different geographical areas of Argentina. The free radicals scavenging capacity, the reducing power, the SOD-like activity, and the ability to diminish the production of NO in lipopolysaccharide (LPS)-stimulated macrophages were studied. The in vitro anti-inflammatory activity in relation to ROS generation was also studied. Finally, polyphenols such as flavonoids and tannins were quantified to relate their presence with the activities mentioned.

Methods

The minimum standards of reporting checklist contains details of the experimental design, and resources used in this study (Additional file 1).

Plant material

Urera aurantiaca Wedd. (Urticaceae) obtained in the province of Salta was collected in Orán, Salta, Argentina (23°07′01.0″S, 64°18′40.2″W) in April 2013 by P. Mercado. A voucher specimen (no. 212) was deposited at Herbario LIL Fundación Miguel Lillo, San Miguel de Tucumán, Argentina.

Urera aurantiaca Wedd. (Urticaceae) obtained in the province of Misiones province was collected in Eldorado, Misiones, Argentina (26°24′23.4″S, 54°41′37.3″W) in April 2013 by H.A. Keller. A voucher specimen (no. 11330) was deposited at Herbario del Instituto de Botánica del Nordeste (CTES), Corrientes, Argentina.

Extraction

The dried aerial parts of the specimens obtained Salta and Misiones were ground to a fine powder and extracted sequentially by maceration with solvents of different polarity. Briefly, the plant powder was first extracted with dichloromethane, then with ethyl acetate, and finally, the marc was extracted with methanol. Solvents were put in contact with the plant material overnight in order to obtain an extract enriched in polyphenols. After extraction, the methanol extracts were lyophilised. Yields were 4.4% for the Salta extract and 4.6% for the Misiones extract.

Phytochemical analysis

Total phenol content

The total phenol content in the extracts was determined by the Folin–Ciocalteu's colorimetric method, as described by Singleton et al. [16]. The absorbance was measured at 760 nm and compared with a gallic acid calibration curve. Results were expressed as mg of gallic acid equivalents per gram of extract (GAE/g).

Flavonoids determination

The total flavonoids content was determined in the extracts by the aluminum chloride colorimetric method, as described by Chang et al. [17]. Briefly, the diluted standard solutions or the extract (0.5 ml) were mixed with 1.5 ml 95% ethanol, 0.1 ml 10% aluminum chloride, 0.1 ml 1 M potassium acetate and 2.8 ml distilled water. After incubation at room temperature for 30 min, the absorbance was measured at 415 nm. Dilutions of quercetin in ethanol were used to generate the calibration curve (125, 250, 500 and 1000 μg/ml).

Tannins determination

The tannin content was calculated as the difference between the contents of total phenols and the non-complex residual phenols [18] after the removal of tannins from the medium by complexation with casein, as described by Amorim et al. [19] with slight modifications. Briefly, 500 mg of casein were transferred into a 25 ml Erlenmeyer flask. Five ml of the extract and 5 ml of distilled water were then added. After 2 h, which is the time period required for the complexing of the tannins to the protein, the extract was filtered into a 10 ml volumetric flask and the volume was then adjusted to 10 ml with distilled water. The tannin content was expressed as the percentage of the total phenols that were complexed with casein.

High performance liquid chromatography

The HPLC method was developed and validated according to Filip et al. [20] and performed in a Varian 9000 instrument equipped with a diode array detector and a Rheodyne injector fitted with a 20 μl loop. A C18 column (Kinetex 5 μm, 150 mm × 4.6 mm) was employed. As mobile phase, solvent A: H_2O/AcOH (98:2) and solvent B: MeOH/AcOH (98:2) were used. The elution gradient was: from 15 to 40% B in 30 min; from 40 to 75% B in 10 min; from 75 to 85% B in 5 min. The elution was performed at flow rate of 1.2 ml/min. Detection was done at 325 nm.

Cell suspensions and culture conditions

The American Type Culture Collection (ATCC) RAW264.7 murine macrophage cell line was cultured in corlorless Dulbecco's Modified Eagle's medium supplemented with 10% FBS, 2 mM glutamine and 100 IU/ml penicillin and 100 μg/ml streptomycin and kept in a humidified incubator at 5% CO_2 and 37 °C.

Cell proliferation and nitric oxide determination

To determine cell proliferation rate and NO production, macrophages were incubated for 24 h without any treatment (basal conditions) or with LPS (1 μg/ml) alone or in the presence of different concentrations of the extracts. After incubation, the supernatant was separated to determine the NO levels and the cells were used to determine proliferation. The nitrite accumulated in the culture medium, which is an indicator of NO production, was measured by the Griess' reaction [21]. Briefly, 100 μl of each supernatant were mixed with 50 μl of a 1% sulfanilamide solution in 5% phosphoric acid and 50 μl of a 0.1% naphthylene diamine dihydrochloride solution. The mixture was incubated at room temperature for 20 min, and the absorbance was read at 540 nm. As standard curve, serial dilutions of a $NaNO_2$ solution were employed.

Results were expressed as mean ± SEM of three determinations performed in triplicate.

Cell proliferation was determined by the reduction of 3-(4,5-dimethylthiazol-2-yl)-2,5-diphenyltetrazolium bromide (MTT) (Sigma). Briefly, cells were incubated for 4 h in 100 μl RPMI 1640 and 10 μl of 5 mg/ml MTT (Sigma, St. Louis, MO, USA). After incubation, the formazan formed was dissolved in acidified isopropanol (0.04 N HCl in isopropanol) and read at 540 nm.

2,2-Diphenyl-1-picrylhydrazyl (DPPH) radical scavenging activity

The scavenging activity of the extracts on the stable free radical DPPH was assayed by the modified method described by Blois [22]. The bleaching rate of DPPH is monitored at a characteristic wavelength in the presence of the sample. Briefly, a volume of 0.1 ml of an aqueous dilution of the extract was mixed with 0.5 ml of a 500 μM DPPH solution in absolute ethanol and 0.4 ml of a 0.1 M Tris–HCl buffer, pH 7.4. The mixture was kept for 20 min in the darkness, and then the absorbance was read at 517 nm. The percentage of decrease of DPPH absorbance was calculated by measuring the absorbance of the sample and applying the following equation:

$$\% \text{ of inhibition} = [1 - (As/A0)] \times 100,$$

where As is absorbance of sample and A0 is the absorbance of the DPPH solution.

Superoxide dismutase (SOD)-like activity

To determine the SOD activity, the inhibitory capacity of the extracts on the adrenaline autoxidation was evaluated. Briefly, 50 μl of the extract were treated with 910 μl of sodium phosphate buffer (0.05 M) pH: 10.7 and 1 mM adrenaline. Under these conditions, adrenaline rapidly undergoes autoxidation to produce the adrenochrome, which is a pink coloured product that can be measured at 480 nm using a UV/visible spectrophotometer in kinetic mode. The antioxidant activity of sample was evaluated as the % of epinephrine autoxidation inhibition. The absorbance was monitored at 480 nm, and the Δ absorbance/min was determined to calculate the % of inhibition as: [(Abs/min control − Abs/min sample)/Abs/min control] × 100 [23].

Reducing power assay

The reducing power was determined according to Ferreira et al. [24], with slight modifications. Different concentrations of the extract (2.5 ml) were mixed with 2.5 ml of 200 mM sodium phosphate buffer (pH 6.6) and 2.5 ml of 1% potassium ferricyanide. The mixture was incubated at 50 °C for 20 min. After adding 2.5 ml of 10% trichloroacetic acid (w/v), the mixture was centrifuged at 3500 rpm for 10 min. The upper layer (2.5 ml) was mixed with 2.5 ml deionised water and 1 ml of 0.1% ferric chloride, and the absorbance was measured at 700 nm. The reducing power is directly proportional to the mixture absorbance.

Inhibition of lipid peroxidation of egg yolk

The lipid peroxidation assay was done according to Dissanayake et al. [25], with minor modifications. The egg yolk was separated from the albumen and the yolk membrane was removed. A 10% v/v yolk solution was prepared in 1.15% of KCl. The solution was homogenized for 30 s and ultra sonicated for 5 min.

A 1% (w/v) of thiobarbituric acid solution was then prepared in 1.1% (w/v) SDS.

The reaction mixture contained 25 μl of the extract, 125 μl of egg yolk solution and 100 μl of distilled water. Distilled water (125 μl) was used as the control. Acetic acid (20%, 375 μl) and 1% thiobarbituric acid (375 μl) were then added. These mixtures were vortexed for 5 s and kept in a water bath 95 °C for 60 min. Butanol (1.25 ml) was added to each tube and vortexed for 5 s. After centrifuging at 3000*g* for 10 min, the butanol layer was separated. Absorbance values were measured at 532 nm.

Inhibition of albumin denaturation

The method was performed according to Kumari et al. [26] and Sakat et al. [27], with minor modifications. The reaction mixture (0.5 ml) consisted of 0.40 ml bovine serum albumin (1% aqueous solution), 0.05 ml of the extract at different concentrations (1000, 800, 600, and 400 μg/ml), and 0.05 ml of salicylic acid (inductor of protein denaturation). As positive control, distilled water (0.05 ml) was used instead of the extracts while as negative control, no salicylic acid was employed. Samples were incubated at 37 °C for 20 min and then heated at 57 °C for 20 min. After cooling the samples, 2.5 ml phosphate buffer saline (pH 6.3) were added to each tube. Turbidity was measured spectrophotometrically at 660 nm. The percentage inhibition of protein denaturation was calculated as follows:

$$\text{Percent inhibition} = \frac{\text{Abs}_{\text{control}} - \text{Abs}_{\text{treated}}}{\text{Abs}_{\text{Control}}} \times 100$$

where $\text{Abs}_{\text{control}}$ represents 100% protein denaturation.

Proteinase inhibitory action

The antitryptic activity of the extract was assayed as described by Oyedapo and Famurewa [28], with minor modifications. The reaction mixture (1.0 ml) contained 0.03 ml trypsin (0.3 μg), 0.5 ml of the extract at different concentrations (10, 25, 50, and 100 μg/ml) and 0.5 ml of 20 mM Tris–HCl buffer (pH 7.4). The mixture was incubated at 37 °C for 5 min and then, 0.5 ml of 0.8% (w/v) casein was added. The mixture was further incubated for 20 min and 1 ml of 70% perchloric acid was added to terminate the reaction. The cloudy suspension was clarified by centrifugation and the absorbance of the supernatant was read at 280 nm against buffer as blank.

Statistical analysis

Data were expressed as the average of triplicate values of three independent experiments. To compare two values, the Student's *t* test was used. Multiple comparisons were performed by analysis of variance (ANOVA) and the Dunnett's test. A $p<0.05$ was considered statistically significant.

Results

Firstly, the extracts were obtained and their chemical composition was determined. The objective of the extraction was to obtain polyphenolic compounds. Once the extracts were prepared, the total polyphenols, flavonoids, and tannins were quantified. Table 1 shows that the Salta extract rendered the highest total phenolic and flavonoids content, meanwhile the Misiones extract presented a higher amount of tannins than the Salta

Table 1 Quantitative determination of polyphenols, flavonoids, and tannins in Salta and Misiones extracts

Urera aurantiaca extracts	Total polyphenols (GAE/g)	Flavonoids (%)	Tannins (%)
Salta	30.90 ± 1.8^a	2.10 ± 0.015^a	39.7 ± 0.2^a
Misiones	14.05 ± 2.60^b	1.49 ± 0.052^b	48.2 ± 1.1^b

Statistical differences were determined by *t*-Student test ($a \neq b$: $p < 0.05$)

extract. Furthermore, a chromatographic profile was also obtained by HPLC analysis. Figure 1 shows that the differences in the extracts appeared to be quantitative and not qualitative.

Secondly, the antioxidant activity of the extracts was measured with the DPPH test. Both extracts presented a polyphenol concentration-dependent antioxidant activity (Fig. 2a). The EC_{50} obtained with the Salta extract was fourfold lower than that of Misiones extract (Fig. 2b–d).

Furthermore, the reducing power of the extracts was studied. A concentration-dependent reducing power was demonstrated in both extracts (Fig. 3a). However, the Salta extract reached an inhibition of 100% at 1000 μg/ml, meanwhile for the Misiones extract, the maximum inhibition achieved was 33.7% at the same concentration. In addition, the Salta extract presented a lower EC_{50} value. In Fig. 3b–d the EC_{50} values for this activity in comparison with the polyphenols, flavonoids and tannins content is shown.

The SOD-like activity was then used as a more specific method for the measurement of the antioxidant activity. Both extracts presented a concentration-dependent SOD-like activity; however, the EC_{50} for the Misiones extract was lower than that exhibited by the Salta extract (363 vs. 537 μg/ml, Fig. 4a). In Fig. 4b–d the EC_{50} values for this activity in comparison with the polyphenols, flavonoids and tannins content is shown.

To complete the antioxidant activity profile, the inhibition of lipid peroxidation of egg yolk was assayed. Results indicated that the Salta extract exerted an inhibitory

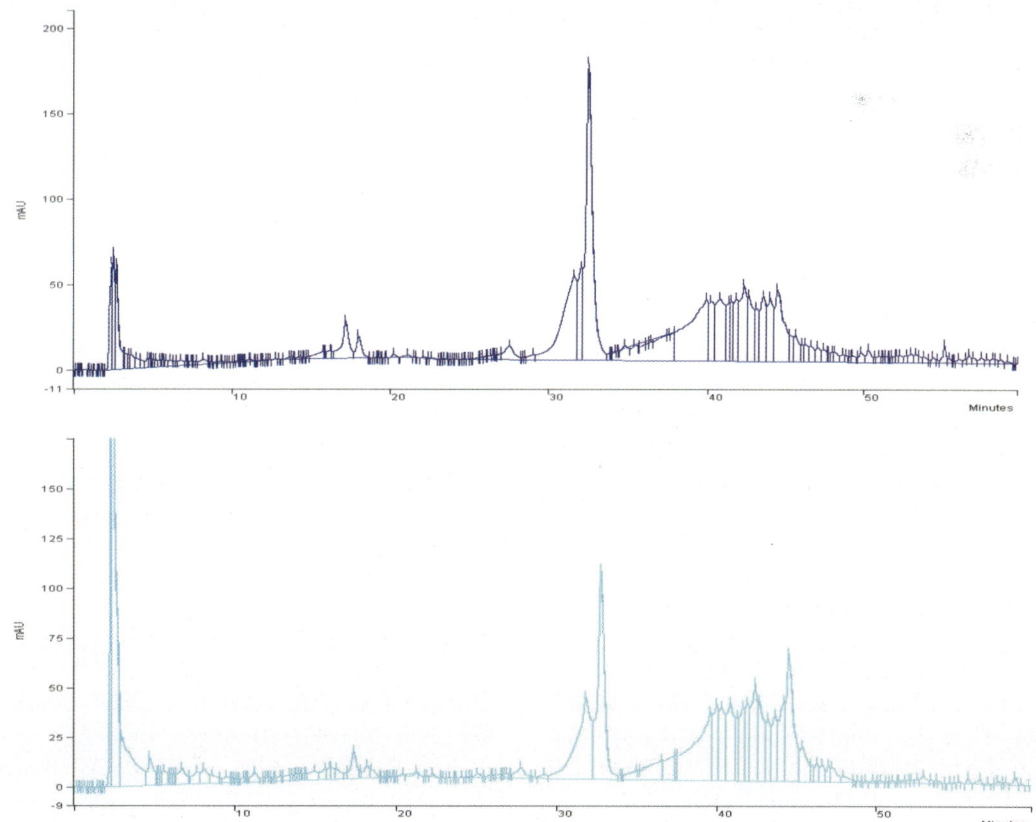

Fig. 1 HPLC profiles: **a** Salta extract, **b** Misiones extract

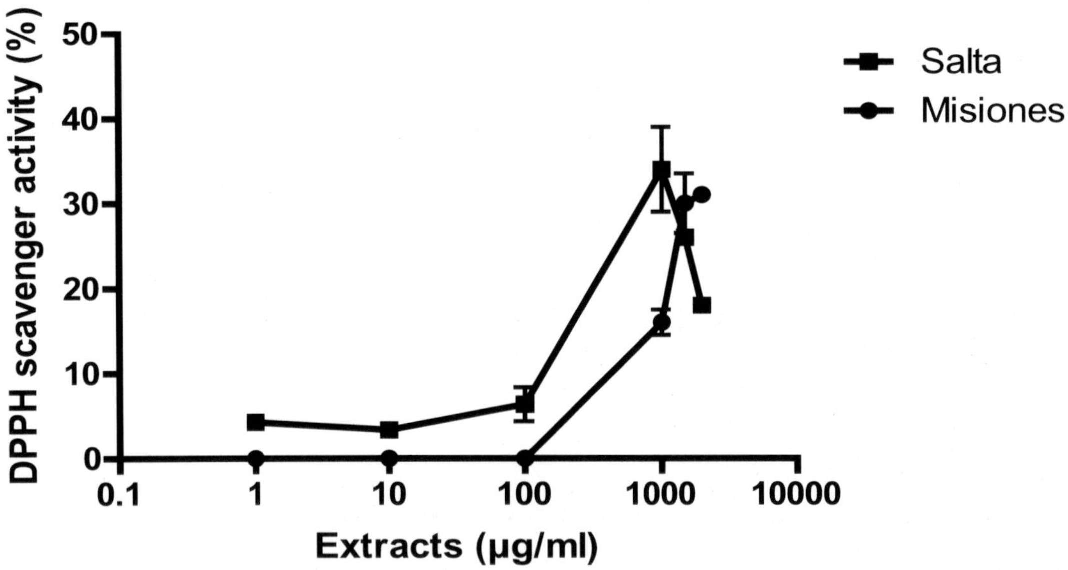

Extracts	DPPH scavenger activity EC50 (μg/ml)
Misiones	977 ± 40
Salta	245 ± 20

Fig. 2 DPPH scavenger activity. **a** DPPH antioxidant activity as a function of the extract concentration. **b–d** Comparison between the DPPH activity and the polyphenols, flavonoids and tannins content and EC_{50} for Salta and Misiones extracts. Results represent mean ± SEM of three experiments performed in triplicate. ***$p < 0.001$ significant differences between extracts EC_{50}

effect that was higher than that of the Misiones extract, exhibiting a lower EC_{50} value (1862 μg/ml) and a maximum effect of 52% of inhibition at 2 mg/ml. On the other hand, the Misiones extract also inhibited lipid peroxidation (EC_{50}: > 2000; maximum inhibition: 16.7%, Fig. 5a). It noteworthy that the Misiones extract, at 100 μg/ml, exerted a pro-oxidant action, while the Salta extract, at 100 μg/ml, caused an inhibition of lipid peroxidation of 12%. Figure 5b–d show the EC_{50} value for this activity in comparison with the polyphenols, flavonoids and tannins content.

The in vitro anti-inflammatory activity was studied in relation with the antioxidant activity by two methods: the inhibition of albumin denaturation and the proteinase inhibitory action. As shown in Fig. 6a, both extracts inhibited the heat-induced albumin denaturation; however, the Salta extract presented a maximum inhibition of 64.4% at 1000 μg/ml, as compared to the Misiones extract with which the maximum inhibition achieved was 11.2%, at the same concentration. In addition, the Salta extract exhibited a lower EC_{50}. In Fig. 6b–d, the EC_{50} values are shown in comparison with each compound content.

Finally, the trypsin inhibitory capacity was higher for the Salta extract than for the Misiones extract, showing a lower EC_{50} value (Fig. 7a). In Fig. 7b–d, the relationship between this activity and the compounds content is shown.

Finally, the effect on the nitrosative stress was studied on macrophages stimulated or not with LPS, which is an inductor of NO. The percentage of NO produced and the effect on cell proliferation were studied.

Figure 8a shows that in unstimulated macrophages, low concentrations of the Salta extract decreased the NO production, while higher concentrations increased

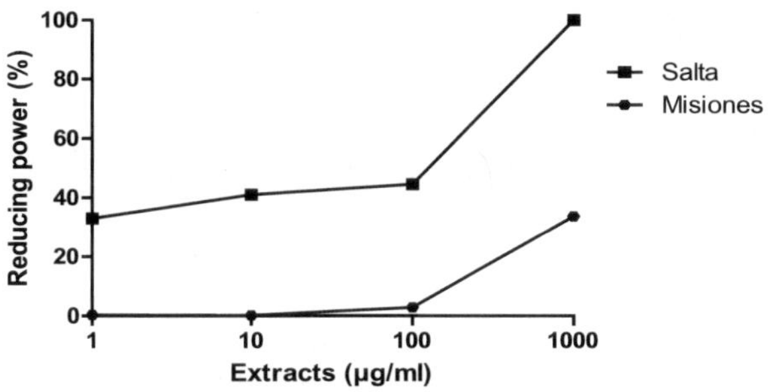

Extracts	Reducing power activity EC50 (µg/ml)
Misiones	>1000
Salta	126 ± 30

Fig. 3 Reducing power determination. **a** Reducing power as a function of the extract concentration. **b–d** Comparison between the reducing power and the polyphenols, flavonoids and tannins content and EC_{50} for Salta and Misiones extracts. Results represent mean ± SEM of three experiments performed in triplicate. Significant differences between extracts EC_{50} values were determined by the *t*-Student test (***$p < 0.001$)

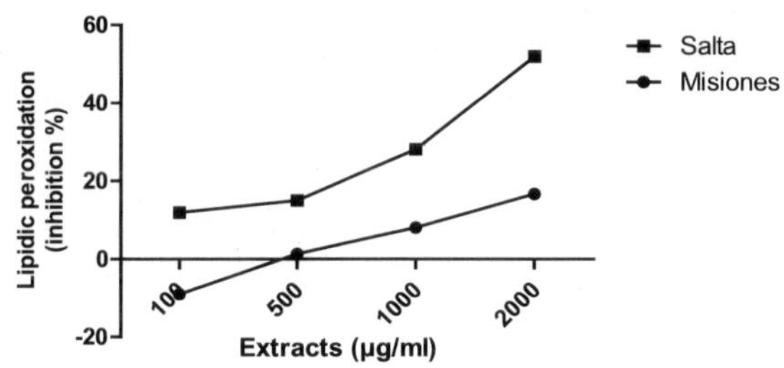

Extracts	Inhibition of lipid peroxidation EC50 (µg/ml)
Misiones	>2000(µg/ml)
Salta	1862 ± 20

Fig. 4 Lipid peroxidation. **a** Percentage of inhibition of lipid peroxidation as a function of the extract concentration. **b–d** Comparison between the lipid peroxidation inhibitory activity and the polyphenols, flavonoids and tannins content and EC_{50} for Salta and Misiones extracts. Results represent mean ± SEM of three experiments performed in triplicate. Significant differences between extracts EC_{50} were determined by the *t*-Student test (**$p < 0.01$)

the production of this mediator. On the other hand, the Misiones extract increased the NO production at all the concentrations assayed. LPS increased the NO release by macrophages (data not shown). Neither the Salta nor the Misiones extract modified cell proliferation at any

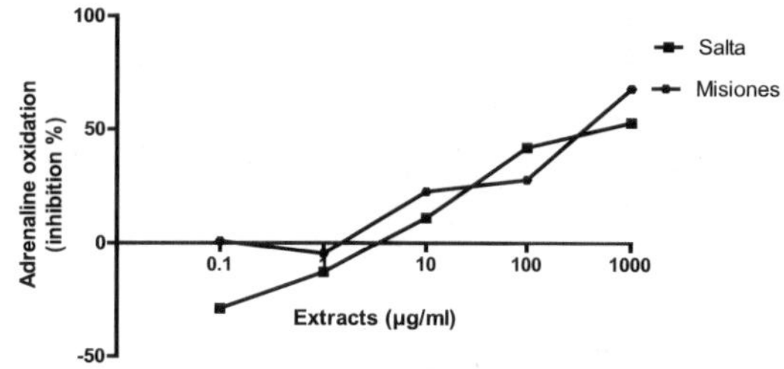

Extracts	Inhibition of adrenaline oxidation EC50 (µg/ml)
Misiones	363 ± 24
Salta	537 ± 59

Fig. 5 SOD like activity. **a** Percentage of inhibition of adrenaline oxidation as a function of the extract concentration. **b–d** Comparison between the adrenaline oxidation inhibition (SOD-like activity) and the polyphenols, flavonoids and tannins content and EC_{50} for Salta and Misiones extracts. Results represent mean ± SEM of three experiments performed in triplicate. Significant differences between extracts EC_{50} values were determined by the *t*-Student test (*$p < 0.05$)

concentration, but LPS was capable of decreasing cells proliferation. Under LPS stimulation, the Salta and Misiones extracts presented a biphasic effect, increasing the NO production at low concentrations and decreasing it at higher ones. The effect exerted by the Salta extract at high concentrations was higher than that of the Misiones extract (Fig. 8b). Moreover, the Salta extract, at 100 µg/ml, and the Misiones extract, at 100 and at 250 µg/ml were capable of reversing the antiproliferative effect exerted by LPS.

Discussion

In this work the polyphenol-related antioxidant activity of two extracts of *Urera aurantiaca* from different geographical zones form Argentina was demonstrated.

DPPH.is a stable free radical with a maximum absorbance at 517 nm. This free radical can readily be scavenged by an antioxidant to be transformed into 1,1-diphenyl-2-picrylhydrazine. The degree of bleaching indicates the scavenging power of the extract. In this assay, the Salta extract presented higher scavenging activity and potency than the Misiones extract.

The extracts also proved to have reducing power. This effect was assessed by direct electron donation in the reduction of $[Fe(CN)_6]^{3-}$ to $[Fe(CN)_6]^{4-}$ [29]. The product was visualized by the appearance of the intense Prussian blue coloured complex, whose absorbance was measured at 700 nm. The Salta extract had a higher capacity (lower EC_{50}) than the Misiones extract in reducing the complex Fe^{3+}/ferricyanide, reaching

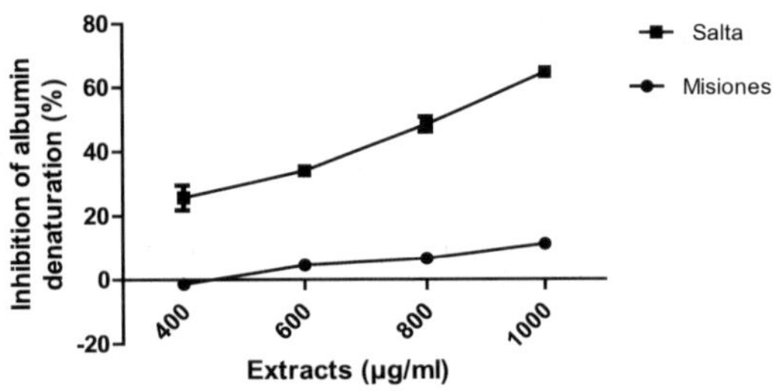

Extracts	Inhibition of albumin denaturation EC50 (µg/ml)
Misiones	>1000
Salta	812 ± 59

Fig. 6 Inhibition of albumin denaturation. **a** Percentage of inhibition of albumin denaturation as a function of the extract concentration. **b–d** Comparison between the albumin denaturation inhibitory action and the polyphenols, flavonoids and tannins content and EC_{50} for Salta and Misiones extracts. Results represent mean ± SEM of three experiments performed in triplicate. Significant differences between extracts EC_{50} values were determined by the *t*-Student test (*p < 0.05)

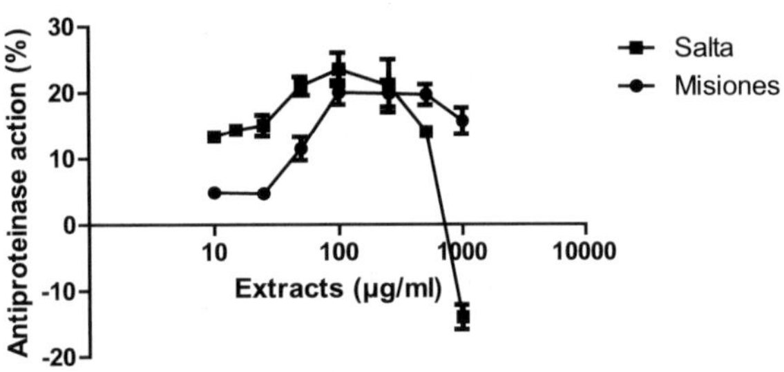

Extracts	Antiproteinase action EC50 (µg/ml)
Misiones	42 ± 4
Salta	< 10

Fig. 7 Proteinase inhibitory action. **a** Percentage of trypsin inhibition as a function of the extract concentration. **b–d** Comparison between the proteinase inhibitory action and the polyphenols, flavonoids and tannins content and EC_{50} for Salta and Misiones. Results represent mean ± SEM of three experiments performed in triplicate. Significant differences between extracts EC_{50} were determined by the *t*-Student test (**p < 0.01)

the highest inhibitory activity. The antioxidant effect exerted by reductants is based on the interruption of free radical chain reaction by donation of a hydrogen atom. Reductants also react with certain precursors of peroxide, thus preventing peroxide formation and lipid peroxidation. Our results indicate that the marked reducing power and DPPH scavenger activities exerted by the Salta extract seem to be due to the presence of polyphenols, such as flavonoids, whose content was directly proportional to such biological activity. The reducing power of these compounds is achieved through electron donation to free radicals to convert them into more stable products thus terminating the free radical chain reaction. The scavenging activity and the reducing power are known to be related to the nature of the phenolic compounds, which contribute to their electron transfer/hydrogen donating ability [30]. Thus, flavonoids generally have higher antioxidant activity because of the double bonds present in ring C, and their antioxidant ability depends on their hydroxyl group arrangement [31]. On the contrary, tannins did not appear not to be related to these effects since the Salta extract presented a higher potency than the Misiones extract and a lower tannins content.

The Salta extract showed scavenger activity and reducing power that were directly proportional to the inhibition on lipid peroxidation. Moreover, the inhibition of lipid peroxidation correlated positively with the presence of flavonoids and not with the presence of tannins. The inhibition of lipid peroxidation might be due to the hydrogen-donating capacity of phenolic derivatives and subsequent radical stabilization.

On the other hand, the SOD-like activity was higher in the Misiones extract, and such activity correlated with a higher tannin content, as compared to the Salta extract. The SOD-like activity exerted by the extract is highly desirable, since such activity would contribute to the elimination of the superoxide radical, which causes tissue injury, including carcinogenesis, inflammation, and aging. Many clinical trials have been carried out to assess the efficacy of SOD to treat several diseases caused by the generation of high levels of superoxide. However, the treatment must be administered by the parenteral route, since SOD is inactivated by digestive enzymes and gastric juices. An alternative approach is to find low molecular weight compounds that mimic SOD or which can enhance its enzymatic activity. Such mimicry was achieved by the Misiones extract.

It is known that oxidative stress induces inflammation and vice versa. In this regard, the denaturation of proteins is a well-documented cause of inflammation, and ROS are known to stimulate this process. Salicylic acid has been demonstrated to have a dose-dependent ability to induce thermal protein denaturation by ROS generation. Proteolytic enzymes, such as trypsin, which are essential modulators of the inflammatory response [32], are also activated by ROS. To complete the study of antioxidant activity, the effect of the extracts was assayed on albumin denaturation and on tryptic casein hydrolysis. As

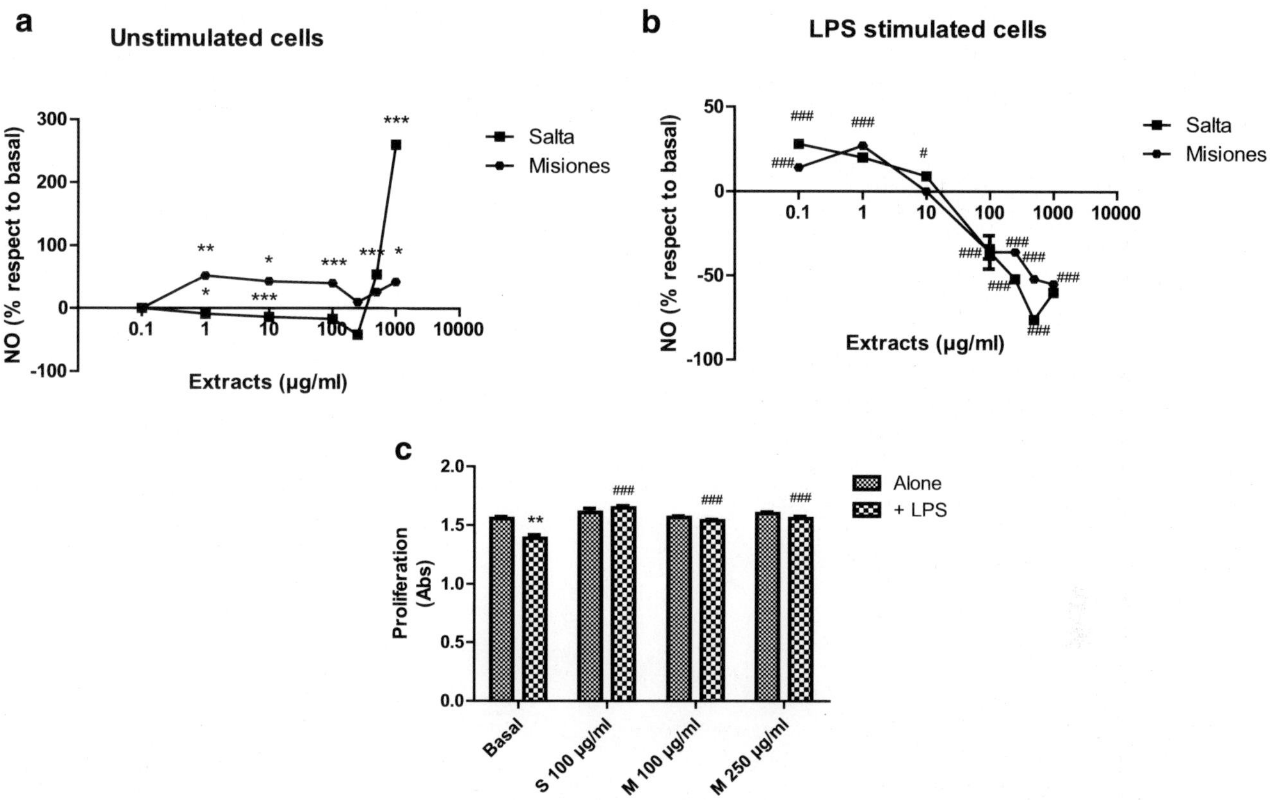

Fig. 8 Effect of the extracts on RAW264.7 macrophages. Cells were incubated for 24 h in the presence of the extracts alone or with LPS. **a** Effect of different concentrations of the extracts on NO production without LPS stimulation. **b** Effect of different concentrations of the extracts on NO production in the presence of LPS. **c** Effect of the extracts on macrophages proliferation in the absence or the presence of LPS. Results represent mean ± SEM of three experiments performed in triplicate. Statistical differences from the control group were determined by ANOVA + Dunnett's test (*$p < 0.05$; **$p < 0.01$; ***$p < 0.001$ vs. control group; #$p < 0.05$; ###$p < 0.001$ vs. LPS group)

expected, the Salta extract exerted a higher antioxidant activity, as evidenced by the lower EC_{50} on both models. These effects were related to the polyphenol content, especially flavonoids. The EC_{50} of the extracts for the DPPH scavenger, reducing power and SOD like activities were lower or equal (depending on the extract) than the EC_{50} for lipid peroxidation, inhibition of albumin denaturation and protease inhibition. These results may suggest that an antioxidant activity is required to induce the anti-inflammatory actions.

Nitric oxide is a diffusible free radical that plays many roles as an effector molecule in diverse biological systems, including neuronal messenger, vasodilatation and antimicrobial and antitumor activities [33]. It is a potent pleiotropic inhibitor of physiological processes such as smooth muscle relaxation, neuronal signaling, inhibition of platelet aggregation, and regulation of cell mediated toxicity. It is known that NO induces cell death by apoptosis. Macrophages can produce high amounts of NO upon activation by cytokines and LPS. After stimulation with LPS, macrophages secrete several pro-inflammatory products such as TNF-α, interleukins, and NO. Many transcriptor factor families, including NF-kB, activator protein 1 (AP-1), among others, are considered critical regulators of gene expression in the setting of the inflammatory process. Although these factors play an essential beneficial role in physiological processes, the deregulation of NF-kB activity and the sustained production of pro-inflammatory cytokines and NO are involved in the pathogenesis of several diseases [34].

In LPS-stimulated macrophages, both extracts were capable of decreasing the production of NO only at high concentrations, thus blunting the effect of LPS. Moreover, the extracts were able to revert the antiproliferative effect of LPS. All these effects suggested an antioxidant and anti-inflammatory activity at high concentrations. Low concentrations of the extracts had the opposite effect in NO production, increasing it without modification of cell proliferation. This protective effect of the extracts could be related to their antioxidant activity and to the presence of polyphenols. Many studies have shown that many flavonoids and related polyphenols contribute

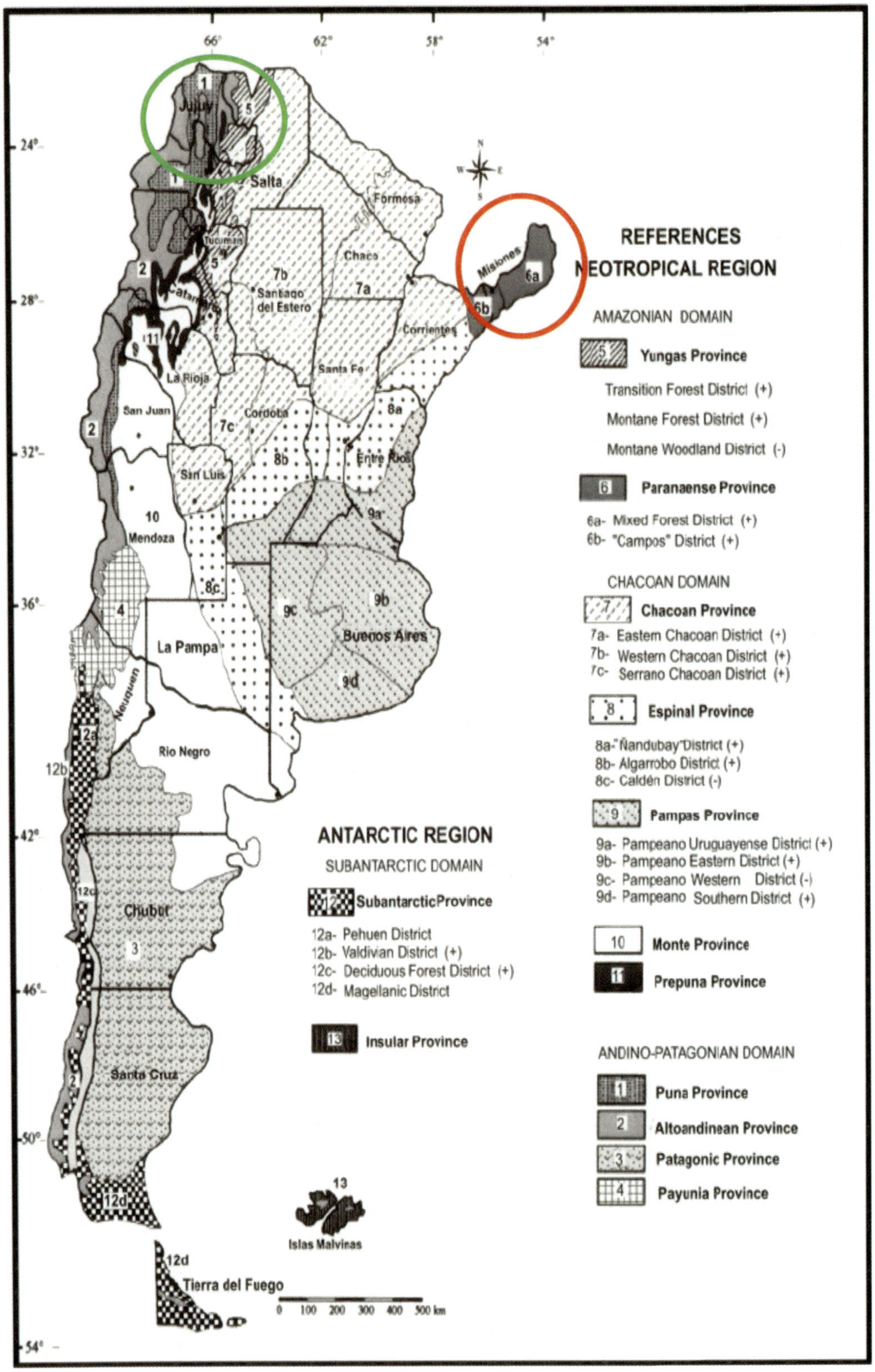

Fig. 9 Phytogeographic Argentinean provinces and *Urera aurantiaca* distribution. Paranaense phytogeographic Province and Yungas phytogeographic province are marked in red and green, respectively

significantly to the anti-inflammatory activities exerted by many plants [35, 36].

In relation to NO production, it can be suggested that the extracts also exert an immunomodulatory activity on cells without LPS activation, demonstrating a pro-oxidant activity at low and high concentrations. The Salta extract appeared to be more effective in reducing the production of NO.

The differences observed in the antioxidant activities of the extracts could be related to a quantitative rather to a qualitative difference in the polyphenols content. These quantitative differences observed between both extracts could be a consequence of genotypic, developmental and environmental factors. It is known that specimens of same plant species growing under different environmental conditions show significant differences in the production and accumulation the primary and secondary metabolites [37]. Influenced by environmental factors, secondary metabolites act as a chemical interface between the plant and its environment. The chemical interaction between plants and their environment is mediated mainly by the biosynthesis of secondary metabolites, which exert their biological roles as a plastic adaptive response to their environment.

The Salta specimen was collected in the Oran zone (phytogeographic province of the Yungas) and the Misiones specimen was collected in Eldorado (Paranaense phytogeographic province) [38] (Fig. 9). These phytogeographic zones differ in climate, temperature and precipitations, factors which can influence the production of primary and secondary metabolites. In this sense, the Paranaense province is a moist forest with subtropical climate, whereas the Yungas is a rain mountain forest which constitutes a subtropical complex biome with extreme temperatures that range from 50 °C in summer to 10 °C in winter. The climate is wet and hot, with summer precipitations and winter frost. In fact, it is a very rainy and foggy zone. These differences between the biomes could explain the differences observed in the specimens.

Conclusion

The present study demonstrated the in vitro antioxidant and anti-inflammatory activities of two methanol extracts of *U. aurantiaca*. The presence of flavonoids and other polyphenols in the extracts may be responsible for the biological activity observed. The differences found between the extracts effectiveness are probably related to ambient conditions: temperature, rain, soil composition and ecosystem.

Abbreviations

DPPH: 2,2-diphenyl-1-picrylhydrazyl; LPS: lipopolysaccharide; MTT: 3-(4,5-dimethylthiazol-2-yl)-2,5-diphenyltetrazolium bromide; NO: nitric oxide; RNS: reactive nitrogen species; ROS: reactive oxygen species; SOD: superoxide dismutase.

Authors' contributions

CM and IP performed the experimental procedures. CA coordinated the work. All authors analysed the results. All authors read and approved the final manuscript.

Acknowledgements

Not applicable.

Competing interests

The authors declare that they have no competing interests.

Consent for publication

Not applicable.

Funding

This work was supported by Grant PIP 0007 from the National Research Council (CONICET).

References

1. Kaplan M, Mutlu E, Benson M, Fields J, Banan A, Keshavarzian A. Use of herbal preparations in the treatment of oxidant mediated inflammatory disorders. Complement Ther Med. 2007;15:207–16.
2. Chatterjee S. Chapter two—oxidative stress, inflammation, and disease Oxidative stress and biomaterials. New York: Academic press Elsevier; 2016. p. 35–58.
3. Lee J, Koo N, Min DB. Reactive oxygen species, aging, and antioxidative nutraceuticals. Compr Rev Food Sci Food Saf. 2004;3:21–33.
4. Gou Z, Jiang S, Zheng C, Tian Z, Lin X. Equol inhibits LPS-induced oxidative stress and enhances the immune response in chicken HD11 macrophages. Cell Physiol Biochem. 2015;36:611–21.
5. Halliwell B. Free radicals and antioxidants: a personal review. Nutr Rev. 1994;52:253–65.
6. MartínezCrovetto R. Plantas utilizadas en medicina en el noroeste Corrientes. Corrientes: Miscelanea; 1981. p. 37.
7. Riedel R, Marrassini C, Anesini C, Gorzalczany S. Anti-inflammatory and antinociceptive activity of *Urera aurantiaca*. Phytother Res. 2015;2015(29):59–66.
8. Marrassini C, Anesini C. Modulatory effect of an *Urera Aurantiaca* extract on immune and tumoral cells during inflammation. Phytother Res. 2016;31:265–73.
9. Kasote DM, Jagtap SD, Thapa D, Khyade MS, Russell WR. Herbal remedies for urinary stones used in India and China: a review. J Ethnopharmacol. 2017;203:55–68.
10. Weckerle CS, Ineichen R, Huber FK, Yang Y. Mao's heritage: medicinal plant knowledge among the Bai in Shaxi, China, at a crossroads between distinct local and common widespread practice. J Ethnopharmacol. 2009;123:213–28.
11. Li DL, Xing FW. Ethnobotanical study on medicinal plants used by local Hoklos people on Hainan Island, China. J Ethnopharmacol. 2016;194:358–68.
12. Zheng XL, Wei JH, Sun W, Li RT, Liu SB, Dai HF. Ethnobotanical study on medicinal plants around Limu Mountains of Hainan Island, China. J Ethnopharmacol. 2013;148:964–74.
13. Au DT, Wu J, Jiang Z, Chen H, Lu G, Zhao Z. Ethnobotanical study of medicinal plants used by Hakka in Guangdong, China. J Ethnopharmacol. 2008;117:41–50.
14. Telascrea M, de Araujo CC, Marques MOM, Facanali R, de Moraes PLR, Cavalheiro AJ. Essential oil from leaves of *Cryptocarya mandioccana* Meisner

(Lauraceae): composition and intraspecific chemical variability. Biochem Syst Ecol. 2007;35:222–32.

15. Rahimmalek M, Tabatabaei BES, Etemadi N, Goli SAH, Arzani A, Zeinali H. Essential oil variation among and within six *Achillea* species transferred from different ecological regions in Iran to the field conditions. Ind Crops Prod. 2009;29:348–55.
16. Singleton VL, Orthofer R, Lamuela-Raventós RM. Analysis of total phenols and other oxidation substrates and antioxidants by means of Folin–Ciocalteu reagent. Methods Enzymol. 1999;299:152–78.
17. Chang CC, Yang MH, Wen HM, Chern JC. Estimation of total flavonoid content in propolis by two complementary colorimetric methods. J Food Drug Anal. 2002;10:178–82.
18. Santos SC, Mello JCP. Farmacognosia da planta ao medicamento. 5th ed. Porto Alegre: Editora da URFGS/UFSC; 2004. p. 615–56.
19. Amorim ELC, Nascimento JE, Monteiro JM, Peixoto Sobrinho TJS, Araujo TAS, Albuquerque UP. A simple and accurate procedure for the determination of tannin and flavonoid levels and some applications in ethnobotany and ethnopharmacology. Functional ecosystems and communities. Funct Ecosyst Commun. 2008;2:88–94.
20. Filip R, Lopez P, Giberti G, Coussio J, Ferraro G. Fitoterapia. 2001;72:774–8.
21. Becherel PA, Chosidow O, LeGoff L, Frances C, Debre P, Mossalayi MD. Inducible nitric oxide synthase and proinflammatory cytokine expression by human keratinocytes during acute urticaria. Mol Med. 1997;3:686–94.
22. Blois MS. Antioxidant determination by the use of a stable free radical. Nat Geosci. 1958;181:1199–200.
23. Carrillo MC, Kanai S, Nokubo M, Kitani K. Der-prenyl induces activities of both superoxide dismutase and catalase but not glutathione peroxidase in the striatum of young male rats. Life Sci J. 1991;48:517–21.
24. Ferreira ICFR, Baptista P, Vilas-Boas M, Barros L. Free radical scavenging capacity and reducing power of wild edible mushroom from northeast Portugal: individual cap and stipe activity. Food Chem. 2007;100:1511–6.
25. Dissanayake DP, Abeytunga D, Vasudewa NS, Ratnasooriya WD. Inhibition of lipid peroxidation by extracts of *Pleurotus ostreatus*. Phcog Mag. 2009;5:266–71.
26. Kumari CS, Yasmin N, Hussain MR, Babuselvam M. *In vitro* anti-inflammatory and anti-arthritic property of *Rhizopora mucronata* leaves. Int J Pharm Sci Res. 2015;6:482–5.

(Lauraceae): composition and intraspecific chemical variability. Biochem Syst Ecol. 2007;35:222–32.

27. Sakat SS, Juvekar AR, Gambhire MN. In vitro antioxidant and anti-inflammatory activity if methanol extract of *Oxalis corniculata* Linn. Int J Pharm Pharm Sci. 2010;2:146–55.
28. Oyedapo OO, Famurewa AJ. Antiprotease and membrane stabilizing activities of extracts of *Fagara zanthoxyloides*, *Olax subscorpioides* and *Tetrapleura tetraptera*. Int J Pharmacogn. 1995;33:65–9.
29. Yen GC, Chen HY. Antioxidant activity of various tea extracts in relation to their antimutagenicity. J Agric Food Chem. 1995;43:27–32.
30. Brand-Williams W, Cuvelier ME, Berset C. Use of a free radical method to evaluate antioxidant activity. Lebenson Wiss Technol. 1995;28:25–30.
31. Kondo K, Kurihara M, Fukuhara K, Tanaka T, Suzuki T, Miyata N, Toyoda M. Conversion of procyanidin B-type (catechin dimer) to A-type: evidence for abstraction of C-2 hydrogen in catechin during radical oxidation. Tetrahedron Lett. 2000;41:485–8.
32. Alam MB, Hossain MS, Haque ME. Antioxidant and anti-inflammatory activities of the leaf extract of *Brassica nigra*. IJPSR. 2015;2:303–10.
33. Hagerman AE, Riedl KM, Jones GA, Sovik KN, Ritchard NT, Hartzfeld PW. High molecular weight plant polyphenolics (tannins) as biological antioxidants. J Agric Food Chem. 1998;46:1887–92.
34. Marrassini C, Davicino R, Acevedo C, Anesini C, Gorzalczany S, Ferraro G. Vicenin-2, a potential anti-inflammatory constituent of *Urtica circularis*. J Nat Prod. 2011;74:1503–7.
35. Luo XD, Basile MJ, Kennelly EJ. Polyphenolic antioxidants from the fruits of *Chrysophyllum cainito* L. (star apple). J Agric Food Chem. 2002;50:1379–82.
36. Okoli CO, Akah PA. Mechanism of the antiinflammatory activity of the leaf extracts of *Culcasia scandens* P. beauv (Araceae). Pharmacol Biochem Behav. 2004;79:473–81.
37. Sampaio BL, Edrada-Ebel R, Da Costa FB. Effect of the environment on the secondary metabolic profile of *Tithonia diversifolia*: a model for environmental metabolomics of plants. Sci Rep. 2016;6:1–11.
38. Cabrera AL. Regiones fitogeográficas argentinas. Enciclopedia argentina de agricultura y jardinería. Buenos Aires: Acme; 1976. p. 85.

6

A simple method for HPLC retention time prediction: linear calibration using two reference substances

Lei Sun[1,2], Hong-yu Jin[1], Run-tao Tian[3], Ming-juan Wang[1], Li-na Liu[1], Liu-ping Ye[4], Tian-tian Zuo[1] and Shuang-cheng Ma[1*]

Abstract

Background: Analysis of related substances in pharmaceutical chemicals and multi-components in traditional Chinese medicines needs bulk of reference substances to identify the chromatographic peaks accurately. But the reference substances are costly. Thus, the relative retention (RR) method has been widely adopted in pharmacopoeias and literatures for characterizing HPLC behaviors of those reference substances unavailable. The problem is it is difficult to reproduce the RR on different columns due to the error between measured retention time (t_R) and predicted t_R in some cases. Therefore, it is useful to develop an alternative and simple method for prediction of t_R accurately.

Methods: In the present study, based on the thermodynamic theory of HPLC, a method named linear calibration using two reference substances (LCTRS) was proposed. The method includes three steps, procedure of two points prediction, procedure of validation by multiple points regression and sequential matching. The t_R of compounds on a HPLC column can be calculated by standard retention time and linear relationship.

Results: The method was validated in two medicines on 30 columns.

Conclusion: It was demonstrated that, LCTRS method is simple, but more accurate and more robust on different HPLC columns than RR method. Hence quality standards using LCTRS method are easy to reproduce in different laboratories with lower cost of reference substances.

Keywords: RP-HPLC, Retention time, Relative retention, Linear calibration using two reference substances, Multi-component analysis, Traditional Chinese medicines

Background

Multi-components analysis is an effective strategy for quality control of traditional Chinese medicines (TCMs), which have complex chemical profiles. But the classic external standard method was severely confined in its application due to the high cost of reference substances. As a consequence, substitute reference substance methods such as extractive reference substance (ERS) method and single standard to determine multi-components (SSDMC) method for overall quality control of TCMs have emerged, and widely used in Chinese pharmacopoeia 2015 edition, the United States Pharmacopoeia (USP39-NF34) and literatures [1–10]. In general, ERS method provides only one reference chromatogram in the pharmacopoeias, instructions of ERS and literatures. But there are hundreds of brands of C_{18} columns in the market. It means that the reference chromatogram may be different from the actual chromatogram. Due to the column types and other various factors, the error between measured retention time (t_R) and predicted t_R by the relative retention (RR) method cannot be ignored sometimes.

In order to improve the reproducibility of chromatographic separation and RR, the method of classification of C_{18} columns has been proposed [11–15]. The columns were divided into three types: A, B and EP. Although the

*Correspondence: masc@nifdc.org.cn
[1] National Institutes for Food and Drug Control, No. 2 Tiantan Xili, Dongcheng District, Beijing 100050, People's Republic of China
Full list of author information is available at the end of the article

same type of columns was used to repeat the analytical methods, the differences in the performance and the separation effects were still large. And then the methods for selecting columns with equivalent selectivity, such as the USP approach [16], the PQRI approach [17, 18] and Katholieke Universiteit Leuven column classification system [19–21] were proposed. Take PQRI approach [17, 18] as an example, hydrophobicity (H), steric interaction (S), hydrogen-bond acidity (A), hydrogen-bond basicity (B) and ion-exchange capacity (C), were used to describe the performance of the column. And the similarity between a column and the reference column was calculated by these five parameters. When the similarity was less than three, the two columns were regarded to be equivalent. Using the equivalent column, the reproducibility of separation and RR could be improved to some extent. However, in addition to column, many other factors also have great influences on the chromatograms, such as the dead volume of chromatographic system, the different structure of analytes, the complexity of the chromatographic conditions, and so on. Therefore, it is necessary to develop a method that takes all aforementioned factors into account to reduce the prediction error of the t_R.

According to the thermodynamic theory of liquid chromatography, there is a linear relationship between the t_R of the compounds on two different HPLC systems (including chromatographs and columns) [22]. For better understanding, the pdf of reference 22 (in Chinese, Additional file 1) and the English version of reference 22 (only the section of theory was translated, Additional file 2) are provided. Combined with the above principle and previous studies [23–25], a novel method using two reference substances for predicting HPLC t_R has been proposed (linear calibration by two reference substances, LCTRS). The St_R (arithmetic average of t_R for the same compound on different HPLC system under the same chromatographic conditions) is used as the reference value, and the linear regression is used as the basic algorithm for t_R prediction. In this study, the method was validated in two medicines on 30 C_{18} columns. Compared with the RR method, LCTRS method is proved to be more accurate, and more robust on different HPLC columns. Hence, it provides a good prospective application in quantification of multi-components in TCMs as well as related substances in pharmaceutical chemicals.

Methods

The Minimum Standards of Reporting Checklist contains details of the experimental design, and statistics, and resources used in this study (Additional file 3).

Instruments and reagents

Waters e2695 HPLC (2998PDA detector), Agilent 1260 HPLC (DAD detector), and Shimadzu LC-2010A HT HPLC (UV–Vis detector) were used. Matlab software was provided by Math Works Inc. USA. 30 C_{18} columns (shown in Table 1), from 13 manufacturers, included A, B, and EP types were used. And most columns belong to type B according to the previous study [11–15]. According to the PQRI approach [17, 18] and using the data from the USP website (http://www.usp.org/USPNF/columns.html), the similarity of columns were calculated using col1 as the reference column. The similarity (0–13.18) showed that the differences among the columns were large, which indicated that the selected columns are in a wide range and have good representative trait.

Reference substances of psoralen, isopsoralen, Chonglou saponin I, Chonglou saponin II, Chonglou saponin VI, Chonglou saponin VII, ethinylestradiol, and herbal reference substances including Psoraleae Fructus (Psoraleae) and Paridis Rhizome (Paridis), were supplied by the National Institutes for Food and Drug Control, China. Methanol, acetonitrile, and phosphoric acid were HPLC graded and supplied by the Fischer Company, USA. Ammonium nitrate (analytical grade) was supplied by Beijing Chemical Works. Water was prepared by Milli-Q system, Millipore Company, USA.

Preparation of sample solution

Psoraleae [26]: weigh 0.5 g of the powder and place it in a 50-mL stopper conical flask, then add 25 mL of ethanol. Sonicate the mixture for 30 min and centrifuge for 5 min. Filter the supernatant through a 0.45-μm PTFE filter.

Paridis [27]: weigh 0.5 g of the powder to a stopper conical flask, add 25 mL of ethanol, heat under reflux on a water bath for 30 min, cool and filter the supernatant through a 0.45-μm PTFE filter.

Chromatographic conditions

Psoraleae [26]: mobile phase A was water and mobile phase B was methanol. The elution procedure was shown below: 0–20 min, 50%B→70%B; 20–45 min, 70%B→85%B; 45–50 min, 85%B→90%B; 50–60 min, 90%B. Detection wavelength was 308 nm. Paridis [27]: mobile phase A was water and mobile phase B was acetonitrile. The elution procedure was shown below: 0–40 min, 30%B→60%B; 40–50 min, 60%B→30%B; 50–60 min, 30%B. Detection wavelength was 203 nm. Column temperatures were both set at 30 °C and flow rate was 1.0 mL/min.

Results

HPLC chromatogram of samples

The typical chromatograms of Psoraleae and Paridis were shown in Fig. 1. The peaks were mainly identified by the reference substances. For those peaks without reference substances, UV–Vis spectrum and mass spectrum were used for identification.

Table 1 t_R (min) of four saponins in Paridis on different columns

No.	Brand	Chonglou saponin VII	Chonglou saponin VI	Chonglou saponin II	Chonglou saponin I
col1	Discovery C_{18}^{a}	21.234 ± 0.021	23.001 ± 0.006	32.773 ± 0.007	35.118 ± 0.004
col2	Discovery C_{18}^{b}	16.555 ± 0.010	17.989 ± 0.006	27.161 ± 0.011	29.154 ± 0.002
col3	Xbridge C_{18}^{a}	21.101 ± 0.004	23.070 ± 0.027	32.483 ± 0.021	34.963 ± 0.006
col4	BDS HypersilC_{18}^{a}	21.014 ± 0.011	22.898 ± 0.018	32.679 ± 0.032	35.170 ± 0.036
col5	Inertsil ODS-2[a]	22.132 ± 0.009	24.502 ± 0.004	33.176 ± 0.017	35.936 ± 0.003
col6	Kromasil C_{18}^{a}	21.276 ± 0.012	23.693 ± 0.016	32.618 ± 0.006	35.929 ± 0.007
col7	Luna C_{18}(2)[a]	20.760 ± 0.018	23.362 ± 0.008	30.941 ± 0.011	33.813 ± 0.003
col8	Luna C_{18}(2)[b]	16.551 ± 0.008	18.865 ± 0.023	25.923 ± 0.016	28.310 ± 0.011
col9	Inertsil ODS-3[b]	17.225 ± 0.006	19.640 ± 0.005	26.754 ± 0.013	29.471 ± 0.005
col10	Alltima C_{18}^{a}	20.856 ± 0.008	23.752 ± 0.021	31.687 ± 0.011	34.872 ± 0.004
col11	Symmetry C_{18}^{a}	21.016 ± 0.015	22.076 ± 0.016	32.470 ± 0.023	35.476 ± 0.010
col12	Gemini C_{18}^{a}	21.300 ± 0.014	23.756 ± 0.007	31.599 ± 0.003	34.337 ± 0.015
col13	CapcellpakC_{18}MG[a]	21.076 ± 0.012	23.828 ± 0.004	31.627 ± 0.006	34.695 ± 0.001
col14	Zorbax Extend-C_{18}^{a}	17.201 ± 0.022	19.731 ± 0.003	27.525 ± 0.009	30.504 ± 0.005
col15	Sunfire C_{18}^{a}	21.652 ± 0.013	24.065 ± 0.024	32.375 ± 0.010	35.197 ± 0.006
col16	Sunfire C_{18}^{b}	17.501 ± 0.006	19.571 ± 0.018	27.401 ± 0.004	29.826 ± 0.010
col17	Nucleosil C_{18} HD[a]	21.452 ± 0.013	23.735 ± 0.006	32.747 ± 0.019	35.513 ± 0.011
col18	ODS Hypersil[a]	19.669 ± 0.010	21.583 ± 0.022	30.361 ± 0.007	32.657 ± 0.005
col19	CapcellpakC_{18}AQ[a]	20.092 ± 0.013	22.560 ± 0.010	29.568 ± 0.006	32.218 ± 0.005
col20	Spherisorb ODS2[a]	18.684 ± 0.006	21.334 ± 0.021	28.580 ± 0.008	31.385 ± 0.004
col21	Zorbax SB-C_{18}^{a}	18.438 ± 0.015	20.986 ± 0.010	28.085 ± 0.008	30.849 ± 0.007
col22	DiamonsilC_{18}^{a}	22.082 ± 0.021	25.078 ± 0.005	32.475 ± 0.020	35.721 ± 0.023
col23	DiamonsilC_{18}^{b}	16.769 ± 0.007	19.154 ± 0.008	26.240 ± 0.011	28.935 ± 0.004
col24	Diamonsil C_{18}(2)[a]	19.296 ± 0.016	22.819 ± 0.004	31.192 ± 0.019	34.710 ± 0.009
col25	Kromasil Eternity C_{18}^{a}	19.732 ± 0.017	22.099 ± 0.018	29.535 ± 0.004	32.153 ± 0.021
col26	Shim-pack VP-ODS[b]	19.015 ± 0.007	21.059 ± 0.014	29.401 ± 0.002	31.845 ± 0.001
col27	Agilent HC-C_{18}^{a}	23.492 ± 0.247	25.839 ± 0.250	34.884 ± 0.344	37.637 ± 0.330
col28	Agilent TC-C_{18}^{a}	20.609 ± 0.003	22.574 ± 0.005	30.806 ± 0.003	32.783 ± 0.002
col29	Venusil MP C_{18}^{b}	17.970 ± 0.007	20.468 ± 0.011	27.287 ± 0.031	29.985 ± 0.007
col30	Nucleosil C_{18} AB[a]	18.348 ± 0.012	20.209 ± 0.017	29.233 ± 0.011	31.893 ± 0.014
	St_R (Average t_R)	19.803	22.110	30.319	33.035

[a] 4.6 mm × 250 mm × 5 μm
[b] 4.6 mm × 150 mm × 5 μm

Standard retention time (St_R)

Under the same chromatographic conditions, measured retention time ($t_R$mea) of the four saponins in Paridis on different chromatographic systems (which includes HPLC instruments and columns, hereinafter referred to as columns due to the differences of t_R mainly caused by columns) were shown in Table 1. The arithmetic average of t_R for the same compound on different columns is called St_R, formula (1). Just like RR, St_R is the reference value for calculating the predicted retention time ($t_R$pre) of analyte in the samples. Theoretically, under the same chromatographic condition, the RR calculated by different columns is constants, but St_R is not. It will be discussed in Section "Minimum number of columns for St_R calculation" that the advantages of using St_R was better than t_R of any single column. In this paper, the deviation (Δt_R) of $t_R$mea and $t_R$pre (formula 2) was used to evaluate the merits and defects of RR method and LCTRS method.

$$St_R = \sum_{i=1}^{n} t_{Ri}/n \quad (n \geq 1) \tag{1}$$

$$\Delta t_R = |t_R mea - t_R pre| \tag{2}$$

Linear principle of LCTRS

According to the chromatographic thermodynamic theory, Wang et al. proved that there was a linear relationship between the t_R of the same compounds on different

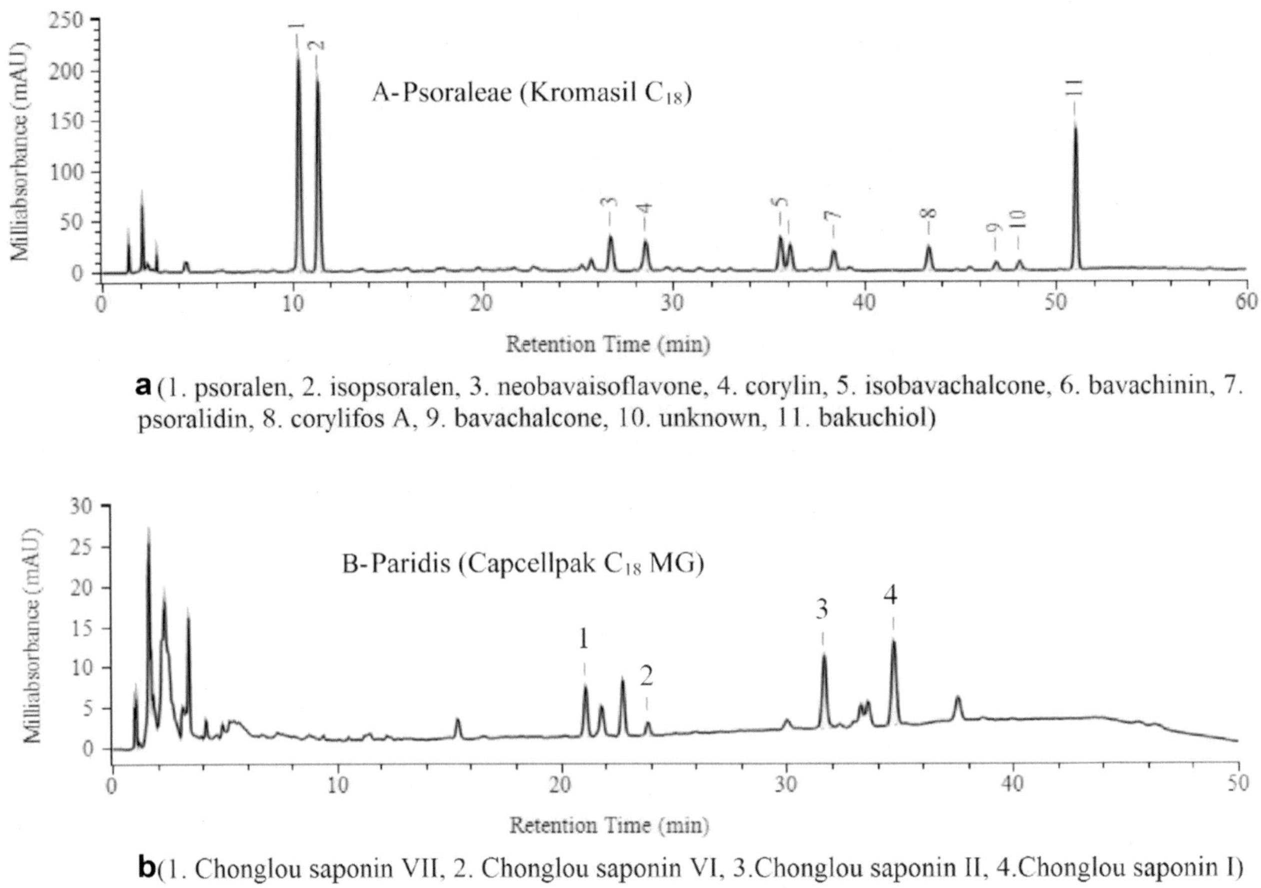

Fig. 1 HPLC chromatograms of samples

HPLC system (mainly considered as columns) under the same chromatographic conditions [22], as expressed in formula (3) and Fig. 2a, b.

$$t_R coli = a \times t_R colj + b \tag{3}$$

Since formulas (1) and (3) are both linear, thus there is a linear relationship between t_R and St_R for each compound, as shown in formula (4) and Fig. 2c, d. It is noteworthy that the correlation coefficient of the linear regression is higher than that shown in Fig. 2a, b.

$$t_R coli = a \times St_R + b \tag{4}$$

Minimum number of columns for St_R calculation

Theoretically, t_R on any column can be used as reference value for linear fitting. But the Δt_R calculated with random column were instable. Thus, the reasonable number of columns for St_R calculation was thoroughly investigated by random sampling. St_R was calculated based on 1, 5, 10, 15, 20, 25, and 30 columns combined with non-replicate random sampling times of 30, 100, 100, 100, 100, 100, and 1, respectively. The value of St_R with $t_R$mea on 30 columns was used to fit multiple point linear equation. The averages of Δt_R (average ± standard deviation) were calculated, as shown in Fig. 3. For both medicines, the prediction deviation was reduced with increasing number of columns. However, the prediction accuracy will not be significantly improved when the number of columns reaches five, which is considered as a low-cost and reasonable limit. It is recommended to choose five–fifteen columns for St_R calculation.

Even for the columns with same type of packing material, there are still some differences among the column stationary phase, packing techniques and errors in the process of chromatographic analysis. Those differences will cause deviation of t_R. The physical explanation of St_R calculation was to evenly mix and refill the stationary phase of the columns selected. Because of reducing the random and system errors, the prediction result was accurate and robust.

Procedure of two points prediction

For RR method, only one compound was chosen as reference compound (reference substance required), and RR

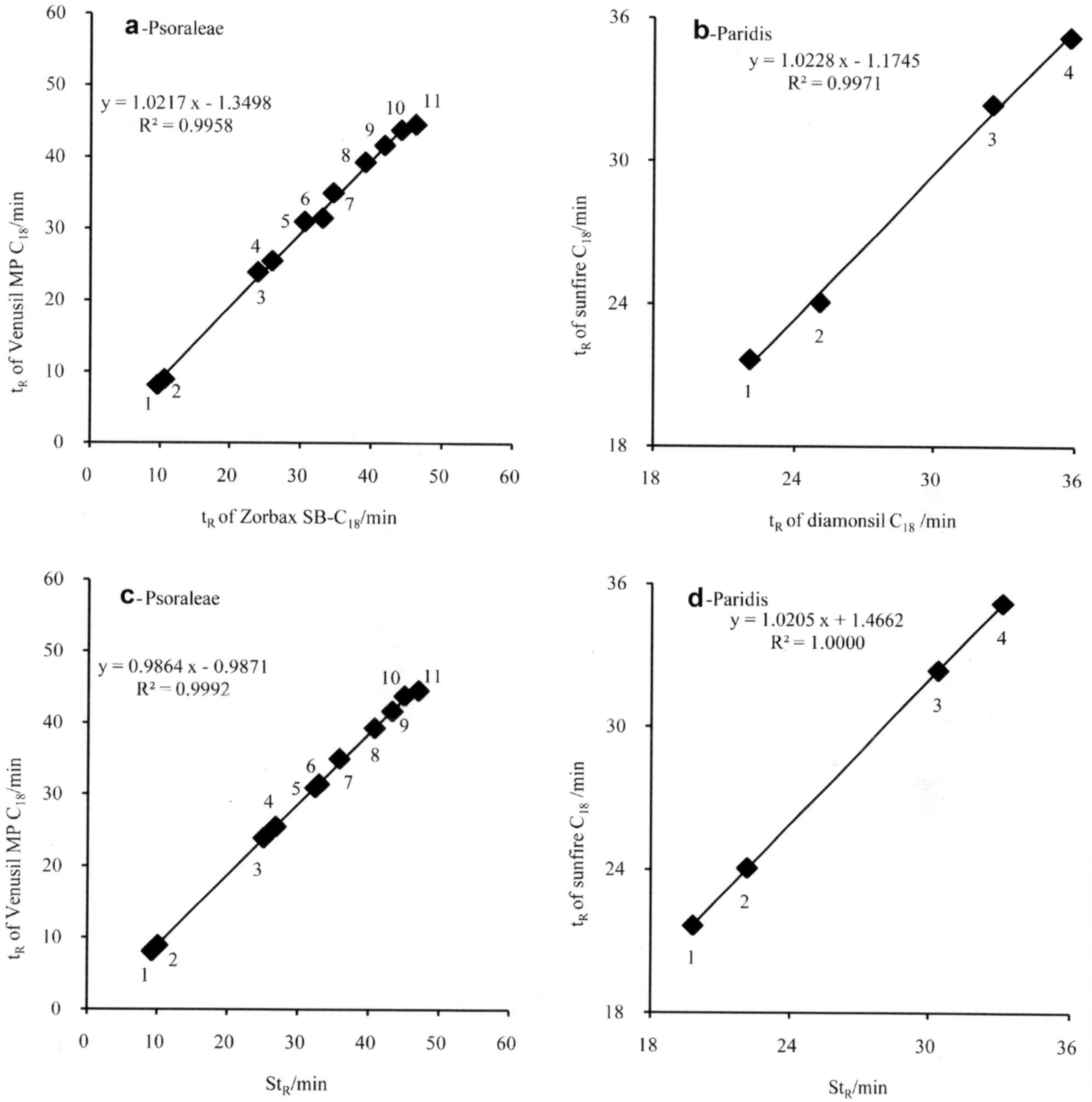

Fig. 2 Linear fitting results of Psoraleae and Paridis, code No. is the same as that in Fig. 1

of all other compounds were used as reference value for calculating $t_R$pre. For LCTRS method, two compounds were chosen as reference compounds (reference substances required), and St_R of all other compounds were used as reference value for calculating $t_R$pre. The reference compounds, the value of RR and St_R were shown in Tables 2 and 3.

Take Paridis as an example. First of all, reference substances solution of two reference compounds (Chonglou saponin VII and Chonglou saponin I) and sample solution were performed on a C_{18} column (col4: BDS Hypersil C_{18}). The $t_R$mea (21.014 and 35.170 min) of two reference compounds in the sample solution were obtained by the reference substances solution (Fig. 4a). Then two points, Chonglou saponin VII (19.803, 21.014) and Chonglou saponin I (33.035, 35.170), could be determined in the coordinate using St_R as abscissa and $t_R$mea as ordinate. Based on the two points, the following linear equation

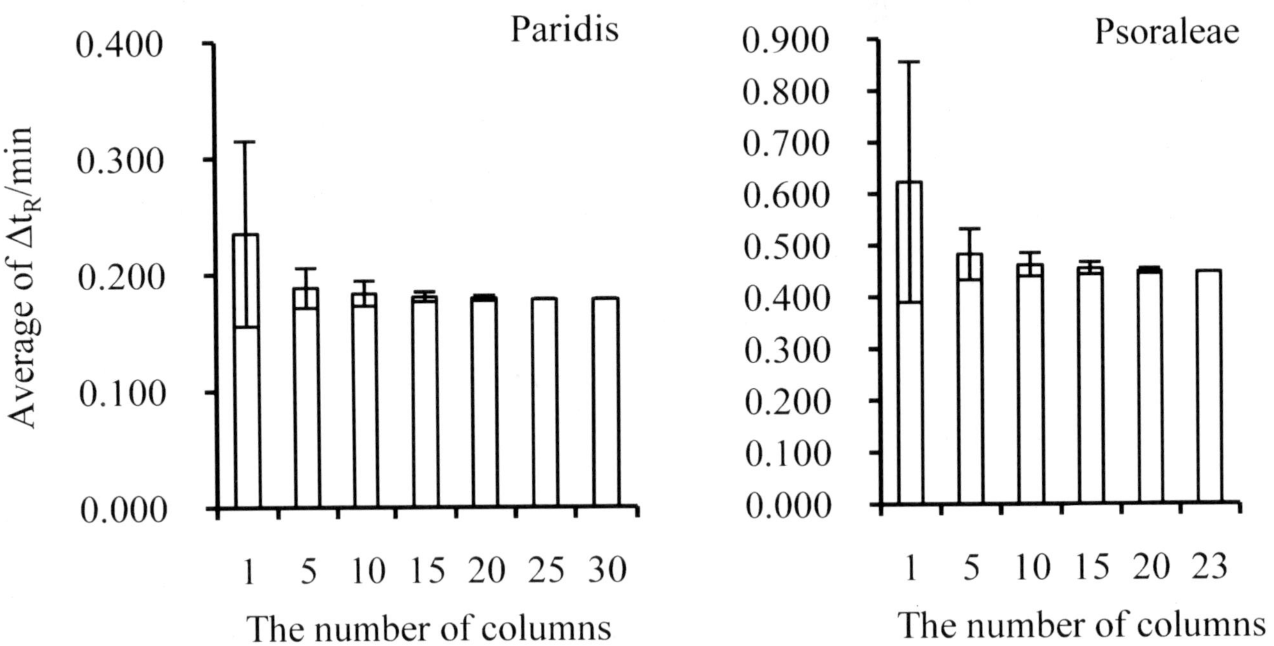

Fig. 3 Prediction results of different number of columns for S_{tR} calculation

Table 2 RR and reference compound for RR method

	Peak 1	Peak 2	Peak 3	Peak 4	Peak 5	Peak 6	Peak 7	Peak 8	Peak 9	Peak 10	Peak 11
Psoraleae (n = 23)	0.226	0.247	0.615	0.657	0.794	0.808	0.878	1.000[a]	1.061	1.103	1.152
Paridis (n = 30)	0.652	0.729	1.000[a]	1.090							

[a] Reference compound

Table 3 St_R (min) and reference compound for LCTRS method

	Peak 1	Peak 2	Peak 3	Peak 4	Peak 5	Peak 6	Peak 7	Peak 8	Peak 9	Peak 10	Peak 11
Psoraleae (n = 23)	9.271	10.122[a]	25.143	26.854	32.437	32.951	35.843	40.793[a]	43.254	44.950	46.937
Paridis (n = 30)	19.803[a]	22.156	30.319	33.035[a]							

[a] Reference compound

was given: $y = 1.0698x - 0.1719$ (Fig. 4b). Taking St_R of analytes (Chonglou saponin VI and Chonglou saponin II) into equation, the $t_R$pre of Chonglou saponin VI (23.481 min) and Chonglou saponin II (32.263 min) were attained, respectively. Finally, in the chromatogram of the sample solution, the corresponding peaks of Chonglou saponin VI and Chonglou saponin II can be found within the range of $t_R\text{pre} \pm t_R\text{W}$ (t_RW is abbreviation of t_R window, in this case is 0.6 min), as shown in Fig. 4c. It can be seen that Δt_R of analytes calculated by prediction of two points were 0.583 min and 0.416 min (The $t_R$mea of analytes were 22.898 min and 32.679 min).

Procedure of multiple points regression

After assignment of the peaks of analytes in the sample solution by prediction of two points regression, the $t_R$mea of those peaks should be validated by multiple points regression. In this procedure, $t_R$mea and St_R of reference compounds and analytes were used to fit a multiple points linear regression: $Y = 1.1038x - 1.1075$ (Fig. 4d). Taking St_R of analytes (Chonglou saponin VI and Chonglou saponin II) into new equation, the new $t_R$pre of Chonglou saponin VI (23.297 min) and Chonglou saponin II (32.358 min) were calculated. If Δt_R of all analytes were less than the given t_RL (t_RL: t_R limit, in this case

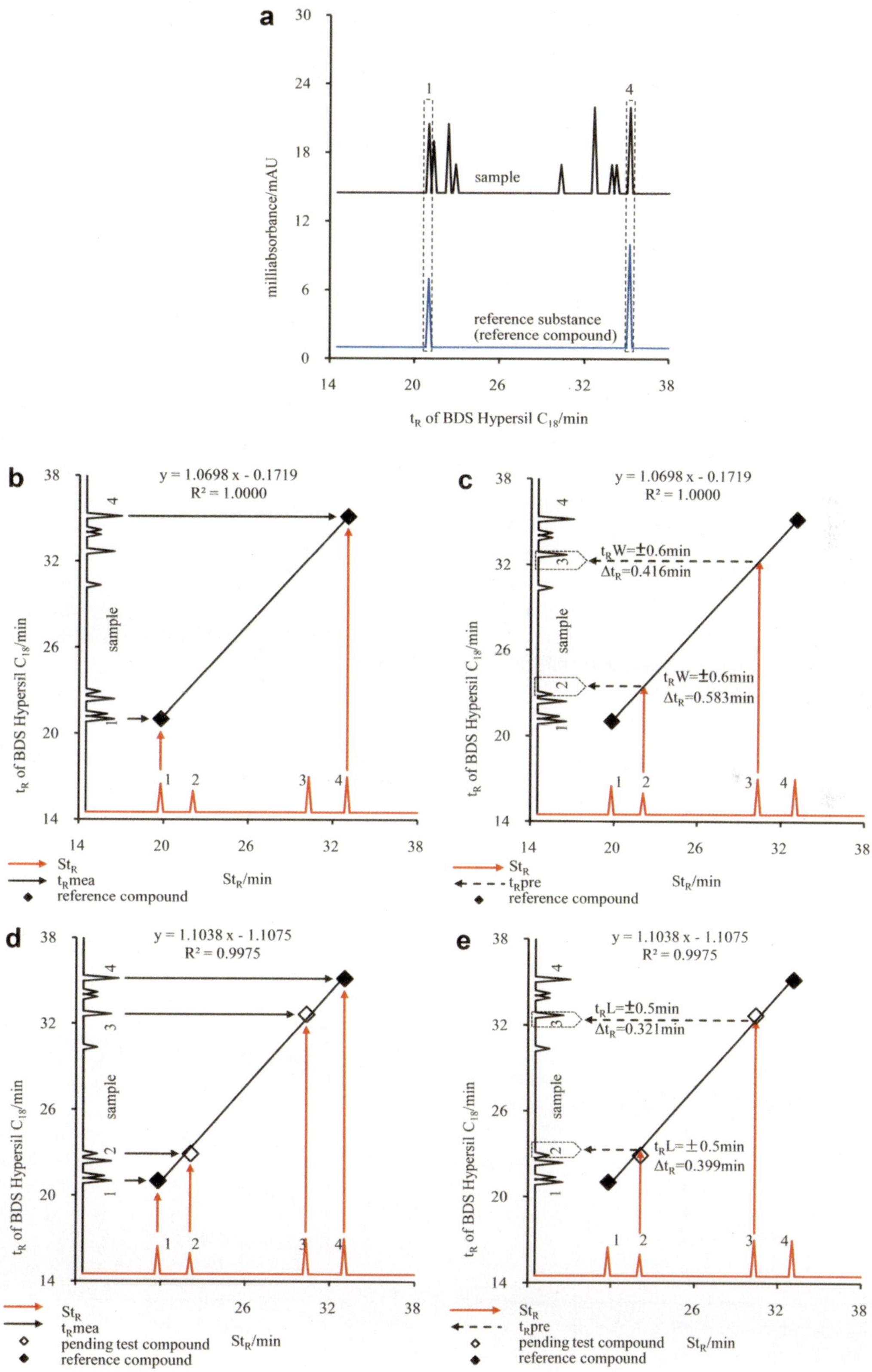

Fig. 4 Flow chart of LCTRS (Paridis, code No. is the same as that in Fig. 1)

is 0.5 min), the prediction was success, otherwise failure (Fig. 4e). In this case, Δt_R were 0.399 and 0.321 min, respectively. The step of validation by multiple points was based on the principle of stepwise linear regression, which can further improve the prediction accuracy.

The purpose of setting that the t_RW is larger than t_RL is to increase the amount of suitable columns and to improve the accuracy of prediction. Generally, the recommended ranges of t_RW and t_RL are 0.8–2.0 and 0.5–1.5 min, respectively. If necessary, the values can be adjusted in accordance with different samples under different chromatographic conditions. If the Δt_R of some compounds are large, their t_RW and t_RL can be set individually.

Sequential matching rule

If the t_R of two peaks are too close, e.g. less than 2 min, there would be a mistake for peak matching by the least Δt_R rule. Take Psoraleae for example, as shown in Fig. 5a, peak #6 was assigned to peak A in the sample solution on col6 (Kromasil C_{18}) with a small Δt_R of 0.515 min. However, peak #5 was not found and peak B in the sample solution was not matched. When t_RW was set as 1.2 min, $t_R$mea of peak A was within the window of $t_R$pre of peak #5. $t_R$mea of the peaks A and B would both fall into the window of $t_R$pre of peak #6. Because of the existence of one common peak (peak A), peaks #5 and 6 should be treated as peak series for sequential matching. That is, the earlier $t_R$pre will be matched to the peak with the earlier $t_R$mea. Although Δt_R of peak #6 increased to 1.036 min, the match results were correct, as shown in Fig. 5b. This rule can be further applied to multiple-peak series, which has a close t_R.

Comparison between LCTRS method and RR method

The comparison among unadjusted RR method, adjusted RR method (dead time was measured by ammonium nitrate as probe compound), prediction by two points, and validation by multiple points was summarized in Tables 4 and 5. The results showed that the unadjusted RR method and adjusted RR method were similar, their prediction accuracy were bigger and suitable for less positive columns. But the prediction deviation was reduced and the number of positive columns was increased by LCTRS method. The best was validation by multiple points which was based on the prediction by two points.

Exclusion of column and compound by linear fitting

Nonlinear shift of t_R for a compound on different columns could be caused either by different column packing materials and use of other packing techniques, or by the different compound structure. In order to exclude the columns and compounds with relatively large nonlinear shift, linear fitting of $t_R$mea and St_R were performed. The

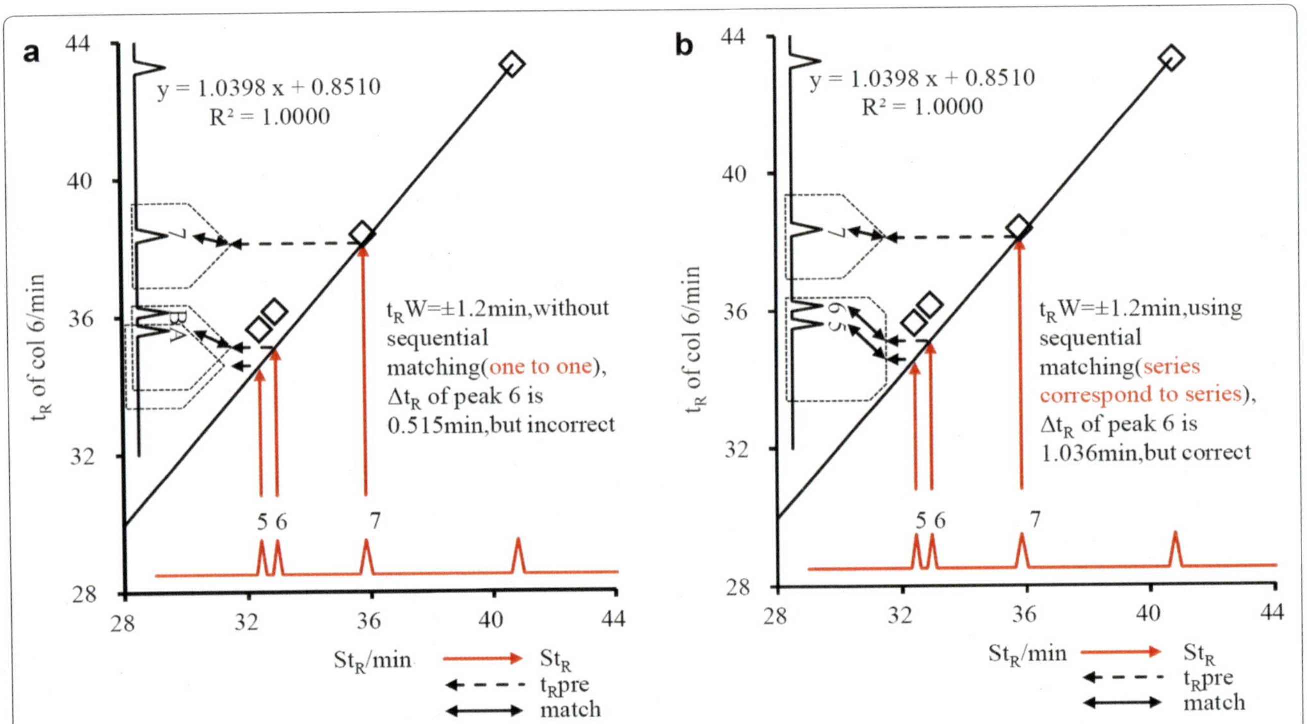

Fig. 5 Advantage of sequential matching (Psoraleae, code No. is the same as that in Fig. 1)

following rules were used to identify the outlier column and compound. (1) In a regression scatter plot, the compounds obviously deviated from a regression line (the correlation coefficient is usually less than 0.99). (2) Δt_R was usually larger than 1–2 min. The excluded columns and compounds would not be used for St_R calculating.

For Psoraleae: no obvious nonlinear deviation was observed of all 11 compounds. 23 columns met the requirements (the average of correlation coefficient was 0.9989). The outlier columns were col2, 8, 12 (Fig. 6a), 16, 19, 20 and 30. For Paridis: no obvious nonlinear deviation was observed of four saponins. All 30 columns met the requirement with average correlation coefficient of 0.9993.

In order to simulate t_R of compound with large structural difference, reference substances solution of

Table 4 Comparison result by four methods (Psoraleae)

Method	Maximum of Δt_R/min	Average of Δt_R/min	Number of positive columns[a]
Unadjusted RR	3.494	0.804	2
Adjusted RR	3.001	0.886	3
Prediction by two points	2.194	0.599	5
Validation by multiple points	1.689	0.465	9

[a] The columns which meet the following requirements are called positive column, (1) the resolution of peaks meets the requirements; (2) Δt_R of all pending test compounds are no more than t_RL (for Psoraleae is 1.2 min)

Table 5 Comparison of prediction result in four methods (Paridis)

Method	Maximum of Δt_R/min	Average of Δt_R/min	Number of positive columns[a]
Unadjusted RR	1.811	0.420	12
Adjusted RR	1.562	0.410	9
Prediction by two points	0.836	0.283	25
Validation by multiple points	0.545	0.204	30

[a] $t_RL = 0.5$ min

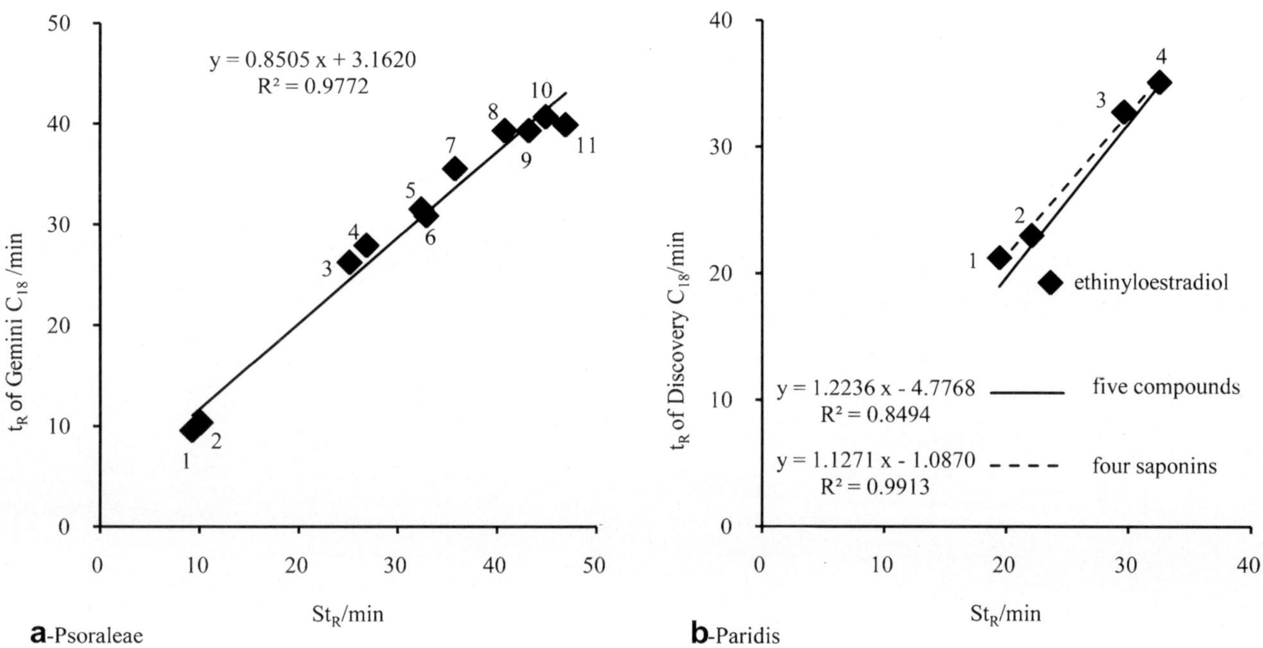

Fig. 6 Outlier column (**a**) and Outlier compounds (**b**), code No. is the same as that in Fig. 1

ethinylestradiol mixing with four Chonglou saponins were used to measure t_R of those five compounds on 30 columns. Nonlinear shift of ethinylestradiol was observed on col1 (Fig. 6b), 2–6, 8, 11, 15–18, 26–28 and 30. It appears that the HPLC retention behaviors of ethinylestradiol and four Chonglou saponins were significantly different on this chromatographic condition. It further indicated that the classification and similarity evaluation of columns should be based on the characteristics of columns as well as analytes.

If the outlier compounds cannot be excluded. The following approaches could be used: (1) specify one or more suitable columns; (2) provide reference substances for those compounds; (3) use UV–Vis spectrum and/or mass spectrum for assistant peak identification.

Selection of two reference compounds

Ideally there should be no difference in selecting any of the two compounds as reference compounds. However, because of the difference of HPLC instruments, columns, compounds structure, complexity of elution condition, and accidental error of analysis, different selection of reference compound pairs will make differences. In order to find out the rule for reference compounds selection, each combination of possible reference compound pairs for the two medicines was studied. The average of Δt_R corresponding to each reference compound pair were calculated and shown in Fig. 7. It can be seen that, for the two medicines, the Δt_R of prediction by two points step would be decreased with increasing coverage of t_R [as shown in formula (5). The coverage of t_R is a reflex of the relative position of the two reference compounds. The first compound is at one end (with smaller t_R), the last compound is at the other end (with bigger t_R). If the coverage is high, the two reference compounds are near both ends, otherwise they are in the middle or near the same end]. The coverage corresponding to the smallest Δt_R was 80–100%.The results of Psoraleae (Fig. 7a) showed the advantage of choosing reference compounds with smaller linear deviation, when the coverages of t_R were similar. Therefore, the optimized reference compounds for Psoraleae were peak #2 and peak #8, rather than peak #1 and peak #11 which had a maximum coverage of t_R but with more deviation from linearity. The selection rule decreases the randomness of choosing reference compounds and the amount of calculation (or the Δt_R of all possible reference compound pairs will be calculated every time). The accurate and simple selection procedures were as follows. Firstly, Select two reference compound pairs with large t_R coverage (80–100%). Secondly, exclude compounds with large linear deviation based on the linear fitting results. Thirdly, calculate the Δt_R of the rest reference compound pairs and select reference compound pairs with the smallest Δt_R.

$$\textit{Coverage of } t_R = \frac{t_{R2} - t_{R1}}{t_{Rlast} - t_{Rfirst}} \quad (5)$$

t_{R2} is t_R (or St_R) of second reference compound; t_{R1} is t_R (or St_R) of first reference compound; t_{Rlast} is t_R (or St_R) of last compound; t_{Rfirst} is t_R (or St_R) of first compound.

In summary, the establishment procedures of LCTRS were as follows. Firstly, select five–fifteen different brands of C_{18} columns, and record the HPLC chromatograms of reference substances and sample on all columns. Secondly, calculate initial St_R by using all columns, and perform linear fitting of t_R on each column with St_R. Exclude outlier columns and compounds, and recalculate final St_R using remaining columns. Finally, select two reference compounds with large t_R coverage and low linear deviation.

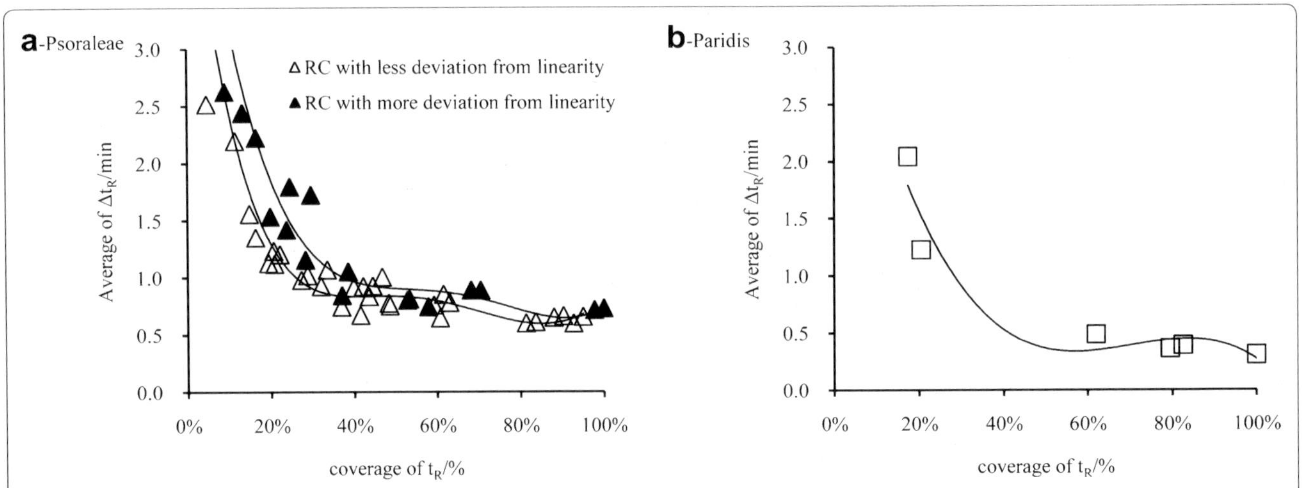

Fig. 7 Selection of two reference compound (abbreviated as RC)

Discussion

Advantages of LCTRS method

According to the study of Wang et al. [22], t_R of the compounds on different HPLC system follows the linearity principle. The RR method can be regarded as external standard one point method, which means the regression line is forced to pass origin. However, most of the linear equations have intercepts, which is why the deviation of unadjusted RR method was large. For considering the dead time, adjusted RR method should be better than unadjusted RR method in theory. But the probe compound for dead time measurement would be interacted with mobile phases and stationary phases of the columns. The interaction would increase the error in dead time measurement. So the prediction accuracy of this method was not improved in practice. For prediction by two points and validation by multiple points, dead time, gradient delay, volume exclusion effect of stationary phase, retention behavior of homologous compounds and so forth, were fully considered. Thus, the prediction accuracy was significantly improved. Stepwise linear regression was used in the validation by multiple points step, which further improved the prediction effect.

Compatibility of LCTRS method and RR method

Both LCTRS method and RR method are equivalent in mathematics. Formulas can be expressed in the same form. In the LCTRS, calibrated retention (CR) is defined as the ratio of St_R of analytes to reference compounds, as shown in formula (6). Different from RR, CR is based on statistics of St_R. Thus, its prediction accuracy was equal to LCTRS (only equal to prediction by two points).

$$CR = RR = \frac{t_{Ri} - t_{R1}}{t_{R2} - t_{R1}} \tag{6}$$

where t_{Ri} is St_R of analytes in CR, or t_R of analytes in RR; t_{R1} is St_R of the first reference compound in CR, or dead time in adjusted RR, or zero in unadjusted RR; t_{R2} is St_R of the second reference compound in CR, or t_R of reference compound in RR.

Conclusion

A new method for t_R prediction of HPLC chromatographic peaks was proposed. 16 compounds in two medicines under isocratic or gradient elution conditions were tested through three brands of HPLC instruments with 30 different brands of C_{18} columns. It is demonstrated that the method is simple, accurate, and robust for more HPLC columns. Furthermore, the calculation approach of St_R and the selection rule of the two reference compounds were discussed.

Both multi-components analysis in TCMs and determination of related substances in pharmaceutical chemicals need lots of reference substances for peak identification. But it may be not affordable for routine analysis and research using all reference substances. LCTRS is a simple and low-cost alternative method for peak identification. Compared with RR method, it need one more reference substance but is more accurate and suitable for more HPLC columns. LCTRS method provides a good prospective application for overall quality evaluation of TCMs and impurities analysis in pharmaceutical chemicals.

Abbreviations

TCMs: traditional Chinese medicines; RR: relative retention; LCTRS: linear calibration using two reference substances; t_R: retention time; SSDMC: single standard to determine multi-components; St_R: arithmetic average of t_R; Δt_R: deviation of t_R; $t_R$pre: predicted retention time; $t_R$mea: measured retention time; CR: calibrated retention.

Authors' contributions

LS and SCM conceived the study. LS and HYJ designed the study. LS and LPY conducted the experiments. LS, RTT, MJW, LNL and TTZ analyzed the data. LS wrote the manuscript. RTT and SCM revised the manuscript. All authors read and approved the final manuscript.

Author details

[1] National Institutes for Food and Drug Control, No. 2 Tiantan Xili, Dongcheng District, Beijing 100050, People's Republic of China. [2] Xinjiang Institute for Food and Drug Control, Urumqi 830004, China. [3] Chemmind Technologies Co., Ltd., Beijing 100085, China. [4] Huainan Food and Drug Inspection Center, Huainan 232007, China.

Acknowledgements

We would like to thank Ms. Yu Pang from Center for Drug Reevaluation and Mr. Chao Zhang from Suzhou Institute for Drug Control for the useful suggestions on this paper.

Competing interests

The authors declare that they have no competing interests.

Funding

This project was financially supported by Youth Development Research Foundation of NIFDC (2013WA8), National Natural Foundation of China (81303214) and National Major Scientific and Technological Special Project for "Significant New Drugs Development" (2014ZX09304307-002).

References

1. Gao XY, Jiang Y, Lu JQ, Tu PF. One single standard substance for the determination of multiple anthraquinone derivatives in rhubarb using high-performance liquid chromatography-diode array detection. J Chromatogr A. 2009;1216(11):2118–23.
2. Hou JJ, Wu WY, Da J, Yao S, Long HL, Yang Z, Cai LY, Yang M, Liu X, Jiang BH, Guo DA. Ruggedness and robustness of conversion factors in method of simultaneous determination of multi-components with single reference standard. J Chromatogr A. 2011;1218(33):5618–27.
3. Hou JJ, Wu WY, Liang J, Yang Z, Long HL, Cai LY, Fang L, Wang DD, Yao S, Liu X, Jiang BH, Guo DA. A single, multi-faceted, enhanced strategy to quantify the chromatographically diverse constituents in the roots of *Euphorbia kansui*. J Pharm Biomed Anal. 2014;88(88C):321–30.
4. Wu X, He J, Xu H, Bi K, Li Q. Quality assessment of Cinnamomi Ramulus by the simultaneous analysis of multiple active components using high-performance thin-layer chromatography and high-performance liquid chromatography. J Sep Sci. 2014;37(18):2490–8.

5. Liao H, Li Q, Liu R, Liu J, Bi K. Fingerprint analysis and multi-ingredient determination using a single reference standard for Saposhnikoviae Radix. Anal Sci. 2014;30(12):1157–63.
6. Zhong JS, Wan JZ, Liu YP, Ding WJ, Wu XF, Xie ZY. Simultaneous HPLC quantification of seven chromones in *Aloe barbadensis* Miller using a single reference standard. Anal Methods. 2014;6(12):4388–95.
7. Du YY, Li Q, Liu JJ, Yin YD, Bi KS. Combinative method using multi-components quantitation by single reference standard and HPLC fingerprint for comprehensive evaluation of *Rhodiola crenulatav* H. Ohba. Anal Methods. 2014;6(15):5891–8.
8. Da J, Cheng CR, Yao S, Long HL, Wang YH, Khan LA, Li YF, Wang QR, Cai LY, Jiang BH, Liu X, Wu WY, Guo DA. A reproducible analytical system based on the multi-component analysis of triterpene acids in *Ganoderma lucidum*. Phytochemistry. 2015;114:146–54.
9. Lu WY, Liu YG, Yang HS, Sheng Y, Shi HM, Yu LL. Simultaneous HPLC quantification of five major triterpene alcohol and sterol ferulates in rice bran oil using a single reference standard. Food Chem. 2014;148(4):329–34.
10. Zhang YW, Li Q, Lv CX, Liu XJ, Chen XH, Bi KS. Simultaneous determination of four active components in *Alisma orientale* (Sam.) Juz. by HPLC–DAD using a single reference standard. J Pharmaceut Anal. 2015;5(2):85–92.
11. Gilroy JJ, Dolan JW, Snyder LR. Column selectivity in reversed-phase liquid chromatography: IV type-B alkyl-silica columns. J Chromatogr A. 2003;1000:757–78.
12. Gilroy JJ, Dolan JW, Carr PW, Snyder LR. Column selectivity in reversed-phase liquid chromatography: V. Higher metal content (type-A) alkyl-silica columns. J Chromatogr A. 1026;2004(1026):77–89.
13. Wilson NS, Gilroy J, Dolan JW, Snyder LR. Column selectivity in reversed-phase liquid chromatography: VI. Columns with embedded or end-capping polar groups. J Chromatogr A. 2004;1026(1–2):91–100.
14. Visky D, Vander Heyden Y, Iványi T, Baten P, De Beer J, Kovács Z, Noszál B, Dehouck P, Roets E, Massart DL, Hoogmartens J. Characterisation of reversed-phase liquid chromatographic columns by chromatographic tests: rational column classification by a minimal number of column test parameters. J Chromatogr A. 2003;1012(1):11–29.
15. Dehouck P, Visky D, Vander Heyden Y, Adams E, Kovács Z, Noszál B, Massart DL, Hoogmartens J. Characterisation of reversed-phase liquid-chromatographic columns by chromatographic tests: comparing column classification based on chromatographic parameters and column performance for the separation of acetylsalicylic acid and related compounds. J Chromatogr A. 2004;1025(2):189–200.
16. Bidlingmeyer B, Chan CC, Fastino P, Henry R, Koerner P, Maule AT, Marques MRC, Neue U, Ng L, Pappa H, Sander L, Santasania C, Snyder L, Wozniak T. HPLC column classification. Pharm Forum. 2005;31(2):637–45.
17. Dolan JW, Maule A, Bingley D, Wrisley L, Chan CC, Angod M, Lunte C, Krisko R, Winston JM, Homeier BA, McCalley DV, Snyder LR. Choosing an equivalent replacement column for a reversed-phase liquid chromatographic assay procedure. J Chromatogr A. 2004;1057(1–2):59–74.
18. Snyder LR, Dolan JW, Carr PW. The hydrophobic-subtraction model of reversed-phase column selectivity. J Chromatogr A. 2004;1060(1–2):77–116.
19. Visky D, Haghedooren E, Dehouck P, Kovács Z, Kóczián K, Noszál B, Hoogmartens J, Adams E. Facilitated column selection in pharmaceutical analyses using a simple column classification system. J Chromatogr A. 2006;1101(1–2):103–14.
20. Kóczián K, Haghedooren E, Dragovic S, Noszál B, Hoogmartens J, Adams E. Column selection for pharmaceutical analyses based on a column classification using four test parameters. J Pharm Biomed Anal. 2007;44(4):894–905.
21. Dragovic S, Haghedooren E, Németh T, Palabiyik IM, Hoogmartens J, Adams E. Evaluation of two approaches to characterise liquid chromatographic columns using pharmaceutical separations. J Chromatogr A. 2009;1216(15):3210–6.
22. Wang LX, Xiao HB, Liang XM. A new method to improve the reproducibility of retention time on reversed phase C_{18} columns in different laboratories. Chin J Anal Chem. 2003;31(10):1232–6.
23. Sun L, Jin HY, Pang Y, Ma SC. Two reference substances for determination of multiple components (1): linear calibration using two reference substances for identification of chromatographic peaks. Chin J Pharm Anal. 2013;33(8):1424–30.
24. Sun L, Pang Y, Jin HY, Liu LN, Ma SC. Two reference substances for determination of multiple components II influence of detection wavelength selection on quantitative analysis. Chin J Pharm Anal. 2013;33(9):1578–86.
25. He B, Yang SY, Zhang Y. A new method of calibration and positioning in quantitative analysis of multi components by single marker[J]. Acta Pharm Sin. 2012;12:1653–9.
26. Department of Health Hong Kong Special Administrative Region The People's Republic of China. Hong Kong Chinese Materia Medica Standards, vol. 3, Government Logistics Department. Beijing; 2012. p. 101.
27. National Commission of Chinese Pharmacopoeia. Pharmacopoeia of People's Republic of China, vol. I, China Medical Science Press. Beijing; 2015. p. 260.

7

Bioaccessibility and risk assessment of heavy metals, and analysis of arsenic speciation in *Cordyceps sinensis*

Li Zhou[1,2], Sheng Wang[1], Qingxiu Hao[1], Liping Kang[1], Chuanzhi Kang[1], Jian Yang[1], Wanzhen Yang[1], Jingyi Jiang[1], Lu-Qi Huang[1*] and Lanping Guo[1,2*]

Abstract

Background: *Cordyceps sinensis* (*C. sinensis*) is a famous and precious Traditional Chinese Medicine (TCM), while frequent reports of heavy metals, especially arsenic, exceeding standards in *C. sinensis* in recent years have raised concerns of its safety. Therefore, it is urgent for a research on heavy metals (Cu, Pb, As, Cd, Hg) in *C. sinensis*, of its bioaccessibility, dietary exposure estimation, arsenic speciation analysis and health risks assessment to human body.

Methods: Three 30 g batches of mixed wild growth *C. sinensis* samples were collected from Qinghai Province and each batch were divided into three parts: the whole *C. sinensis*, the stroma and the caterpillar body. The in vitro gastrointestinal method was used to evaluate the bioaccessibility of the heavy metals in the samples. The arsenic speciation analysis in the in vitro gastrointestinal solutions and dilute nitric acid extracted solutions were conducted using high performance liquid chromatography–inductively coupled plasma mass (HPLC–ICP-MS) method. Finally, the target hazard quotient (THQ) developed by the US EPA (1989) was used to assess the health risks of heavy metals in *C. sinensis*.

Results: The contents of Cu, Pb, Cd and Hg in the stroma were higher than those in the caterpillar body. In contrast, As was mainly found in the caterpillar body. In the whole *C. sinensis*, the average bio-accessibilities of Cu, Pb, As, Hg and Cd were 41.29, 40.11, 64.46, 18.91, and 81.14%, respectively. While in the caterpillar body, the corresponding bio-accessibilities values were 48.26, 42.92, 66.15, 12.86, 87.07%, respectively, and were 38.30, 30.53, 30.18, 7.46, and 82.30%, respectively in the stroma part. Different arsenic speciations of arsenite [As(III)], arsenate [As(V)] and trace amounts of methylarsonic acid [MMA] were detected. Of the total As, 8.69% was in inorganic form, which was also the major form of dissolved As. Among the extracted inorganic species, the concentrations of As(III) and As(V) were 0.56 ± 0.16 and 0.29 ± 0.06 mg kg^{-1}, respectively. In the gastrointestinal solutions, only As(III) and As(V) could be detected; the sum content of the two species was 2.00–2.73%. The bioaccessibility target hazard quotient (BTHQ) values for Cu, Pb, As, Cd and Hg in *C. sinensis* were 0.0041, 0.0040, 0.5334, 0.0020 and 0.0005, respectively, all less than 1.

*Correspondence: huangluqi01@126.com; glp01@126.com
[1] National Resource Center for Chinese Materia Medica, State Key Laboratory Breeding Base of Dao-di Herbs, China Academy of Chinese Medical Sciences, Beijing 100700, People's Republic of China
Full list of author information is available at the end of the article

Conclusion: None of the five heavy metals in *C. sinensis* can be 100% absorbed by human body. The content of arsenic in *C. sinensis* is high, but the strong toxic inorganic arsenic accounted for only 8.69%. The heavy metals in *C. sinensis* presented no obvious risks to human health in a reasonable taking way.

Keywords: *Cordyceps sinensis*, Heavy metals, As, Gastrointestinal digestion, Risk assessment

Background

With the rapid development of modern industry, a large number of heavy metals are discharged into the environment along with waste water, waste residue and waste gas from industrial and agricultural activities, resulting in environmental heavy metal contamination [1]. Heavy metals in the natural environment could enter human body via a variety of ways and can accumulate in the body [2–4], affecting normal organism physiological functions and causing inflammation and a variety of diseases, including cancer [5].

Cordyceps sinensis (BerK). Sacc is a parasitic fungus that grows on the larva of Lepidoptera. It is a Traditional Chinese Medicine known as DongChong-XiaCao (winter worm-summer grass) [6, 7]. It can effectively regulate the immune system and protect the nervous system, with anti-tumour properties [7, 8]. In recent years, the price of *C. sinensis* has risen dramatically [9], due to its efficacy and the scarcity of resources, and at present, the price of *C. sinensis* in different specifications ranges from $30,000 to $100,000 per kilogram. At the same time, concerns about the heavy metal As in *C. sinensis* have also grown with reports of high As content in *C. sinensis.* Our previous study found that contents of arsenic in 20 batches of *C. sinensis* were 2.59–12.56 mg kg^{-1} [10]. The excess rate of As was 88.24% based on the international standards of Chinese Medicine-Chinese Herbal Medicine Heavy Metal Limit (4 mg kg^{-1} for As) [11].

Chemical speciations of arsenic in nature include arsenate [As(V)], arsenite [As(III)], methylarsonic acid (MMA), dimethylarsinic acid (DMA), arsenobetaine (AsB), and arsenocholine (AsC), etc. [12]. Studies have shown that inorganic arsenic species are the most dangerous species of arsenic, and As(III) is more toxic than As(V), with the toxicity of As(III) almost 60 times that of As(V). MMA and DMA are considered to be hypotoxic; however, arsenosugars and arsenic greases are believed to be non-toxic [13, 14]. As(III) has a strong affinity with enzymes and the SH and NH groups of proteins in the body, and it can combine with thiols to form stable complexes that can hinder the cell's normal metabolism and inhibit some enzymes [15, 16].

At present, the heavy metal problem of *C. sinensis* has received extensive attention. Previous researches on the heavy metal of *C. sinensis* mainly focused on its determination method and content, while researches on the species of As contained and the bioaccessibilities and health risk of heavy metals of *C. sinensis* considering its usage were rarely reported. In this study, we focused on the dietary exposure and bioaccessibilities of As, Cu, Pb, Cd and Hg and the variety of As species present in *C. sinensis* [17, 18], aiming to assess the risks of heavy metals and supplement the research on the safety of *C. sinensis*.

Methods

The Minimum Standards of Reporting Checklist contain details of the experimental design, and statistics, and resources used in this study (Additional file 1).

Instrumentation

An ICP-MS (ICAP-Q, Thermo Fisher Scientific, Analytical System, United States, Massachusetts) operating under normal multi-element tuning conditions was used to determine the total levels of As, Cu, Pb, Cd and Hg. The main analytical parameters were as follows: RF forward power, 1550 W; plasma argon flow rate, 13.98 L min^{-1}; auxiliary argon flow rate, 0.80 L min^{-1}; nebulizer argon flow rate, 1.10 L min^{-1}; integration time, 0.02 s per point; and points per peak, 3.

An ICP-MS was used as the detector system following species separation by HPLC for arsenic speciation analysis, and the column effluent was directly introduced into a nebulizer and spray chamber. Data were collected by single ion monitoring at m/z 75. For chromatographic separation, a high-pressure pump (Ultimate 3000 RSLCnano, Thermo Fisher Scientific, United States, Massachusetts) was used as the sample delivery system. A Dionex IonPacTM AS7 column (2 × 250 mm Thermo Fisher Scientific, United States, Massachusetts) was used for arsenic speciation analysis. The mobile phases were 0.1 mol L^{-1} ammonium carbonate (A) and 4 nmol L^{-1} ammonium carbonate (B). The elution gradient system was 0% B (0–2.5 min), 0–100% B (2.5–8 min), 100% B (8–10 min), 100–0% B (10–10.01 min), 0% B (10.01–20 min). The flow rate was 0.25 mL min^{-1}. The injection volume was 20 μL.

Calibration standards and reagents

The single-element standard solutions (1000 mg L^{-1}) of Cu, Pb, As, Cd, and Hg, purchased from the National Standard Material Center (Beijing, China), were used as the standard calibration solutions. Standard solutions of As As(III), As(V), MMA, AsC and AsB, purchased from the National Standard Material Center (Beijing, China) were used as the standard source solutions, with their concentrations guaranteed. DMA certified reference material was prepared from commercially available reagents, with its purity evaluated before use. Working mixture standard solutions were prepared daily by diluting the source standard solutions to proper concentrations with pure water. Deionized water (18.2 MΩ) purified with a Milli-Q system (Millipore, Inc, Spain) was used for all solution preparation. Plasticware and glassware were maintained in 15% HNO_3 for 24 h before use.

Simulated gastrointestinal juices

Simulated gastric juice (pH 1.8 ± 0.1) was prepared by dissolving 10.0 g of pepsin in 800 mL deionized water, then 16.4 mL of dilute hydrochloric acid (prepared by diluting 234 mL of concentrated hydrochloric acid to 1000 mL with deionized water) was added, and finally, additional deionized water was added to bring the total volume up to 1000 mL.

Simulated intestinal juice was prepared just before use by mixing equal volumes of A and B solutions. (Solution A was 6.8 g of potassium dihydrogen phosphate dissolved in 500 mL of water, and 0.1 mol L^{-1} NaOH was used to adjust the pH to 6.8. Solution B was 10 g of pancreatin dissolved in water up to 500 mL) [19].

***Cordyceps sinensis* samples**

Three 30 g batches of *C. sinensis* samples were collected from Qinghai Province and were numbered 1, 2, and 3. All samples were dried at 40 °C and stored at 4 °C before analysis [20].

Sample preparation for contents determination of Cu, Pb, As, Cd, and Hg by ICP-MS

Each batch of *C. sinensis* samples were equally divided into two parts. One part, the whole *C. sinensis* (W), was ground with a mortar and passed through a 50-mesh sieve and numbered W_1, W_2, and W_3, respectively. The other part was separated into stroma (S) and caterpillar body (C), and those two portions were separately ground with a mortar and passed through a 50-mesh sieve and numbered S_1, S_2, S_3 and C_1, C_2, C_3, respectively.

The whole *C. sinensis* samples, stroma samples and caterpillar body samples were digested with a microwave digestion system. Approximately 0.2 g of each sample was precisely weighed and transferred in PTEF vessels with 5 mL of concentrated HNO_3 and 1 mL of H_2O_2. The operating procedure of the microwave system was as follows: the samples were heated at 100 °C for 3 min in the 1st step, 160 °C for 8 min in the 2nd step, and 190 °C for 30 min in the 3rd step, and then cooled to room temperature. The sample solutions were diluted to 50 mL with pure water. The blank and reference materials (carrots) were prepared at the same time under the same procedure.

Method validation

The method was fully validated by characteristic indices including linearity, limit of detection (LOD), limit of quantitation (LOQ), accuracy, and stability.

Extraction procedures for arsenic speciation analysis in the whole *C. sinensis*, stroma and caterpillar body by HPLC–ICP-MS

Dilute nitric acid solution extraction

5 mL of dilute nitric acid solution (HNO_3: water = 2: 98) was added to precisely weighed 0.2 g samples of whole *C. sinensis*, stroma and caterpillar body, respectively. The mixtures were soaked overnight, then heated in a thermostatic water bath for 120 min at 90 °C and shaken for 1 min every 30 min. The mixture was cooled to room temperature and centrifuged at 11.5*g* for 10 min after extraction. The supernatants were removed, and 5 mL of dilute nitric acid solution was added to the remaining pellets. The extraction was repeated using procedure described above. The combined supernatants from the two rounds of extraction were analysed immediately after filtration. The procedure was performed in triplicate [21].

In vitro gastrointestinal digestion of whole *C. sinensis*, stroma and caterpillar body for arsenic speciation analysis

Gastric digestion

The prepared gastric juice (5 mL) was added to 0.5 g of precisely weighted whole *C. sinensis*, stroma and caterpillar body samples, respectively. Then the samples were heated for 1 h in a water bath, shaken for 30 min in a shaker (250 r min^{-1}), and heated for an additional 3 h at 38 °C. The mixture was centrifuged at 11.5*g* for 10 min, and the collected supernatant was used as gastric digestion extract solution.

Intestinal digestion

The prepared intestinal juice (5 mL) was added to the solid fraction obtained in the gastric digestion, following the digestion procedure as above. The residue was discarded.

The supernatant was passed through a 0.45 μm PVDF syringe-type filter before analysis. The procedure was performed in triplicate [22].

Preparation of in vitro gastrointestinal solution samples for determination of Cu, Pb, As, Cd and Hg content by ICP-MS

After digestion, the two liquid extracts were mineralized in a microwave oven. The samples were appropriately diluted before analysis.

Health risk assessment of heavy metals

To evaluate the potential acute or long-term hazards from exposure to heavy metals in *C. sinensis*, the DI, DE, and THQ of heavy metals were calculated using the following formulas [23].

$$DI = C \times FIR$$

where DI is the dietary intake of the heavy metal (μg person^{-1} day^{-1}), C is the measured concentration of the heavy metal in the samples and FIR is the daily dose (g), which was taken as the maximum daily dose (9 g) recommended by the "Chinese Pharmacopoeia" standard.

$$DE = DI / WAB$$

where DE is the dietary exposure (μg kg^{-1} body weight day^{-1}) and WAB is the average individual body weight (62 kg).

For noncancerous effects, the target hazard quotient (THQ) developed by the US EPA (1989) has been used to evaluate potential health risks associated with long-term exposure to chemical pollutants in foodstuffs and was therefore used to assess the health risks from heavy metals in *C. sinensis* over a lifetime in this study. A THQ value higher than 1 indicates that those ingested *C. sinensis* are affecting health adversely to some extent. And if the THQ value is less than 1, it suggests that the amount of heavy metal exposed to the body has no significant effect on human health.

$$THQ = \frac{C \times FE \times ED \times FIR}{WAB \times AT \times RFD \times 1000}$$

$$BTHQ = THQ \times \text{Bio} - \text{accessibility}_{HM}$$

where C is the measured concentration of heavy metal in *C. sinensis*; EF is the exposure frequency (90 day per year); ED is the exposure duration (50 years); FIR is the daily dose (9 g); AT is the averaging time for non-carcinogens (70 × 365 day); RFD is the oral reference dose provided by the US EPA (Cu = 0.04 μg g^{-1} day^{-1} body weight, Pb = 0.0035 μg g^{-1} day^{-1} body weight, As = 0.0003 μg g^{-1} day^{-1} body weight, Cd = 0.001 μg g^{-1} day^{-1} body weight, Hg = 0.0005 μg g^{-1} day^{-1} body weight); 10^{-3} is the unit conversion factor; WAB is the average individual body weight (62 kg).

It has been observed that using the total concentrations of heavy metals may overestimate the amount absorbed through oral ingestion; the oral bioaccessibility is defined as the fraction of a compound that is released from its matrix in the gastrointestinal tract, and thus becomes available for intestinal absorption, i.e., enters the blood stream [24]. The bioaccessibility value is used to avoid overestimating risk.

Results

Method validation for quantitative analysis of Cu, Pb, As, Cd and Hg

Performance parameters of the analytical method were evaluated, and the detection limits (DL) for the elements (expressed in μg L^{-1}) were as follows: Cu: 0.007; Pb: 0.026; As: 0.010; Cd: 0.005; and Hg: 0.006. The quantification limits (QL) for the elements (expressed in μg L^{-1}) were Cu: 0.020; Pb: 0.100; As: 0.030; Cd: 0.020; and Hg: 0.020. The standard curve prepared for each element was linear. The relative standard deviations (RSDs) were less than 3% (Table 1). The results of the reference material were in good consistence with the certified values (Table 2).

The bioaccessibility of heavy metals in different parts of *C. sinensis*

The average bioaccessibilities of Cu, Pb, As, Hg and Cd were 41.29, 40.11, 64.46, 18.91, and 81.14% in whole *C. sinensis*, respectively; 48.26, 42.92, 66.15, 12.86, and 87.07% in caterpillar body; and 38.30, 30.53, 30.18, 7.46, and 82.30% in stroma (Table 3). The bioaccessibilities of Cu, As, Hg and Cd in each part in the gastric extract were higher than those in the intestinal extract, and the vast majority of Cu and Cd were dissolved by the gastric juice. While the bioaccessibility of Pb in gastric juice was lower than that in intestinal juice. The dissolved quantity of each heavy metal is proportional to its total content of the sample. However, the bioaccessibilities of different heavy metals sometimes varies based on their binding forms and properties. The average contents of Cu, Pb, As, Hg and Cd were 15.02, 1.39, 13.47, 0.06, and 0.08 mg kg^{-1} in caterpillar body and 18.63, 2.06, 1.49, 0.07, and 0.22 mg kg^{-1} in stroma, respectively. The contents of Cu, Pb, Hg, and Cd content in the stroma were greater than those in the caterpillar body. The As content was substantially higher in the caterpillar body than it was in the stroma.

Arsenic speciation analysis in whole *C. sinensis*, stroma and caterpillar body

In some parts of the samples, only As(III), As(V) and MMA were found, and MMA was only present in trace

Table 1 Regression equations, correlation coefficients, linear ranges and detection limits

Analyte	Linear equation	R^2	Linear range (μg L^{-1})	LOD (μg L^{-1})	LOQ (μg L^{-1})
Cu	Y = 38371.1x + 1119.4	0.9999	0.02–200	0.007	0.020
Pb	Y = 230129.3x + 32337.6	0.9996	0.10–20	0.026	0.100
As	Y = 2504.2x + 32.7	0.9999	0.02–20	0.010	0.030
Cd	Y = 30243.4x + 300.6	0.9998	0.02–20	0.005	0.020
Hg	Y = 34165.1x + 84.7	0.9973	0.02–5	0.006	0.020

Table 2 The content of heavy metals in standard reference material for carrot

Analyte	Carrot (reference material)	
	Reference value (mg kg^{-1})	Measured value (mg kg^{-1})
Cu	4.1 ± 0.3	3.89
Pb	0.43 ± 0.07	0.39
As	0.11 ± 0.02	0.11
Cd	0.034 ± 0.004	0.036
Hg	0.0032 ± 0.0008	0.0026

amounts (Table 4). The concentration of arsenic in *C. sinensis* was between 9.00 and 10.18 mg kg^{-1}; almost all the dissolved arsenic is inorganic, making up approximately 8.69% of the total arsenic content. Among the extracted inorganic species, the concentrations of As(III) were 0.41–0.73, and the concentrations of As(V) were 0.25–0.35 mg kg^{-1}. The As species that made up approximately 91.31% of the total arsenic were not identified. When the whole *C. sinensis* was divided into stroma and caterpillar body, the concentrations of As(III) were 0.07–0.08 mg kg^{-1} and were 0.39–0.50 mg kg^{-1} of As(V) in stroma, corresponding to a mean value of 34.20% the total arsenic in the stroma. The concentrations of As(III) were 0.48–0.64 and were 0.28–0.32 mg kg^{-1} of As(V) in caterpillar body. The mean value of these two inorganic arsenic forms made up 6.45% of the total arsenic content in the caterpillar body. Studies have shown that in the stroma of the *C. sinensis*, the As(V) content is greater than that of As(III). In contrast, As(III) content is greater than that of As(V) in caterpillar body.

As speciation analysis following in vitro gastrointestinal digestion

In different parts of *C. sinensis*, only As(III) and As(V) were detected in the in vitro digestion solution (Table 5). Inorganic arsenic was mainly dissolved in gastric juice; the average dissolved contents were 0.20 mg kg^{-1} in gastric juice and 0.02 mg kg^{-1} in intestinal juice. The inorganic arsenic in the in vitro digestion solution accounted for 2.33% of the total arsenic content; in which As(III) was accounted for 1.37% of the total and As(V) for 0.96%. The quantities of inorganic arsenic from the caterpillar body and stroma dissolved in the gastric juice and

Table 3 Bioaccessibility of Cu, Pb, As, Cd and Hg in whole *C. sinensis*, stroma and caterpillar body

Part	Index (%)	Cu	Pb	As	Hg	Cd
	Total heavy metal content (mg kg^{-1})	15.21 ± 1.10	1.44 ± 0.46	9.70 ± 0.62	0.06 ± 0.02	0.11 ± 0.02
W	Bioaccessibility (%)	41.29 ± 1.86	40.11 ± 18.18	64.46 ± 6.68	18.91 ± 14.63	81.14 ± 10.66
	Gastric extract (%)	41.00 ± 2.00	11.25 ± 13.10	49.24 ± 3.95	10.09 ± 5.03	76.92 ± 28.31
	Intestinal extract (%)	0.29 ± 0.30	28.87 ± 12.63	15.21 ± 3.02	8.88 ± 9.58	9.53 ± 11.31
	Total heavy metal content (mg kg^{-1})	15.02 ± 0.95	1.39 ± 0.46	13.47 ± 0.84	0.06 ± 0.01	0.08 ± 0.01
C	Bioaccessibility (%)	48.26 ± 3.69	42.92 ± 5.14	66.15 ± 2.19	12.86 ± 3.57	87.07 ± 4.39
	Gastric extract (%)	44.19 ± 1.67	18.24 ± 11.00	52.54 ± 2.10	7.22 ± 1.88	83.94 ± 4.45
	Intestinal extract (%)	4.07 ± 4.06	24.68 ± 8.53	13.61 ± 1.63	5.70 ± 5.40	3.13 ± 0.23
	Total heavy metal content (mg kg^{-1})	18.63 ± 0.57	2.06 ± 0.44	1.49 ± 0.17	0.07 ± 0.01	0.22 ± 0.06
S	Bioaccessibility (%)	38.30 ± 3.80	30.53 ± 10.80	30.18 ± 9.62	7.46 ± 0.10	82.30 ± 0.49
	Gastric extract (%)	35.77 ± 0.90	13.68 ± 6.37	18.70 ± 5.70	3.05 ± 1.95	79.03 ± 0.28
	Intestinal extract (%)	2.53 ± 3.30	16.85 ± 4.49	11.45 ± 4.51	4.56 ± 2.19	3.28 ± 0.24

Results are expressed as mean ± SD, (n = 3)

W whole *C. sinensis*, *C* caterpillar body, *S* stroma

Table 4 The content of arsenic species in the dilute nitric acid solution (HNO_3: H_2O = 2: 98) extract

Sample ID	Total As ($mg\ kg^{-1}$)	Inorganic arsenic ($mg\ kg^{-1}$)[a]			Organic arsenic ($\mu g\ kg^{-1}$)				Unknown ($mg\ kg^{-1}$)
		As(III)	As(V)	Inorganic arsenic extraction efficiency (%)	MMA	DMA	AsC	AsB	
W_1	9.00 ± 0.21	0.41 ± 0.04	0.26 ± 0.01	7.45	N/A	ND	ND	ND	8.33
W_2	9.93 ± 0.09	0.55 ± 0.02	0.35 ± 0.01	9.06	N/A	ND	ND	ND	9.03
W_3	10.18 ± 0.15	0.73 ± 0.02	0.25 ± 0.01	9.56	N/A	ND	ND	ND	9.20
$\overline{W}$	9.70 ± 0.62	0.56 ± 0.16	0.29 ± 0.06	8.69	N/A	ND	ND	ND	8.85
S_1	1.38 ± 0.14	0.08 ± 0.01	0.50 ± 0.01	41.80	N/A	ND	ND	ND	0.80
S_2	1.41 ± 0.06	0.08 ± 0.00	0.39 ± 0.02	32.66	N/A	ND	ND	ND	0.95
S_3	1.68 ± 0.08	0.07 ± 0.01	0.40 ± 0.02	28.14	N/A	ND	ND	ND	1.19
$\overline{S}$	1.49 ± 0.17	0.08 ± 0.01	0.43 ± 0.06	34.20	N/A	ND	ND	ND	0.98
C_1	14.23 ± 0.10	0.59 ± 0.04	0.30 ± 0.01	6.30	N/A	ND	ND	ND	13.34
C_2	13.62 ± 0.48	0.64 ± 0.07	0.28 ± 0.02	6.70	N/A	ND	ND	ND	12.71
C_3	12.57 ± 0.03	0.48 ± 0.02	0.32 ± 0.00	6.35	N/A	ND	ND	ND	11.76
$\overline{C}$	13.47 ± 0.84	0.57 ± 0.08	0.30 ± 0.02	6.45	N/A	ND	ND	ND	12.60

Results are expressed as mean ± SD, (n = 3)

N/A: trace amounts (LOD < N/A < LOQ); ND: not detected

[a] The concentration calculated based on the original samples. $\bar{x}$: the average value

intestinal juice were 0.21 and 0.09 $mg\ kg^{-1}$ and 0.02 and 0.02 $mg\ kg^{-1}$, respectively, in which As(III) and As(V) accounted for 1.15 and 2.18% and 0.54 and 5.48%, respectively. And only parts of total As were dissolved. The results were consistent with the results in Table 4.

Table 5 The content of As species in the in vitro gastrointestinal digestion juice

Sample ID	Inorganic arsenic (mg·kg)[a]		Total As(III) (%)	Total As(V) (%)
	Gastric extract	Intestinal extract		
W_1	0.22 ± 0.01	0.03 ± 0.00	1.55 ± 0.08	1.19 ± 0.04
W_2	0.21 ± 0.01	0.01 ± 0.01	1.28 ± 0.04	0.97 ± 0.05
W_3	0.19 ± 0.00	0.02 ± 0.00	1.29 ± 0.03	0.71 ± 0.01
$\overline{W}$	0.20 ± 0.02	0.02 ± 0.01	1.37 ± 0.15	0.96 ± 0.24
C1	0.30 ± 0.00	0.02 ± 0.00	1.53 ± 0.01	0.69 ± 0.01
C2	0.15 ± 0.05	0.01 ± 0.00	0.78 ± 0.25	0.43 ± 0.10
C3	0.19 ± 0.00	0.02 ± 0.00	1.15 ± 0.09	0.51 ± 0.06
$\overline{C}$	0.21 ± 0.08	0.02 ± 0.00	1.15 ± 0.38	0.54 ± 0.13
S1	0.09 ± 0.00	0.03 ± 0.02	3.04 ± 1.68	5.81 ± 0.04
S2	0.10 ± 0.00	0.02 ± 0.00	2.44 ± 0.19	6.02 ± 0.16
S3	0.09 ± 0.00	0.01 ± 0.01	1.07 ± 0.25	4.62 ± 1.03
$\overline{S}$	0.09 ± 0.01	0.02 ± 0.01	2.18 ± 1.00	5.48 ± 0.76

Results are expressed as mean ± SD, (n = 3)

[a] The concentration calculated based on the original samples

Estimation of health risks of heavy metals in *C. sinensis*

The DEs for Cu, Pb, As, Cd and Hg were 2.21, 0.21, 1.41, 0.02 and 0.01, respectively, which were all far below the corresponding tolerable limits set by the Joint FAO/WHO Expert Committee on Food Additives (JFCFA) (Table 6). The BTHQ values of these heavy metals were 0.0041, 0.0040, 0.5334, 0.0020 and 0.0005, respectively, all less than 1. The total BTHQ of the five heavy metals was 0.5440.

Based on the risk assessment results, As was the greatest contributor to heavy metal-related risks among the five elements, in agreement with previous findings. Other heavy metals in *C. sinensis* had no significant influence on human health.

Discussion

Bioaccessibility for heavy metal in *C. sinensis*

Bioaccessibility is defined as the proportion of a pollutant that can be dissolved in the gastrointestinal environment, indicating the relative amount of the pollutant in the matrix that can be absorbed by the body, and higher bioaccessibilities indicate greater potentials for absorbing pollutants. The heavy metals in Chinese herbal medicines enter the body through gastrointestinal tract, and cannot be 100% absorbed by digestive system. Therefore, the health risk of heavy metal could be overestimated if the total content of the heavy metal is used to carry out risk assessment instead of the total absorption content. Thus, bioaccessibility may be more accurate in assessing risks of heavy metals in Chinese herbal medicine.

Common methods for determining bioaccessibility of heavy metals are in vitro experiments; in this case, a simulated of gastrointestinal method was used for the simple method, short experimental period, and easily controlled experimental conditions. Dynamic in vitro gastrointestinal models mimic the gradual transit of ingested compounds through the digestive tract. In recent years, this method has been widely used to assess the risks of heavy metals in foods [20, 25, 26]. Studies have shown that the biochemical properties of heavy metals at various digestive stages are related to the characteristics of the heavy metals, their existent morphology, the type of matrix, and so on [27]. In this study, the bioaccessibility of heavy metals in *C. sinensis* and the morphology of arsenic in artificial gastrointestinal fluid were evaluated by in vitro experiments. The risks of heavy metals in *C. sinensis* were evaluated scientifically.

As in vitro gastrointestinal digestion

Based on results of in vitro experiments, the bioaccessibility of arsenic in *C. sinensis* was 64.46%, indicating that arsenic in the *C. sinensis* could not be 100% dissolved by the artificial gastrointestinal fluid. And there were still a large number of unidentified arsenic species in the artificial gastrointestinal extract solution.

The health risks of heavy metals in *C. sinensis*

Cordyceps sinensis is usually consumed for a long period of time to improve health. It is generally recommended to take *C. sinensis* for 2–3 months each year. The target hazard quotient (THQ) was used in this research, taking into consideration of daily dose and factors including most commonly consumed dosage forms and duration of consumption to evaluate potential and long-term risk of heavy metals in *C. sinensis* to human body. In the calculation of the THQ value, the duration of consumption was assumed to be 90 days, and the dosage was "the maximum dosage of 9 g recommended in Chinese Pharmacopoeia (2015 version)". However, under actual conditions, the dosage is usually much less than 9 g because of the extremely high cost of *C. sinensis*, so the calculated THQ value is greater than its actual value and suggests an inflated risk. The experimental results suggested that there is no obvious risk from heavy metals in *C. sinensis* to human body. However, it is worth noting that the BTHQ value of arsenic is 0.5334 and the TBTHQ is 0.5440. If the required course of *C. sinensis* is longer than 90 days, the dose of *C. sinensis* needs to be reduced to avoid damage to the body from heavy metals.

The standards of heavy metals in *C. sinensis*

Different medicinal materials grow in different environments with different life cycles and properties, causing variations in heavy metal contents. The unified standards of heavy metals in Chinese herbal medicines ignore some special properties of medicinal herbs. Chinese medicine is different from food in usages and dosages. Mode and frequency of drug use should be taken into consideration to get more equitable results of evaluation and standardization, when evaluating the risks of heavy metals and determining the standards for heavy metals in Chinese herbal medicines. This study showed that the heavy metals in *C. sinensis* present no obvious risks to human health in a reasonable taking way, indicating the excess of heavy metals in *C. sinensis* might be attributed to the unduly strict standard, and the heavy metal standards for *C. sinensis* need to loose properly.

Conclusion

The five heavy metals cannot be 100% absorbed by human body. The content of arsenic in *C. sinensis* is high, but inorganic arsenic of strong toxic accounted for only 8.69% of the total in dilute nitric acid extracted solutions and for merely 2.33% of the total in the in vitro gastrointestinal solutions. The dietary exposure values of Cu, Pb, As, Cd and Hg were lower than the safety limits set by the Joint FAO/WHO Expert Committee on Food Additives (JFCFA) and the BTHQ of these heavy metals were all less than 1. The heavy metals in *C. sinensis* present no obvious risks to human health in a reasonable taking way. Perhaps, it is the time to loose the heavy metal standards for *C. sinensis* properly.

Table 6 Estimated dietary exposures (DE) and BTHQ values of Cu, Pb, As, Cd and Hg in *C. sinensis*

	Cu	Pb	As	Cd	Hg	Total
DE	2.21	0.21	1.41	0.02	0.01	3.86
BTHQ	0.0041	0.0040	0.5334	0.0020	0.0005	0.5440
PTDI	500	3.57	50	1	0.5	

DE is the dietary exposure (μg kg^{-1} body weight day^{-1})

PTDI is the provisional tolerable daily intake suggested by JECFA [28] given in μg kg^{-1} body weight day^{-1}. The value of Hg refers to the limit of methyl mercury suggested by CAC

Authors' contributions

HLQ and GLP substantial contributions to the conception or design of the work. ZL and WS collected the samples. ZL, HQX and KLP performed the ICP-MS and HPLC–ICP-MS analysis experiment and collected data. YWZ and JJY prepared the *Cordyceps sinensis* samples. YJ and KCZ provided a great help and careful guide for the modification of manuscript including the data processing analysis and grammar part. All authors read and approved the final manuscript.

Author details

[1] National Resource Center for Chinese Materia Medica, State Key Laboratory Breeding Base of Dao-di Herbs, China Academy of Chinese Medical Sciences, Beijing 100700, People's Republic of China. [2] College of Traditional Chinese Medicine, Guangdong Pharmaceutical University, Guangdong 510006, China.

Acknowledgements

The authors wish to acknowledge Guang Yang and Wen Sun, National Resource Center for Chinese Materia Medica, China Academy of Chinese Medical Sciences, State Key Laboratory Breeding Base of Dao-di Herbs. Special thanks to Ge Mo for the language help in this article.

Competing interests

The authors declare that they have no competing interests.

Consent for publication

All of authors consent to publication of this study in journal of Chinese Medicine.

Funding

This work was financially supported by the Reform project of review and approval system of pharmaceutical medical instruments in Chinese Pharmacopoeia Commission (ZG2016-1), The National Key Research and Development Program of China (2017YFC1700701) and Key fields of Chinese Academy of traditional Chinese Medicine (ZZ10-27).

References

1. Luo C, Shen ZG. The mechanisms of heavy metal uptake and accumulation in plants. Chin Bull Bot. 2003;20:59–66.
2. Kampa M, Castanas E. Human health effects of air pollution. Environ Pollut. 2008;151:362–7.
3. Robinson BH. E-waste: an assessment of global production and environmental impacts. Sci Total Environ. 2009;408:183–91.
4. Zeng X, Xu X, Boezen HM, Huo X. Children with health impairments by heavy metals in an e-waste recycling area. Chemosphere. 2016;148:408–15.
5. Koedrith P, Kim H, Weon JI, Seo YR. Toxicogenomic approaches for understanding molecular mechanisms of heavy metal mutagenicity and carcinogenicity. Int J Hyg Environ Health. 2013;216:587.
6. Yoshikawa N, Nishiuchi A, Kubo E, Yu Y, Kunitomo M, Kagota S. *Cordyceps sinensis* acts as an adenosine a3 receptor agonist on mouse melanoma and lung carcinoma cells, and human fibrosarcoma and colon carcinoma cells. Pharmacol Pharm. 2011;02:266–70.
7. Zheng LP, Gao LW, Zhou JQ, Sima YH, Wang JW. Antioxidant activity of aqueous extract of a *Tolypocladium* sp. fungus isolated from wild *Cordyceps sinensis*. Afr J Biotech. 2008;7:3004–10.
8. Guo JY. A contemporary treatment approach to both diabetes and depression by *Cordyceps sinensis*, rich in vanadium. Evid Based Complement Alternat Med eCAM. 2010;7:387.
9. Li SP, Yang FQ, Tsim KWK. Quality control of *Cordyceps sinensis*, a valued traditional chinese medicine. J Pharm Biomed Anal. 2006;41:1571–84.
10. Zhou L, Hao QX, Wang S, Yang Q, Kang CZ, Yang WZ, Guo LP. Study on distribution of five heavy metal elements in different parts of *Cordyceps sinensis* by microwave digestion ICP-MS. China J Chin Materia Med. 2017;42:2934–8.
11. Traditional Chinese medicine—determination of heavy metals in herbal medicines used in traditional Chinese medicine ISO 18664 2015.8.1.
12. Lu T, Zhang LL, Zhang GW, Yi WL, Shen Z. Arsenic speciation of dried *Lentinus edodes* by HPLC–ICP-MS. Food Ind. 2015;12:275–9.
13. Chen SZ, Liu LP, Zhen-Xia DU. The presence form and analytic technology of arsenic in food. Chin J Food Hyg. 2014;3:296–303.
14. Li H, Zhang LS. Toxicity and biological function of arsenic. Mod Pre Med. 2000;27:39–40.
15. Li YH, Dang RH, Xia YJ. The damage of arsenic poisoning to nervous system. Chin J Control Endemic Disenaces. 2001;16:354–6.
16. Gong ZL, Lu XF, Ma MS, Watt C, Li CX. Arsenic speciation analysis. Talanta. 2002;58:77–96.
17. Wang GL, Jin HY, Han XP, Shi Y, Tian JG, Lin RC. Quality study and problems of *Cordyceps sinensis*. Chin Tradit Herbal Drugs. 2008;39:115–8.
18. Larsen EH, Hansen M, Gössler W. Speciation and health risk considerations of arsenic in the edible mushroom *Laccaria amethystina* collected from contaminated and uncontaminated locations. Appl Organomet Chem. 1998;2:285–91.
19. Pharmacopoeia Commission of the People's Republic of China. Chinese pharmacopoeia, vol. 3. Beijing: China Medical Science and Technology Press; 2015.
20. Jin FU, Cui YS. In vitro model system to evaluate the influence of ph and soil-gastric/intestinal juices ratio on bioaccessibility of pb, cd and as in two typical contaminated soils. J Agro Environ Sci. 2012;31:245–51.
21. Chen SB, Wen-Jing YU, Zhao YL. Speciation analysis of arsenic and determination of abio-arsenic in food. Acad Period Farm Products Process. 2013;8:86–8.
22. Pizarro I, Gómez-Gómez M, León J, Román D, Palacios MA. Bioaccessibility and arsenic speciation in carrots, beets and quinoa from a contaminated area of chile. Sci Total Environ. 2016;565:557–63.
23. Chien LC, Hung TC, Choang KY, Yeh CY, Meng PJ, Shieh MJ, Ha BC. Daily intake of tbt, cu, zn, cd and as for fishermen in taiwan. Sci Total Environ. 2002;285:177–85.
24. Ramesh A, Walker SA, Hood DB, Guillén MD, Schneider K, Weyand EH. Bioavailability and risk assessment of orally ingested polycyclic aromatic hydrocarbons. Int J Toxicol. 2004;23:301.
25. Lan DZ, Lei M, Zhou S, Liao BH, Cui YS, Yin NY, Shen Y. Health risk assessment of heavy metals in rice grains from a mining-impacted area in south hunan by in vitro simulation method. J Agro Environ Sci. 2014;33:1897–903.
26. Huang L, Zhou CY, Chen ZL, Zhang JS, Su YM, Peng XC. Advances in the study of in vitro simulation of bioavailability of heavy metals in soil and crops. J Yangtze Univ. 2016;3:42–7.
27. Oomen AG, Hack A, Minekus M, Zeijdner E, Cornelis C, Schoeters G, Verstraete W, Vande WT, Wragg J, Rompelberg CJ, Sips AJ, Van Wijnen JH. Comparison of five in vitro digestion models to study the bioaccessibility of soil contaminants. Environ Sci Technol. 2002;36:3326–34.
28. JECFA. Evaluation of certain food additives and contaminants. Thirty-third Report of the Joint FAO/WHO Expert Committee on Food Additives (JECFA). Technical Report Series 776, Geneva. 1989.

8

Extrahepatic cytochrome P450s play an insignificant role in triptolide-induced toxicity

Yuan Wei[1*], Dujun Wang[1], Meng Chen[2], Zhen Ouyang[1], Shuo Wang[1] and Jun Gu[3,4*]

Abstract

Background: Triptolide, an active ingredient of Chinese medicine plant *Tripterygium wilfordii* Hook.f., has been shown to exert anti-tumor, immunosuppressive, anti-inflammatory, and anti-fertility pharmacological effects. However, triptolide also causes severe side effects, which are manifested as toxicities in multiple organs. The aim of this study was to analyze the role of extrahepatic cytochrome P450 enzymes in triptolide-induced toxicity.

Methods: Xh-CL mouse model with normal liver, but low extrahepatic P450 expression levels was used in this study. Xh-CL mice and C57BL/6 (wildtype, WT) mice were treated with 200 µg/kg triptolide intraperitoneally every other day for 30 days. The serum levels of alanine aminotransferase (ALT), aspartate transaminase (AST), creatine (Cre), and blood urea nitrogen (BUN) were detected by kits. The changes of tissue were observed with H&E staining. Two groups of mice (Xh-CL and WT animals), were received a single dose of 1 mg/kg TP by oral gavage for pharmacokinetic analysis.

Results: Xh-CL mice displayed higher serum levels of ALT, AST, Cre, and BUN compared to untreated Xh-CL mice. The organ-to-body weight ratio for spleen was high, while that for testes was low. Histopathological changes were observed in multiple organs. However, compared with triptolide-treated WT mice, no significant differences in either blood chemistry or histopathology were recorded. Furthermore, pharmacokinetic studies showed no significant differences between triptolide-treated Xh-CL and WT mice.

Conclusions: Our findings suggest that sub-chronic triptolide treatment can induce toxicities in mouse kidney, spleen, and testis with or without normal local P450 functions. Therefore, extrahepatic P450s play an insignificant role in triptolide-induced toxicity.

Keywords: Triptolide, Xh-CL mouse model, Extrahepatic toxicity, Cytochrome P450, Pharmacokinetic

Background

Triptolide (TP) is the primary active diterpenoid triepoxide isolated from *Tripterygium wilfordii* Hook.f. ("thunder god vine" in Chinese herbal medicine). TP exhibits anti-inflammatory, immunosuppressive, anti-fertility, and anti-tumor effects [1, 2]. TP has also shown potential in the treatment of autosomal dominant polycystic kidney disease [3]. However, clinical use of TP is limited because of its toxic effects and narrow therapeutic window. The side effects of TP include gastrointestinal discomfort, amenorrhea, kidney dysfunction, leukopenia, thrombocytopenia, and aplastic anemia, and they have been reported to occur in more than 45% of patients [4].

Previous studies have confirmed that cytochrome P450s are responsible for the hydroxylation of TP in vitro [5], and higher expression of hepatic CYP3A can facilitate the biotransformation of TP and decrease its hepatotoxicity in rats [6, 7]. These findings suggested that the decreased activity of hepatic CYP3A was a key factor responsible for the adverse effects associated with TP in vivo. A clinical study assessing 202 Chinese individuals showed that the hepatic CYP3A metabolic activities were normally distributed [8]. In other words, significantly low hepatic CYP3A metabolic activity was found only in a small percentage of the studied group, indicating that low activity of hepatic CYP3A, as a single factor, was not

*Correspondence: ywei@ujs.edu.cn; jungu@wadsworth.org
[1] School of Pharmacy, Jiangsu University, 301 Xuefu Road, Zhenjiang, Jiangsu, People's Republic of China
[3] Wadsworth Center, New York State Department of Health, 1400 Washington Ave, Albany, NY, USA
Full list of author information is available at the end of the article

sufficient to explain why nearly half of patients treated with TP experienced adverse reactions [4]. Therefore, other related factors affecting TP-induced toxicity should be identified. A previous report showed that most of the TP-induced adverse reactions occurred in extrahepatic tissues [6]. We therefore focused on the role of extrahepatic P450 activities.

A recent study with a liver-specific cytochrome P450 reductase knockout mouse model (LCN mouse) [9] confirmed that inactivation of hepatic P450s abolishes metabolism of TP in the liver, resulting in an increase in TP bioavailability and toxicity in vivo. Xue et al. found that while the role of hepatic P450s in TP-induced toxicity was well defined, the function of extrahepatic P450s could not be assessed because TP circulation levels were greatly increased in the LCN mouse model. This problem may be overcome by using a mouse model that expresses only low levels of extrahepatic cytochrome P450 reductase (Xh-CL). The Xh-CL mouse model was generated by crossing a reversible-CL (r-CL) mouse model with the albumin-Cre mouse model. Xh-CL mice show normal cytochrome P450 reductase (CPR) expression in hepatocytes, while the expression levels in other tissues including brain, kidney, lung, OM, testis, and ovary were only 4–24% of the corresponding levels found in wildtype (WT) mice. No significant differences in liver microsomal activities were found between Xh-CL and WT mice [10]. In this study, we treated Xh-CL mice and WT (C57BL/6) mice with TP and compared toxicity and pharmacokinetics.

Methods

Materials and chemicals

TP (>99% purity) was purchased from ChromaDex (Irvine, CA, USA). It was dissolved in Tween80 (Sigma-Aldrich, St. Louis, MO, USA), and then diluted to the required concentration in 0.9% saline, for a final Tween 80 concentration of less than 1% v/v. Alanine aminotransferase (ALT), aspartate transaminase (AST), blood urea nitrogen (BUN), and creatine analysis kits were purchased from Nanjing Jiancheng Bioengineering Institute (Nanjing, China).

Experimental animals and drug administration

Cpr-low (CL) mice were kindly provided by Prof. Xinxin Ding (Wadsworth Center, Albany, NY, USA). Alb-Cre and C57BL/6 mice were purchased from the Model Animal Research Center of Nanjing University (Nanjing, China), permit number SKXK (Su) 2010-0001. Xh-CL mice were produced by the crossing of the Cpr-low (CL) and Alb-Cre mice as reported previously [10]. The animals were provided with a standard laboratory diet and tap water ad libitum during the experiments. 8-week-old male WT mice weighing 20 ± 2 g were used for experiments. In the general toxicological studies, Xh-CL and WT mice ($n = 5$) were administered 0.1 and 0.2 mg/kg TP by i.p. injection, and the control groups received a vehicle [11]. The mice were dosed at approximately 9:00–10:00A.M. every other day for 30 days. For the pharmacokinetic study, the animals were dosed with 1 mg/kg TP by oral gavage. All animal experiments were approved by the Institutional Animal Ethics and Use Committee of Jiangsu University. The minimum standards of reporting checklist contains details of the experimental design, and statistics, and resources used in this study (Additional file 1).

General characterization of TP-induced toxicity

The mice were weighed and euthanized with carbon dioxide 24 h after the last TP treatment. Blood was collected by cardiac puncture. Serum samples were prepared by centrifugation after coagulation for 30 min at room temperature. Serum levels of ALT, AST, BUN, and creatinine were determined using commercial kits. Organs (brain, liver, lung, kidney, spleen, and testes) were weighed at the time of necropsy. The organ: body weight ratios were calculated. Next, partial tissues were fixed in 10% neutral buffered formalin for histological examination, remaining tissues were frozen at −80 °C. The tissue sections (5-μm thickness) were stained with hematoxylin and eosin (H&E) for pathological analysis, which was carried out by Prof. Miao Chen of the Department of Pathology, First People's Hospital, Zhenjiang, China. For semi-quantitative assessment of the extent of tissue toxicity, the severity of tissue lesions was graded as follows: +, moderate; ±, mild; and −, negative [12].

To determine the tissue distribution of TP in mice, frozen tissues were homogenized in saline (1.0 g wet weight/mL) on ice. Triptolide was extracted from the tissue homogenates including liver, kidney, spleen and testes. Each sample was extracted with an equal volume of ethyl acetate for three times, and then dried under nitrogen. The residues were reconstituted in 50 μL methanol for analysis.

TP concentrations were quantified with an Agilent 1260 Infinity Liquid Chromatography system coupled to the Thermo LXQ™ Linear Ion Trap mass spectrometer (Thermo Fisher Scientific, Waltham, MA, USA). The mobile phase consisted of acetonitrile and water (30:70), with a flow rate of 0.2 mL/min. An electrospray interface in negative ionization mode was used. ESI source parameters were as followed: sheath gas flow rate 10.5 L/min, capillary temperature 325 °C, capillary voltage 3500 V, nebulizer pressure 25 psi, quality scan range (*m/z* 100–1200, fragmentor 110 eV, collision energy 70 eV). Xcalibur™ software (Thermo Finnigan) version 1.2 was used to analysis the data (Thermo Fisher Scientific, Waltham, MA, USA).

Pharmacokinetic analysis

Two groups of mice (Xh-CL and WT animals, 24 mice in each group) were used for pharmacokinetic analysis. The mice received a single dose of 1 mg/kg TP by oral gavage. Blood was collected at 5, 10, 15, 20, 30, 45, 60, and 120 min (n = 3 for each time point). Around 0.5 mL blood was collected from the ocular sinus at each time point. The mice were euthanized with CO_2 immediately after blood collection. Plasma was prepared by centrifugation at 900×*g* for 10 min and kept at −80 °C until analysis. TP was then extracted from 200 μL plasma with 2 × 600 μL ethyl acetate and dried under nitrogen. The residues were reconstituted in 100 μL methanol for analysis. TP concentrations were quantified with an Agilent 1290 Infinity Liquid Chromatography system equipped with Agilent ZORBAX Eclipse Plus C18 column (2.1 × 100 mm, 1.8 μm) (Agilent Technologies, Santa Clara, CA, USA) for pharmacokinetic analysis. The mobile phase consisted of acetonitrile and water (30:70), with a flow rate of 0.2 mL/min and a sample volume of 2 μL. The compound was measured at 218 nm, and the column was maintained at 25 °C. The pharmacokinetic parameters were analyzed with the software package DAS 3.2 (Mathematical Pharmacology Professional Committee of China, Shanghai, China).

Statistical analysis

All data are expressed as mean ± standard deviation (SD). Data were evaluated for statistical significance by one-way analysis of variance (ANOVA) or Student's *t* test. SPSS 13.0 (IBM SPSS, Armonk, NY, USA) was used for analysis, and $p < 0.05$ was considered statistically significant.

Results

Blood chemistry parameters

We first measured AST and ALT levels to assess mouse liver function, and creatinine and BUN levels to evaluate renal function in each group. As shown in Fig. 1a, b, the serum ALT and AST levels in Xh-CL mice treated with 0.2 mg/kg TP differed from those in control Xh-CL mice, indicating liver cell damage or abnormal function (likely acute toxic hepatitis). However, Xh-CL mice treated with 0.1 mg/kg TP showed no significant differences in the levels of kidney and liver toxicity markers compared with the control Xh-CL mice (Fig. 1a, b). Similarly, the serum creatinine and BUN levels in Xh-CL mice treated with

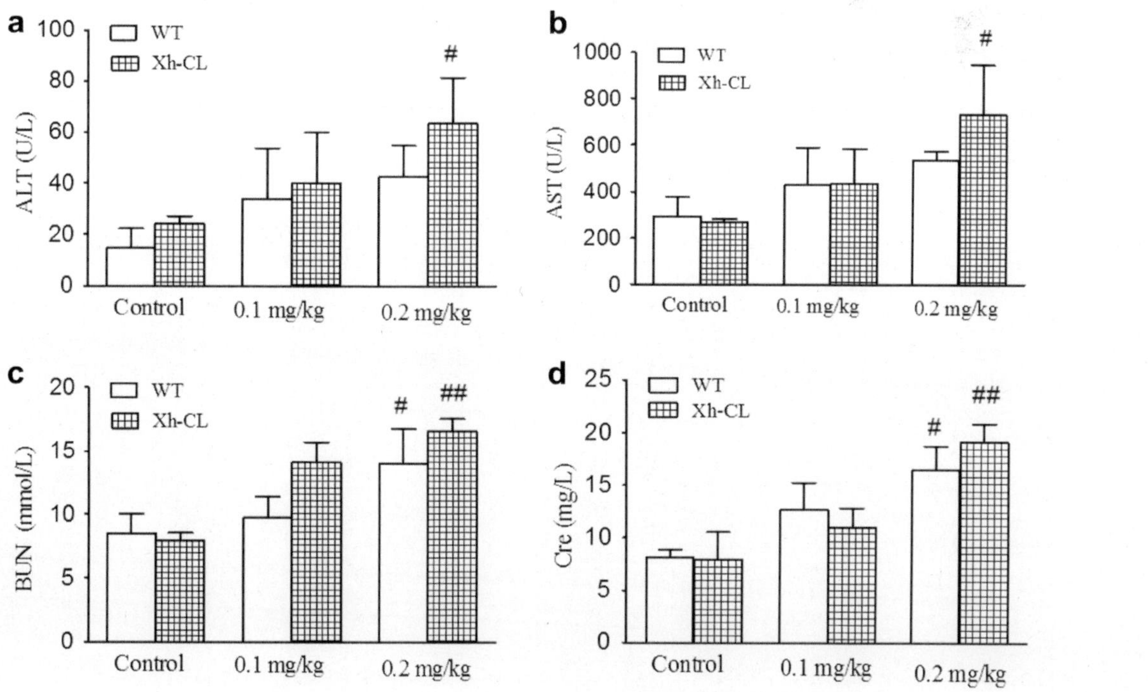

Fig. 1 Effects of triptolide (TP) intraperitoneal (i.p.) injection on serum biochemical parameters in Xh-CL mice and WT mice. TP was administered at doses of 0.1 and 0.2 mg/kg; the control mice were administered with a vehicle, mice were dosed every other day for 30 days. **a** Alanine aminotransferase (ALT); **b** aspartate transaminase (AST); **c** creatinine; **d** blood urea nitrogen (BUN). $^{\#}p < 0.05$, $^{\#\#}p < 0.01$ vs. control

0.2 mg/kg TP differed from those in the control (Fig. 1c, d), indicating renal cell damage or abnormal renal function, and the mice may possibly be suffering from glomerulonephritis. Notably, no significant differences were observed in AST, ALT, creatinine, and BUN levels between Xh-CL mice and WT mice (Fig. 1c, d).

Table 1 Effects of triptolide on organ: body weight ratios

Organ	Mouse group	Organ: body weight ratios (%)		
		Control	0.1 mg/kg	0.2 mg/kg
Brain	Xh-CL	2.01 ± 0.13	2.17 ± 0.19	1.98 ± 0.01
	WT	2.45 ± 0.13	2.44 ± 0.02	2.32 ± 0.06
Liver	Xh-CL	5.67 ± 0.53	5.43 ± 0.13	6.62 ± 0.80
	WT	4.94 ± 0.86	4.54 ± 0.79	7.01 ± 0.25#
Lung	Xh-CL	0.64 ± 0.03	0.73 ± 0.05	0.63 ± 0.01
	WT	0.65 ± 0.01	0.66 ± 0.01	0.64 ± 0.02
Kidney	Xh-CL	1.41 ± 0.06	1.52 ± 0.45	1.54 ± 0.03
	WT	1.40 ± 0.01	1.54 ± 0.08	1.63 ± 0.01
Spleen	Xh-CL	0.34 ± 0.01	0.42 ± 0.02	0.59 ± 0.04#
	WT	0.47 ± 0.02	0.34 ± 0.01	0.61 ± 0.01
Testis	Xh-CL	0.87 ± 0.11	0.63 ± 0.01	0.40 ± 0.03##
	WT	0.74 ± 0.04	0.57 ± 0.03	0.43 ± 0.06#

Xh-CL and WT mice (n = 5 in each group) were administered with 0.1 or 0.2 mg/kg triptolide. The control mice were administered with a vehicle. Mice were dosed every other day for 30 days. Data were shown as mean ± SD

# $p < 0.05$, ## $p < 0.01$ vs. control

Organ: body weight ratios and histopathology analysis

To assess the sub-chronic toxicity of TP, we compared the organ: body weight ratio of various organs between Xh-CL and WT mice. Table 1 shows that Xh-CL and WT mice treated with 0.1 mg/kg TP exhibited no significant differences in organ-to-body weight ratios for any organ compared with the controls. However, significantly increased spleen to body weight ratio was observed in Xh-CL mice treated with 0.2 mg/kg TP ($p < 0.05$) concomitantly with significantly decreased testis weight ($p < 0.01$). In WT mice treated with 0.2 mg/kg TP, liver to body weight ratios were significantly higher ($p < 0.05$), while testis to body weight ratios were significantly lower ($p < 0.05$) when compared with the control mice.

Figure 2 shows the representative images of hepatic lesions in the different exposure groups. Histological analysis revealed some necrotic and swelling hepatocytes in both Xh-CL and WT mice following treatment with 0.2 mg/kg TP (Fig. 2c, f). The representative images of renal lesions in the different groups are shown in Fig. 3. Kidney proximal tubular epithelial cell dilation and some protein casts were found. Glomerular capillary loop lesions were also found in both Xh-CL and WT mice following 0.2 mg/kg TP treatment (Fig. 3c, f). The representative images of lesions in the testes are shown in Fig. 4. In both groups treated with 0.2 mg/kg TP, primary and secondary spermatocytes were reduced (or completely absent) in the seminiferous tubules. In addition,

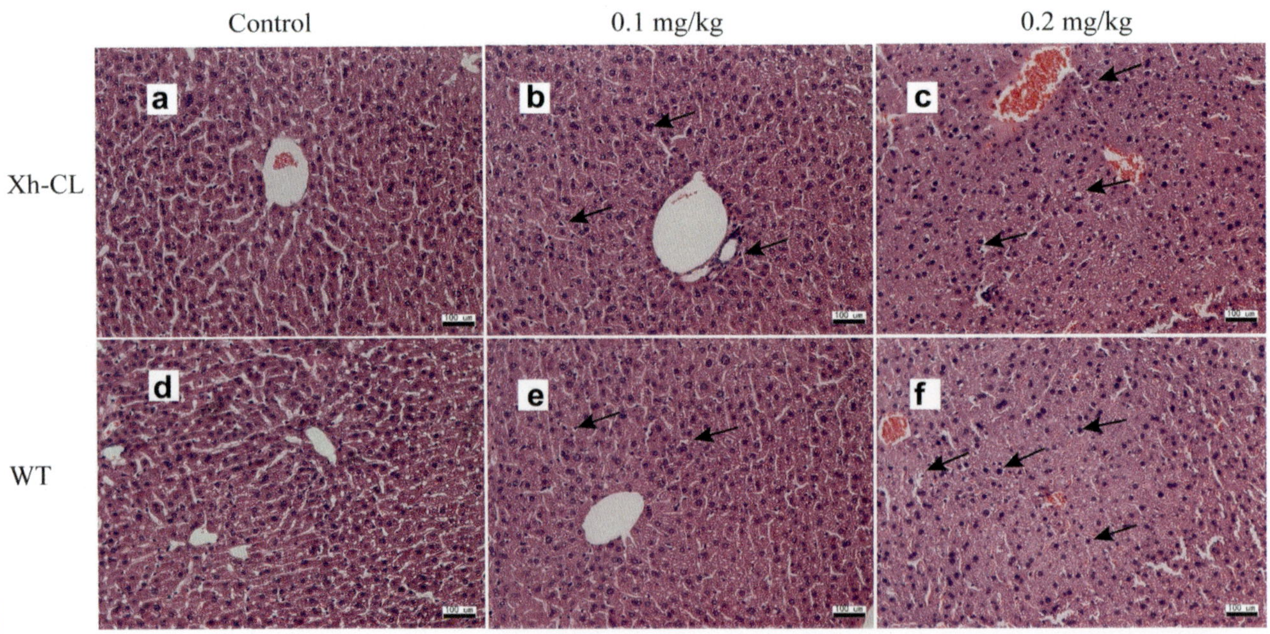

Fig. 2 Comparison of liver lesions in Xh-CL and WT mice following triptolide oral treatment (H&E staining, ×200). The mice were administered with 0.1 mg/kg (**b**, **e**) or 0.2 mg/kg (**c**, **f**) triptolide. The control mice received a vehicle (**a**, **d**). Mice were dosed every other day for 30 days. Arrows indicate necrotic and swollen hepatocytes

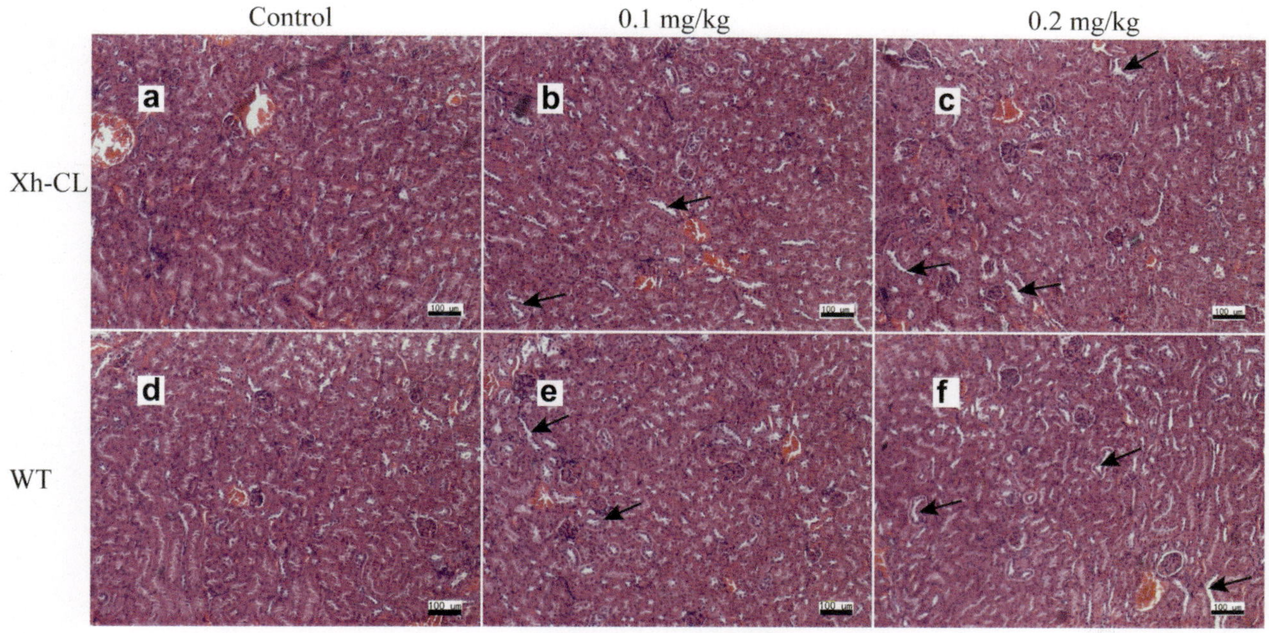

Fig. 3 Comparison of kidney lesions in Xh-CL and WT mice following triptolide oral treatment (H&E staining, ×200). The mice were administered with 0.1 mg/kg (**b**, **e**) or 0.2 mg/kg (**c**, **f**) triptolide. The control mice received a vehicle (**a**, **d**). Mice were dosed every other day for 30 days. Arrows indicate renal proximal tubular dilation; some protein casts are visible

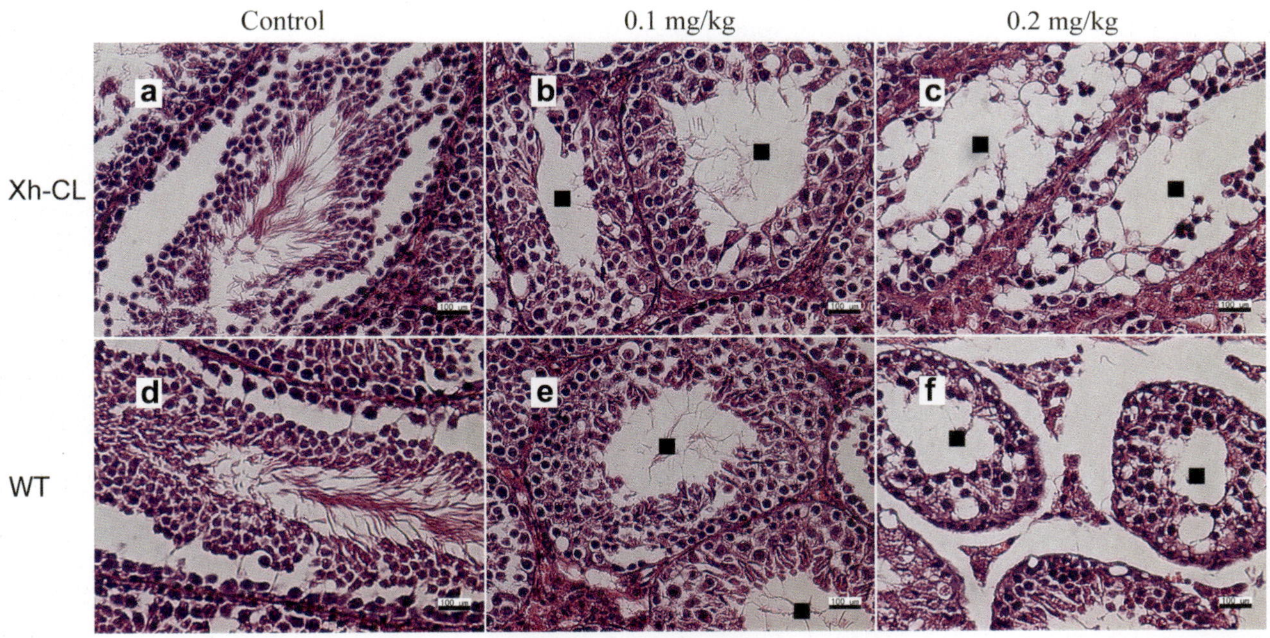

Fig. 4 Comparison of testicular lesions in Xh-CL and WT mice following triptolide oral treatment (H&E staining, ×200). The mice were administered with 0.1 mg/kg (**b**, **e**) or 0.2 mg/kg (**c**, **f**) triptolide. The control mice received a vehicle (**a**, **d**). Mice were dosed every other day for 30 days. Squares indicate reduced primary and secondary spermatocytes in the seminiferous tubules

testicular edema was present (Fig. 4c, f). Figure 5 compares the spleen lesions found in the exposure groups. Splenic sinus dilation and splenic atrophy were observed in both the groups treated with 0.2 mg/kg TP (Fig. 5c, f). These findings suggest that TP induces toxicity in multiple organs in both Xh-CL and WT mice, with similar patterns. The extent of tissue toxicity is shown in Table 2. More severe lesions were found in Xh-CL and WT mice

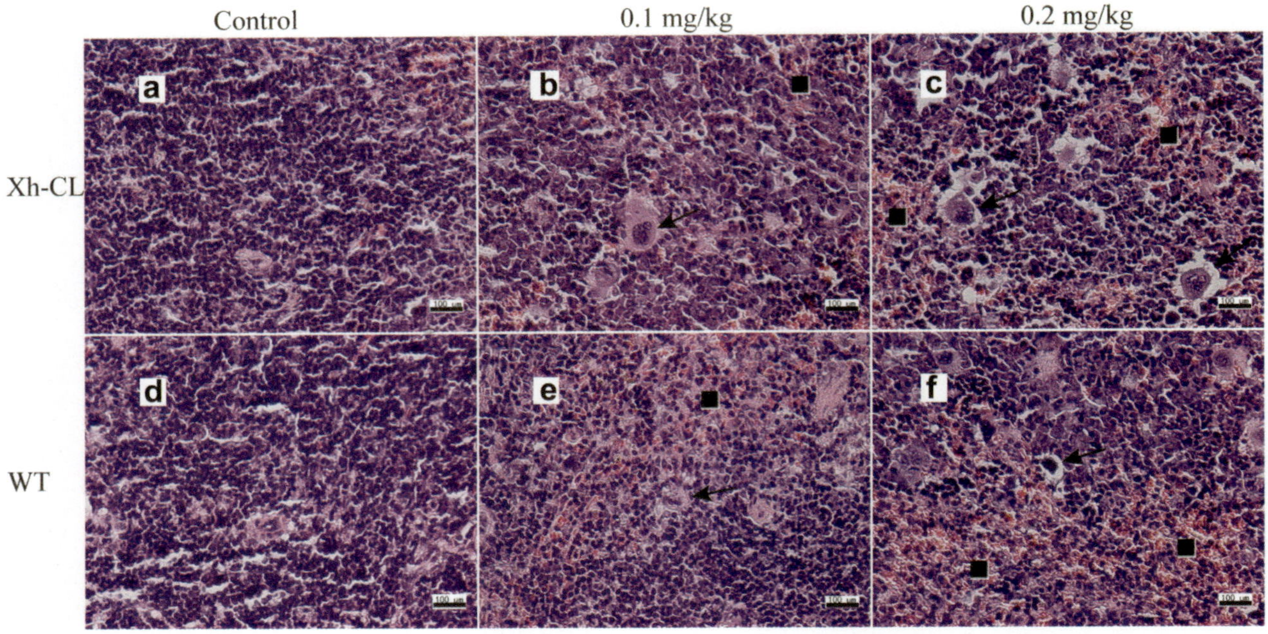

Fig. 5 Comparison of splenic lesions in Xh-CL and WT mice following triptolide oral treatment (H&E, ×200). The mice were administered with 0.1 mg/kg (**b**, **e**) or 0.2 mg/kg (**c**, **f**) triptolide. The control mice received a vehicle (**a**, **d**). Mice were dosed every other day for 30 days. Squares indicate bleeding of dilated splenic sinus. Arrows indicate splenic atrophy

after treatment with 0.2 mg/kg TP. Of the five Xh-CL mice, one exhibited moderate hepatoxicity, while three showed mild liver toxicity, and of the five WT mice, one displayed moderate hepatoxicity, while two showed mild toxicity. Two of the five Xh-CL mice exhibited moderate renal toxicity, while two showed mild toxicity. One of the five WT mice displayed moderate renal toxicity, and two showed mild toxicity. All mice displayed moderate testicular toxicity in both Xh-CL and WT groups. Two of the five Xh-CL mice displayed moderate splenic toxicity, while two showed mild toxicity. One of the five WT mice exhibited moderate splenic toxicity, and three showed mild toxicity. Levels of triptolide in the liver, kidney, testis and spleen of Xh-CL and WT mice were detected, no significant difference was observed between the groups at each dosage (Fig. 6a–d).

Pharmacokinetic analysis

The plasma concentrations of TP were plotted against time curves (Fig. 7). The calculated pharmacokinetic parameters are summarized in Table 3. Plasma TP reached peak levels at 15±0 min in both mouse groups. Other pharmacokinetic parameters, including C_{max}, the area under the curve (AUC), $T_{1/2}$, and CLz/F in the Xh-CL mice were remarkably similar to those in WT mice. These findings indicate that TP was cleared from both Xh-CL and WT mice in a similar manner.

Table 2 Extent of tissue toxicity in Xh-CL and WT mice following triptolide

Organ	Mouse group	Triptolide dose (mg/kg)	Number of mice in each grade		
			+	±	−
Liver	Xh-CL	0.1	0	2	3
		0.2	1	3	1
	WT	0.1	0	1	4
		0.2	1	2	2
Kidney	Xh-CL	0.1	0	2	3
		0.2	2	2	1
	WT	0.1	0	2	3
		0.2	1	2	2
Testis	Xh-CL	0.1	2	3	0
		0.2	5	0	0
	WT	0.1	1	4	0
		0.2	5	0	0
Spleen	Xh-CL	0.1	0	1	4
		0.2	2	2	1
	WT	0.1	1	1	3
		0.2	1	3	1

Xh-CL and WT mice (n = 5 in each group) were treated with 0.1 or 0.2 mg/kg triptolide, mice were dosed every other day for 30 days. The severity of lesions in the tissues was graded as follows: +, moderate; ±, mild; and −, negative

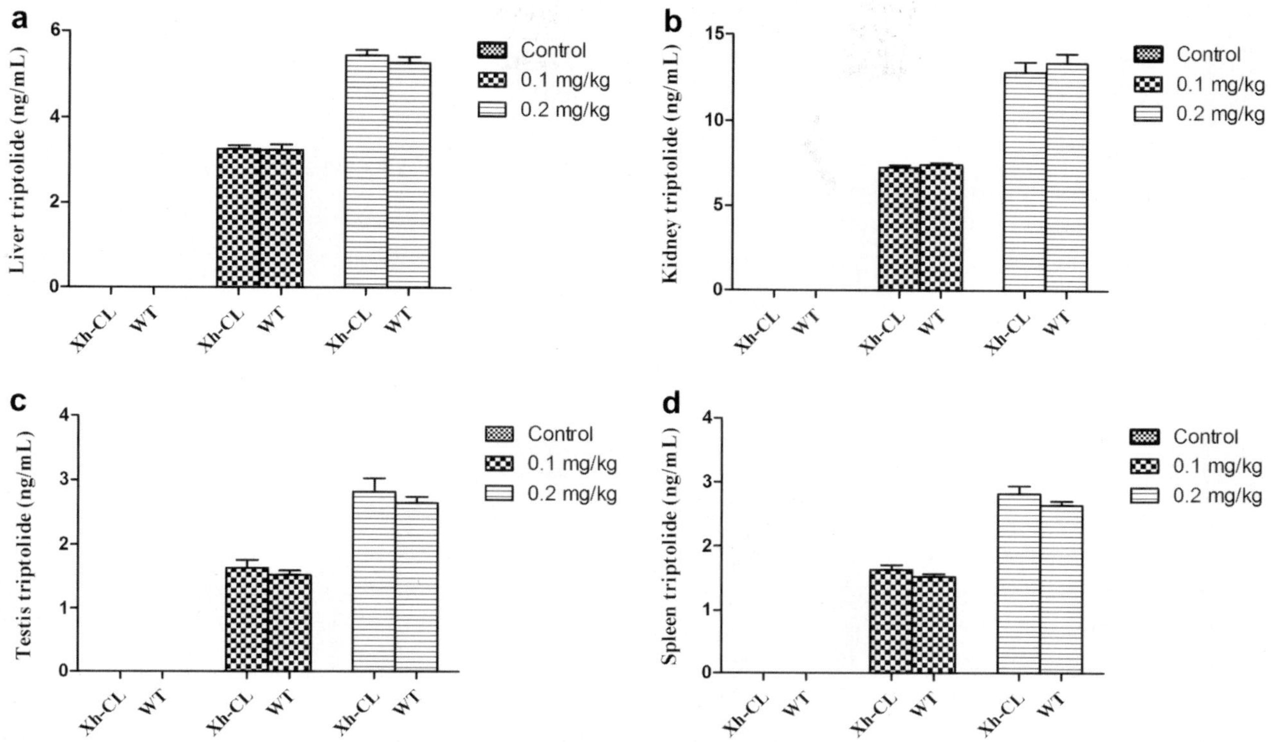

Fig. 6 Levels of triptolide in the liver (**a**), kidney (**b**), testis (**c**) and spleen (**d**) of Xh-CL and WT mice 24 h after oral treatment. The mice were administered with 0.1 or 0.2 mg/kg triptolide. The control mice received a vehicle. Mice were dosed every other day for 30 days. Mean ± standard deviation (indicated by error bars) are shown. No significant difference was observed between the groups at each dosage

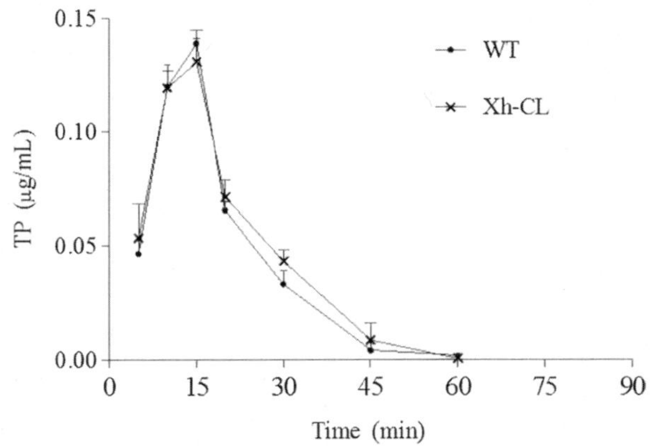

Fig. 7 Triptolide (1.0 mg/kg) clearance in Xh-CL and WT mice. Mean ± standard deviation (indicated by error bars) are shown. No significant difference was observed between the groups at any time point

Discussion

Cytochrome P450 enzymes are involved in the biotransformation of most xenobiotic compounds [13]. The liver is usually regarded as the most important organ in cytochrome P450-mediated drug metabolism, while P450s expressed in various extrahepatic tissues can also contribute to target tissue toxicity induced by tissue-selective toxicants [14].

The mechanism underlying TP-induced toxicity has not yet been elucidated clearly [15]. Theoretically, TP-induced toxicity can be caused either by the parent compound itself or by its reactive metabolites generated through biotransformation reactions. The extrahepatic metabolites can be produced by local P450s or can be generated in the liver or other tissues and then transported to the target tissues by systemic circulation [16]. A study with liver-Cpr-null mouse model reported that inactivation of hepatic P450s suppresses TP metabolism in the liver, leading to an increase in the bioavailability and toxicities of the compound [9]. However, the role of cytochrome P450s in extrahepatic organs was not discussed extensively in the aforementioned study, because extrahepatic toxicity was confounded by the reduced hepatic clearance of TP. This reduction led to greater systemic bioavailability, resulting in possible overestimation of the extrahepatic toxicities. In this study, we evaluated the role of extrahepatic P450 enzymes in triptolide-induced toxicity using Xh-CL mice with normal liver, but low extrahepatic levels of cytochrome P450 enzymes. The knockdown of extrahepatic P450 enzymes in mice could not change either the general toxicities, local tissue levels,

Table 3 Triptolide plasma pharmacokinetic parameters in Xh-CL and WT mice

Group	C_{max} (mg/L)	T_{max} (min)	$AUC_{(0-t)}$ (mg/L min)	$AUC_{(0-\infty)}$ (mg/L min)	$T_{1/2}$ (min)	CLz/F (L/min/kg)
Xh-CL	0.145 ± 0.002	15 ± 0	2.435 ± 0.233	2.445 ± 0.275	6.411 ± 1.41	0.409 ± 0.029
WT	0.139 ± 0.004	15 ± 0	2.579 ± 0.194	2.602 ± 0.198	7.442 ± 1.64	0.384 ± 0.035

Xh-CL and WT mice were administered 1.0 mg/kg triptolide orally. All data are presented as mean ± standard deviation. No significant differences were observed between the groups for any parameter (n = 3). Data were shown as mean ± SD

C_{max} maximum concentration, T_{max} time to reach C_{max}, *AUC* area under the curve, $T_{1/2}$ elimination half-life, *CLz/F* oral clearance

or the pharmacokinetics of TP. Thus, we found that extrahepatic P450 was probably not a significant factor in TP-induced toxicity. Results from the Xh-CL model provided direct evidence for the involvement of extrahepatic CPR-dependent enzymes in extrahepatic tissues, without confounding from reduced hepatic metabolism.

The small intestine is involved in first-pass metabolism of orally ingested xenobiotics, especially the substrates of CYP3A [14, 17]. CYP3A is the predominant cytochrome subfamily in the small intestine, accounting for 70–80% of total intestinal cytochrome content in humans [18]. In mice, intestinal CYP3A was first detected by erythromycin and cyclosporine activities and by immunoblot analysis [19]. The expression of CYP3A in the mouse small intestine was further confirmed by a mouse everted gut sac model [20] and by a systemic analysis of P450s expressed in the mouse small intestine and their inducibility [21]. However, in this study, the reduced CYP3A activity in the small intestine of Xh-CL mice appeared to exert few effects on the pharmacokinetics of TP and TP-induced toxicities.

The TP-induced toxicities were often studied with acute exposures in mice, but liver toxicities were hard to detect in wildtype animals without high doses (e.g. 1.0 mg/kg) close to LD_{50} of TP [6, 22]. In our sub-chronic toxicity study, we generated hepatic toxicological profiles for TP in C57BL/6 mice with moderate doses (0.1 or 0.2 mg/kg). High serum AST and ALT levels were detected, and they were indicatives of liver damage due to liver cell necrosis and cytosol leakage into the serum [23]. Our histological analysis also showed necrotic and swollen hepatocytes in the liver tissue sections. Since *Tripterygium wilfordii* Hook.f. was often used for long-term treatment in traditional Chinese medicine practices [24], data from our sub-chronic study could be helpful to get a better understanding of TP-induced clinical toxicity.

Conclusions

In conclusion, our findings indicate that sub-chronic TP treatment can cause toxic effects in multiple organs in mice, with or without extrahepatic P450 activity. To reduce TP-induced toxicity in clinical settings, related factors other than extrahepatic P450 enzymes should be identified and characterized.

Abbreviations

ALT: alanine aminotransferase; AST: aspartate transaminase; BUN: blood urea nitrogen; Cre: Cre recombinase; CPR: cytochrome P450 reductase; r-CL: reversible-Cpr low; Xh-CL: extrahepatic-CL; TP: triptolide; WT: wild type.

Authors' contributions

Study design and conception: YW; data collection and data analysis: DJW, MC, SW; data interpretation: YW, ZOY; manuscript drafting: YW, DJW; critical revising the manuscript: JG. All authors read and approved the final manuscript.

Author details

[1] School of Pharmacy, Jiangsu University, 301 Xuefu Road, Zhenjiang, Jiangsu, People's Republic of China. [2] Department of Molecular, Cellular and Biomedical Sciences, University of New Hampshire, Durham, NH, USA. [3] Wadsworth Center, New York State Department of Health, 1400 Washington Ave, Albany, NY, USA. [4] School of Public Health, State University of New York at Albany, Albany, NY, USA.

Acknowledgements

We gratefully acknowledge Prof. Xinxin Ding (Wadsworth Center, Albany, NY, USA) for providing the Cpr-low (CL) mice. This work was supported by the National Natural Science Foundation of China (Grant Nos. 81373480, 81102522, and 81573529), the Natural Science Foundation of Jiangsu Province (Grant No. BK2011473), and the Excellent Youth Foundation of Jiangsu University.

Competing interests

The authors declare that they have no competing interests.

Consent for publication

All of authors consent to publication of this study in Journal of Chinese Medicine.

References

1. Li XJ, Jiang ZZ, Zhang LY. Triptolide: progress on research in pharmacodynamics and toxicology. J Ethnopharmacol. 2014;155:67–79.
2. Cheng X, Jing Z, He YH, Jia HW, Zhao LH, Ning Z, Lu AP. Effects of triptolide from Radix *Tripterygium wilfordii* (Leigongteng) on cartilage cytokines and transcription factor NF-κB: a study on induced arthritis in rats. Chin Med. 2009;4(1):1–7.
3. Leuenroth SJ, Okuhara D, Shotwell JD, Markowitz GS, Yu Z, Somlo S, Crews CM. Triptolide is a traditional Chinese medicine-derived inhibitor of polycystic kidney disease. Proc Natl Acad Sci. 2007;104:4389–94.
4. Ming J. Pharmacological and clinical study on polyglycoside of *Tripterygium wilfordii* hook f. Chin Med J. 1996;57:35.
5. Li W, Liu Y, He YQ, Zhang JW, Gao Y, Ge GB, Liu HX, Huo H, Liu HT, Wang LM. Characterization of triptolide hydroxylation by cytochrome P450 in human and rat liver microsomes. Xenobiotica. 2008;38:1551–65.
6. Liu L, Jiang Z, Liu J, Huang X, Wang T, Liu J, Zhang Y, Zhou Z, Guo J, Yang L. Sex differences in subacute toxicity and hepatic microsomal metabolism of triptolide in rats. Toxicology. 2010;271:57–63.

7. Ye X, Li W, Yan Y, Mao C, Cai R, Xu H, Yang X. Effects of cytochrome P4503A inducer dexamethasone on the metabolism and toxicity of triptolide in rat. Toxicol Lett. 2010;192(2):212–20.
8. Zhu B, Liu ZQ, Chen GL, Chen XP, Ou-Yang DS, Wang LS, Huang SL, Tan ZR, Zhou HH. The distribution and gender difference of CYP3A activity in Chinese subjects. Br J Clin Pharmacol. 2003;55:264–9.
9. Xue X, Gong L, Qi X, Wu Y, Xing G, Yao J, Luan Y, Xiao Y, Li Y, Wu X. Knockout of hepatic P450 reductase aggravates triptolide-induced toxicity. Toxicol Lett. 2011;205:47–54.
10. Wei Y, Zhou X, Fang C, Li L, Kluetzman K, Yang W, Zhang QY, Ding X. Generation of a mouse model with a reversible hypomorphic cytochrome P450 reductase gene: utility for tissue-specific rescue of the reductase expression, and insights from a resultant mouse model with global suppression of P450 reductase expression in extrahepatic tissues. J Pharmacol Exp Ther. 2010;334:69–77.
11. Wu N, Liu XY, Wang DJ, Luo P, Wu Y, Wei Y. Sub-chronic toxicities of triptolide to C57BL/6 mice. Chin Tradit Pat Med. 2014;5:004.
12. Gu J, Cui H, Behr M, Zhang L, Zhang QY, Yang W, Hinson JA, Ding X. In vivo mechanisms of tissue-selective drug toxicity: effects of liver-specific knockout of the NADPH-cytochrome P450 reductase gene on acetaminophen toxicity in kidney, lung, and nasal mucosa. Mol Pharmacol. 2005;67:623–30.
13. Porter T, Coon M. Cytochrome P-450. Multiplicity of isoforms, substrates, and catalytic and regulatory mechanisms. J Biol Chem. 1991;266:13469–72.
14. Ding X, Kaminsky LS. Human extrahepatic cytochromes P450: function in xenobiotic metabolism and tissue-selective chemical toxicity in the respiratory and gastrointestinal tracts. Annu Rev Pharmacol. 2003;43:149–73.
15. Xu L, Qiu Y, Xu H, Ao W, Lam W, Yang X. Acute and subacute toxicity studies on triptolide and triptolide-loaded polymeric micelles following intravenous administration in rodents. Food Chem Toxicol. 2013;57:371–9.
16. Anders M, Dekant W, Vamvakas S. Glutathione-dependent toxicity. Xenobiotica. 1992;22:1135–45.
17. Kaminsky LS, Zhang QY. The small intestine as a xenobiotic-metabolizing organ. Drug Metab Dispos. 2003;31:1520–5.
18. Thelen K, Dressman JB. Cytochrome P450-mediated metabolism in the human gut wall. J Pharm Pharmacol. 2009;61:541–58.
19. Berg-Candolfi M, Candolfi E, Benet L. Suppression of intestinal and hepatic cytochrome P4503A in murine Toxoplasma infection. Effects of *N*-acetylcysteine and N G-monomethyl-L-arginine on the hepatic suppression. Xenobiotica. 1996;26:381–94.
20. Emoto C, Yamazaki H, Yamasaki S, Shimada N, Nakajima M, Yokoi T. Use of everted sacs of mouse small intestine as enzyme sources for the study of drug oxidation activities in vitro. Xenobiotica. 2000;30:971–82.
21. Zhang QY, Dunbar D, Kaminsky LS. Characterization of mouse small intestinal cytochrome P450 expression. Drug Metab Dispos. 2003;31:1346–51.
22. Liu M, Dong J, Yang Y, Yang X, Xu H. Progress in research on triptolide. Chin J Chin Mater Med. 2005;30:170–4.
23. Abdel-Fattah SM, Sanad M, Safaa M, Ragaa F. The protective effect of white ginseng against biochemical and pathological changes induced by aflatoxins in rats. J Am Sci. 2010;6:461–72.
24. Shu DF, Song YJ, Li RL. Comparative clinical observation on rheumatoid arthritis treated by triptolide and ethyl acetate extract of *Tripterygium wilfordii*. Chin J Integr Tradit West Med. 1990;10:144–6.

9

The antityrosinase and antioxidant activities of flavonoids dominated by the number and location of phenolic hydroxyl groups

Ai-Ren Zuo[1,2], Huan-Huan Dong[2], Yan-Ying Yu[3], Qing-Long Shu[2*], Li-Xiang Zheng[2], Xiong-Ying Yu[2] and Shu-Wen Cao[1,3*]

Abstract

Background: Compounds with the ability to scavenge reactive oxygen species (ROS) and inhibit tyrosinase may be useful for the treatment and prevention from ROS-related diseases. The number and location of phenolic hydroxyl of the flavonoids will significantly influence the inhibition of tyrosinase activity. Phenolic hydroxyl is indispensable to the antioxidant activity of flavonoids. Isoeugenol, shikonin, baicalein, rosmarinic acid, and dihydromyricetin have respectively one, two, three, four, or five phenolic hydroxyls. The different molecular structures with the similar structure to L-3,4-dihydroxyphenylalanine (L-DOPA) were expected to the different antityrosinase and antioxidant activities.

Methods: This investigation tested the antityrosinase activity, the inhibition constant, and inhibition type of isoeugenol, shikonin, baicalein, rosmarinic acid, and dihydromyricetin. Molecular docking was examined by the Discovery Studio 2.5 (CDOCKER Dock, Dassault Systemes BIOVIA, USA). This experiment also examined the antioxidant effects of the five compounds on supercoiled pBR322 plasmid DNA, lipid peroxidation in rat liver mitochondria in vitro, and DPPH, ABTS, hydroxyl, or superoxide free radical scavenging activity in vitro.

Results: The compounds exhibited good antityrosinase activities. Molecular docking results implied that the compounds could interact with the amino acid residues in the active site center of antityrosinase. These compounds also exhibited antioxidant effects on DPPH, ABTS, hydroxyl, or superoxide free radical scavenging activity in vitro, lipid peroxidation in rat liver mitochondria induced by Fe^{2+}/vitamin C system in vitro, and supercoiled pBR322 plasmid DNA. The activity order is isoeugenol < shikonin < baicalein < rosmarinic acid < dihydromyricetin. The results showed the compounds with more phenolic hydroxyls have more antioxidant and antityrosinase activities.

Conclusion: This was the first study of molecular docking for modeling the antityrosinase activity of compounds. This was also the first study of the protective effects of compounds on supercoiled pBR322 plasmid DNA, the lipid peroxidation inhibition activity in liver mitochondria. These results suggest that the compounds exhibited antityrosinase and antioxidant activities may be useful in skin pigmentation and food additives.

Keywords: Antityrosinase activity, Molecular docking, Antioxidant activity, Phenolic hydroxyl, Isoeugenol, Shikonin

*Correspondence: 276411076@qq.com; Caosw@ncu.edu.cn
[1] State Key Laboratory of Food Science and Technology, Nanchang University, Nanchang 330047, Jiangxi, China
[2] Jiangxi University of Traditional Chinese Medicine, Nanchang, Jiangxi, China
Full list of author information is available at the end of the article

Background

Flavonoids play a key role in the treatment of various diseases. Compounds with the ability to protect against DNA damage caused by reactive oxygen species (ROS) and inhibit tyrosinase may be useful for the treatment and prevention from ROS-related diseases. Flavonoids are a large type of compounds in natural products. Flavonoids already have been used widely as lead compounds or drugs.

Some studies showed that the number and location of phenolic hydroxyl on the flavonoids will significantly influence the inhibition of tyrosinase activity [1–3]. The number of phenolic hydroxyl on the B ring of flavonoids or catechins structure or resorcinol structure, can greatly enhance the inhibition of tyrosinase activity. At present, 4-hexyl resorcinol have been used as commodity in shrimp preservation [4]. The number and position of phenolic hydroxyl on the 1,2-diphenylethene derivatives can greatly effect the inhibition of tyrosinase activity. Two phenol hydroxyls compared to one hydroxyl and phenol hydroxyl replaced methoxyl will significantly enhance the inhibition of tyrosinase activity [5–7].

The tyrosinase inhibition mechanism of phenol hydroxyl compounds was analysed. Because the activity center of tyrosinase is hydrophobic, H^+, combined with Eoxy double oxygen, only come from the hydroxyl of tyrosine and dopamine. Phenol hydroxyl compounds, similar to tyrosine and dopamine, can inhibit the activity of tyrosinase [8].

Phenolic hydroxyl is indispensable to the antioxidant activity of flavonoids. Many studies showed that the antioxidant activity increased with the phenol hydroxyl number in B ring of flavonoids. Seyoum [9] studied the activity of scavenging free radicals of 52 kinds of flavonoids. The result showed that two or three phenol hydroxyls compared to one hydroxyl in A ring or B ring, will greatly enhance the antioxidant activity.

The relationship between phenolic hydroxyl number and antioxidant activity of flavonoids is very significant. The reason may be: (1) the more phenolic hydroxyl number, the more H^+ combined with free radicals; (2) the phenolic hydroxyl has strongly denounce electronic effect, which result to the free radicals reaction; (3) the more phenolic hydroxyl number, the more hydrogen bonding, antioxidant activity is also enhanced obviously [10].

The number and location of phenolic hydroxyl of the flavonoids will significantly influence the inhibition of tyrosinase activity. Phenolic hydroxyl is indispensable to the antioxidant activity of flavonoids. Isoeugenol, shikonin, baicalein, rosmarinic acid, and dihydromyricetin have respectively one, two, three, four, or five phenolic hydroxyls. The different molecular structures with the similar structure to L-3,4-dihydroxyphenylalanine (L-DOPA) were expected to the different antityrosinase and antioxidant activities.

Tyrosinase (EC 1.14.18.1) plays a key role in the biosynthesis of melanin pigment [11]. Under normal physiological conditions, melanin plays a key role in the protection against UV injury, animal mimicry and camouflage [12]. Thus, it has attracted researchers to find efficient tyrosinase inhibitors. Recently, molecular docking for modeling the antityrosinase activity of compounds had been used widely in drug design [13].

Isoeugenol is the major constituent of *Eugenia caryophyllata* Thunb., which has extensive pharmacological activities, such as antimicrobe, stomach-invigorating. The result of Jin [14] indicated that isoeugenol analogs exhibited the cytotoxic activity against A549, KB, and KB-VCR cell lines.

Shikonin is the major constituent of *Arnebia euchroma(Royle)Johnst*, which has extensive pharmacological activities. Shikonin has good antioxidant activities, which supports the use of shikonin as the new anti-aging candidate drug, cosmetic materials and food additives. The results of Chen [15] revealed that SK-Hep-1 cells apoptosis induced by shikonin proceeds by involvement of reactive oxygen species and an oxidative stress-mediated pathway.

Baicalein, a kind of oriental medicine, exhibits antioxidant and anti-inflammatory activities. The results of Li-Weber [16] revealed that baicalein can inhibit several genes of the cell cycle, attenuate NF-κB activity, and scavenge many kinds of oxidative radicals.

Rosmarinic acid, isolated from *Perilla frutescens* (L.) or *Rosmarinus officinalis*, exhibits many potent biological activities. The result of Zhu [17] indicated that rosmarinic acid extract exhibits the high activity of inhibiting á-glucosidase for allergy treatments and diabetes mellitus.

Dihydromyricetin can be used to scavenge the free radicals. It also has the effects of anti-oxidation and anti-tumour. Based on the results of Xin [18], dihydromyricetin was less toxic and highly effective as a good, natural antioxidant for polypropylene.

This investigation tested the antityrosinase activity, the inhibition constant, and inhibition type of compounds. Molecular docking can simulate the binding mode and binding affinity of the tyrosinase and compounds. This investigation also tested the antioxidant effects of isoeugenol, shikonin, baicalein, rosmarinic acid, and dihydromyricetin on supercoiled pBR322 plasmid DNA, lipid peroxidation, and DPPH, ABTS, hydroxyl, or superoxide free radical scavenging activity in vitro.

Methods

Chemicals and reagents

Isoeugenol, shikonin, baicalein, rosmarinic acid, dihydromyricetin, L-3,4-dihydroxyphenylalanine (L-DOPA), tyrosinase (EC 1.14.18.1), phenanthroline, pyrogallol, 2, 2′-azino-bis (3-ethylbenzothiazoline-6-sulfonic acid) (ABTS), diphenyl-2-picrylhydrazyl (DPPH), thiobarbituric acid (TBA), and 2,2′-azobis(2-methylpropionamidine) dihydrochloride (AAPH) were purchased from the Sigma Chemical Company (St. Louis, MO, USA). C3606 reagent kit for organization mitochondria separation was purchased from Shanghai Biyuntian company. Disodium phosphate, sodium dihydrogen phosphate, $K_2S_2O_8$, potassium sulfate, and ferrous sulfate were purchased from Sinopharm Chemical Reagent Co., Ltd (Shanghai, China). All other solvents and chemicals with analytical grade were commercially available. The Minimum Standards of Reporting Checklist contains details of the experimental design, and statistics, and resources used in this study (Additional file 1).

Tyrosinase activity assay

According to the reference of Chen et al. [19], the tyrosinase activity was measured using L-DOPA as a substrate. Dimethyl sulfoxide (DMSO) was used to dissolve the inhibitor samples. L-DOPA in PBS buffer (pH 6.8) was previously incubated at 30 °C. Then, 0.1 mL sample was mixed with 2.8 mL L-DOPA (0.5 mM). After 1 min, the mixture was added to 0.1 mL of tyrosinase solution (5.33 μg/mL) at 475 nm for 400 s, the absorbance was immediately monitored. The relative enzyme activity was regarded as the slope of the linear part. The inhibitory concentration 50 (IC_{50}) was used to examined the antityrosinase activity. Each sample was examined in five times and averaged. The inhibitory rate was examined according to the formula:

$$\text{Inhibitory rate}(\%) = [(S_0 - S_1)/S_0] \times 100\% \qquad (1)$$

where S_1 is the slope value with samples and S_0 is the slope value without samples.

Determination of the inhibition type and inhibition constant

By Lineweaver–Burk plot, the inhibition type was assayed. The inhibition constant was assayed by the second plots of the apparent K_m/V_{mapp} or $1/V_{mapp}$ versus the concentration of the inhibitor.

Molecular docking study

Molecular docking can predict the binding mode and binding affinity of the tyrosinase and compounds. From the Protein Data Bank (UCSD/SDSC and Rutgers, http://www.rcsb.org/), the crystal structure of tyrosinase (PDB code: 2Y9X) was available [20]. The polar hydrogen was added and all ligands and bound water were eliminated. The ligands were used as configuration of each compound. Using Discovery Studio Version 4.5 (CDOCKER Dock, Dassault Systemes BIOVIA, USA), molecular docking was carried out and the interactions were analyzed [21].

DPPH free radical scavenging activity

According to the references of Lee et al. [22], DPPH free radical scavenging capacity was measured. In the tube, 1 mL of tested samples in different concentrations was added in turn. 3.5 mL of ethanol and 0.5 mL of 0.6 mmol/L DPPH methanol solution were added. In room temperature and a dark environment, the reaction lasted 30 min. The wavelength used was 517 nm. Each sample was examined in three times and averaged. The DPPH scavenging activity was examined according to the formula:

$$\text{DPPH scavenging activity } (\%) = [(A_C - A_S)/A_C] \times 100\% \qquad (2)$$

where A_S is the absorbance value with samples and A_C is the absorbance value without samples.

ABTS free radical scavenging activity

According to the references of Wan et al. [23], ABTS free radical scavenging capacity was measured. ABTS was dissolved in water to make 7 mmol/L ABTS water solution. ABTS $^+$ was produced by reacting 2.45 mmol/L potassium persulfate ($K_2S_2O_8$) with the ABTS stock solution. The reaction lasted 12–16 h at room temperature in the dark. The absorbance of $ABTS^+$ stock solution at 734 nm was 0.70 ± 0.02, diluted with methanol.

Samples (0.5 mL) were added to $ABTS^+$ (5 mL) for 6 min. The control group contains 0.5 mL of ethanol and 5 mL of $ABTS^+$ solution. Each sample was examined in three times and averaged. The $ABTS^+$ scavenging activity was examined according to the formula:

$$ABTS^+ \text{ scavenging activity } (\%) = [(A_C - A_S)/A_C] \times 100\% \qquad (3)$$

where A_S is the absorbance value with samples and A_C is the absorbance value without samples.

Hydroxyl free radical scavenging activity

According to the references of De Avellar IGJ et al. [24], hydroxyl free radical scavenging capacity was measured. In the tube, 0.2 mL of samples, 1 mL of PBS buffer (pH = 7.4),0.2 mL of 5 mmol/L phenanthroline, 0.2 mL of 7.5 mmol/L $FeSO_4$, 0.2 mL of 0.05% H_2O_2, 3.2 mL of ethanol were added in turn for 20 min in 37 °C. The wavelength used was 536 nm. Each sample was examined in three times and averaged. The hydroxyl free radical scavenging activity was examined according to the formula:

$$\text{Hydroxyl free radical scavenging activity (\%)} = [(A_C - A_S)/A_C] \times 100\% \quad (4)$$

where A_S is the absorbance value with samples and A_C is the absorbance value without samples.

Superoxide free radical scavenging activity

According to the references of Shen et al. [25], superoxide free radical scavenging capacity was measured using Varioskan Flash multifunction microplate reader (Thermo scientific, USA) and 96 wells plates. Each well was added 264 μL PBS buffer (pH=8.2), 12 μL samples of different concentrations, 25 °C for 10 min. Then 24 μL of 1.25 mmoL/L pyrogallol solution was added and shaken 3 s quickly. The blank group is ethanol. Absorbance values were measured every 30 s. The reaction lasted 5 min in 37 °C. The wavelength used was 320 nm. Each sample was measured in triplicate and averaged. The slope is the self-oxidation rate of pyrogallol. The lower slope indicated the better superoxide free radicals scavenging capacity.

Each sample was examined in three times and averaged. The inhibitory rate was examined according to the formula:

$$\text{Superoxide free radical scavenging activity (\%)} = [(S_C - S_S)/S_C] \times 100\% \quad (5)$$

where S_C is the slope value without samples and S_S is the slope value with samples.

Lipid peroxidation assay in liver mitochondria in vitro

Using the diagnostic kits from Biyuntian (Shanghai, China), liver mitochondria were obtained. The liver mitochondria from Sprague–Dawley (SD) rats were obtained, according to the references of Zuo et al. [26].

In the tubes, 1 mL of mitochondria liquid, 0.5 mL of antioxidant solution, 0.25 mL of 1 mM Vitamin C, and 0.25 mL of 0.1 mM Fe^{2+} were added in turn. The positive control group contains 0.5 mL of 0.05 M PBS buffer, instead of the antioxidant solution. The blank group was added 1 mL of mitochondrial liquid and 1 mL of 0.05 M PBS buffer. The reaction lasted for 1 h at 37 °C. 2.5% hydrochloric acid solution and 2 mL of 20% CCl_3COOH were added for 10 min, followed by 0.3% NaOH solution and 2 mL of 0.67% TBA were added. The test tubes were placed in the water for 30 min at 95 °C, then centrifuged for 10 min at 1372*g*. The wavelength used was 532 nm. Each sample was examined in three times and averaged. The lipid peroxidation inhibition activity was examined according to the formula:

$$\text{Lipid peroxidation inhibition activity (\%)} = [(A_C - A_S)/A_C] \times 100\% \quad (6)$$

where A_S is the absorbance value with samples and A_C is the absorbance value without samples.

Supercoiled pBR322 plasmid DNA assay

According to the references of Lin et al., and Zuo et al. [27, 28], supercoiled pBR322 plasmid DNA assay was measured. Briefly, 10 mM AAPH in PBS (pH 7.4) was added 100 ng of pBR322 DNA to a final volume of 25 μL in microcentrifuge tubes at 37 °C for 1 h. The 25 μL solution contains 15 μL AAPH, 5 μL DNA, 5 μL antioxidants. Five microliter distilled water was used in the absence of antioxidants. After incubation, 2 μL 10× loading buffer were mixed with the samples, loaded into a 0.8% agarose gel. The agarose gel was electrophoresed in 1× TAE gel buffer for 75 min (20 mA, 50 V). Using the Bio-Rad Gel Doc XR system (New York, America), the gels were then photographed under UV transillumination. DNA strand breaks were evaluated. The amount of supercoiled DNA was quantified by the Bio-Rad Quantity One software.

One-way ANOVA was used to analyze the differences among means, and statistically significant was considered by a $P < 0.05$ value (SPSS version 13.0, SPSS).

Results

Tyrosinase activity assay

The substrate of tyrosinase for the diphenolase activity assay was L-DOPA. The results showed that a group of lines with different slopes passing through the origin was the progress curve of enzyme reaction. The slope indicated the diphenolase activity. In the progress of oxidation of L-DOPA, the lag period did not exist. Isoeugenol, shikonin, baicalein, rosmarinic acid, and dihydromyricetin exhibited, with dose dependence, inhibitory effect on tyrosinase diphenolase activity. The IC_{50} values of the five compounds on the tyrosinase diphenolase activity were respectively 33.33 μmol/L, 26.67 μmol/L, 13.33 μmol/L, 6.67 μmol/L, and 3.33 μmol/L ($n=5$, $P<0.05$, Fig. 1; Table 1). The order of activity was: isoeugenol < shikonin < baicalein < rosmarinic acid < dihydromyricetin. Therefore, the five compounds had obvious inhibitory effects on the tyrosinase diphenolase activity. The order of activity was very consistent with the docking score between tyrosinase and compounds.

Inhibition mechanism on the diphenolase activity of tyrosinase

The inhibitory mechanism of isoeugenol, shikonin, baicalein, rosmarinic acid, and dihydromyricetin on tyrosinase for oxidation of L-DOPA was examined. The relationship between the concentration of five compounds and

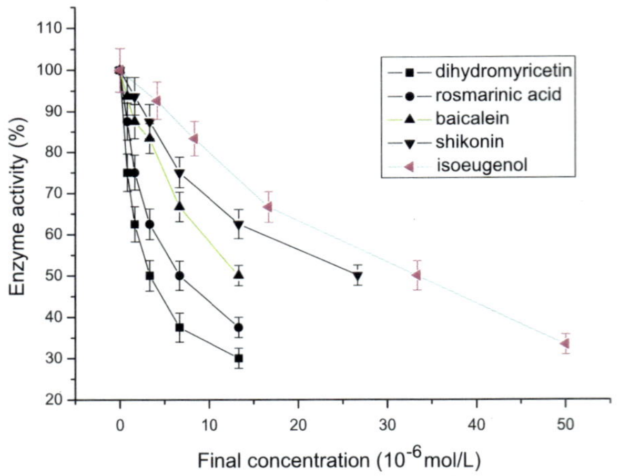

Fig. 1 The inhibition effects of isoeugenol, shikonin, baicalein, rosmarinic acid, and dihydromyricetin on the diphenolase activity of mushroom tyrosinase. The IC_{50} values of the five compounds on the tyrosinase diphenolase activity were respectively 33.33 μmol/L, 26.67 μmol/L, 13.33 μmol/L, 6.67 μmol/L, and 3.33 μmol/L (n = 5, P < 0.05)

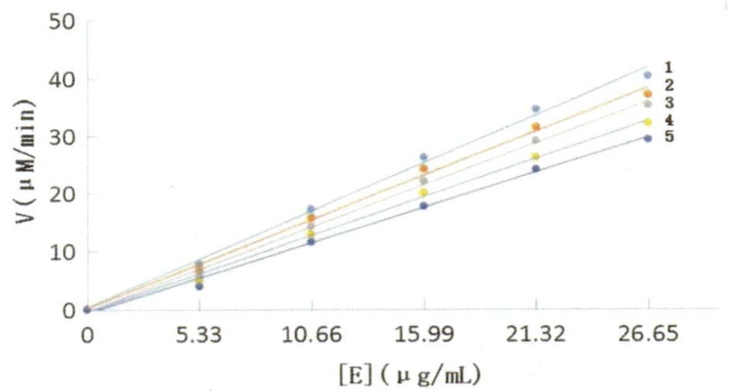

Fig. 2 Determination of the inhibitory mechanism of shikonin on mushroom tyrosinase. The results showed that shikonin was reversible inhibitor of tyrosinase for the oxidation of L-DOPA. L-DOPA = L-3,4-dihydroxyphenylalanine

enzyme activity was examined. The inhibitory mechanism of shikonin on tyrosinase was tested. As shown in Fig. 2, at different inhibitor concentrations, the plots of enzyme activity versus the enzyme concentration gave a family of straight lines, which all passed through the origin. The final concentration of shikonin for curves 1–5 was respectively 0 μmol/L, 3.3 μmol/L, 6.67 μmol/L, 13.33 μmol/L, and 26.67 μmol/L. The presence of an inhibitor resulted in the inhibition of enzyme activity, but did not reduce the amount of enzyme. The inhibitors showed the same behavior. The results exhibited that isoeugenol, shikonin, baicalein, rosmarinic acid, and dihydromyricetin were reversible inhibitors of tyrosinase diphenolase.

By Lineweaver–Burk double-reciprocal plots for the inhibition tyrosinase diphenolase, the inhibition type of the five compounds was examined. The enzyme kinetics in the presence of shikonin are shown in Fig. 3. The final concentration of shikonin for curves 1–6 was respectively 0 μmol/L, 3.3 μmol/L, 6.67 μmol/L, 13.33 μmol/L, 26.67 μmol/Land 33.33 μmol/L. Lineweaver–Burk double-reciprocal plots were the plots of 1/v versus 1/[S]. A family of straight lines intercepted in the second quadrant, which indicated that shikonin was a competitive–uncompetitive mixed type inhibitor (Fig. 3a). It indicated that shikonin can combine with not only enzyme–substrate complexes, but also free enzymes. From a plot of the slope (K_m/V_{mapp}) versus the concentration of the inhibitor, K_I was measured (Fig. 3b). From a plot of the vertical intercept ($1/V_{mapp}$) versus the concentration of inhibitor, K_{IS} was measured (Fig. 3c). The values of K_I and K_{IS} were determined as 19.0 μM and 48.6 μM, respectively. By contrast, isoeugenol was the same inhibitor type as shikonin, and the inhibitor constants (K_I and K_{IS}) were determined as 25.6 μM and 64.7 μM, respectively. Baicalein was the same inhibitor type as shikonin, and the inhibitor constants (K_I and K_{IS}) were determined as 16.5 μM and 38.4 μM, respectively. Rosmarinic acid was the same inhibitor type as shikonin, and the inhibitor constants (K_I and K_{IS}) were determined as 14.3 μM and 29.8 μM, respectively. Dihydromyricetin was the same inhibitor type as shikonin, and the inhibitor constants (K_I and K_{IS}) were determined as 10.26 μM and 23.6 μM, respectively.

Table 1 The IC_{50} values of flavonoids

	Isoeugenol	Shikonin	Baicalein	Rosmarinic acid	Dihydromyricetin
Tyrosinase diphenolase activity (μmol/L)	33.33	26.67	13.33	6.67	3.33
DPPH free radical (μmol/L)	101.6	83.2	58.6	28.5	12.4
ABTS free radical (μmol/L)	36.36	27.27	9.09	6.82	3.41
Hydroxyl free radical (μmol/L)	32.5	18.3	11.6	8.3	4.2
Superoxide free radical (μmol/L)	38.2	31.5	16.1	12.3	7.6
Lipid peroxidation (μmol/L)	25.1	16.67	12.5	8.33	6.25

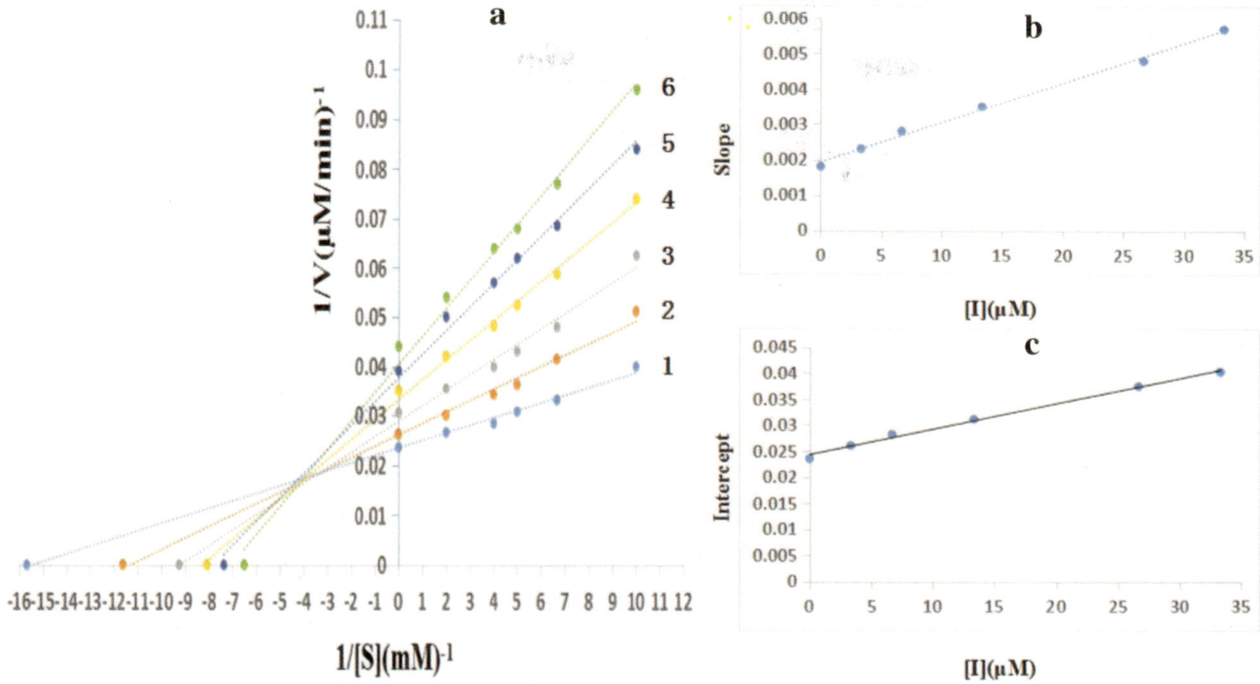

Fig. 3 **a** Lineweaver–Burk plots for the inhibition of shikonin on mushroom tyrosinase for the oxidation of L-DOPA. **b** The plot of slope versus the concentration of shikonin for determining the inhibition constants K_I. $K_I = 19$ μmol/L. **c** The plot of intercept versus the concentration of shikonin for determining the inhibition constants K_{IS}. $K_{IS} = 48.6$ μmol/L. K_I = equilibrium constant for inhibitor binding with free enzyme; K_{IS} = enzyme–substrate complex; L-DOPA = L-3,4-dihydroxyphenylalanine

Molecular docking

Figure 4 shows that docking simulations colored 2D-representations of binding mode and binding position between tyrosinase and compound isoeugenol (a), shikonin (b), baicalein (c), rosmarinic acid (d), and dihydromyricetin (e), respectively. The binding interactions between tyrosinase and compound include mainly the pi–pi stacked, conventional hydrogen bond, pi–alkyl, and alkyl. Molecular docking results implied that the compounds could interact with the amino acid residues in the active center of tyrosinase.

The docking score between tyrosinase and compound isoeugenol, shikonin, baicalein, rosmarinic acid, and dihydromyricetin was 33.14, 36.13, 37.93, 44.56, 50.98, respectively. The order of activity was: isoeugenol < shikonin < baicalein < rosmarinic acid < dihydromyricetin. The order of activity was very consistent with the experimental results (Fig. 1). Docking score indicates the interaction affinity between enzyme and ligand by the optimized algorithm, which helps to speculate the scope of inhibitory activity. The main significance of docking score is the evaluation index for quick preliminary screening compounds. In this paper, based on the docking score, the inhibit tyrosinase activity of five typical compounds was verified by the experiments in vitro.

Figure 5 shows that docking simulations of conformational changes and binding position between tyrosinase and inhibitors. Colored 3D-representations of the protein–ligand complex showed that surface and conformation changes of compounds before (a) and after (b) docking into tyrosinase. Docking simulations of binding position of compound isoeugenol (A), shikonin (B), baicalein (C), rosmarinic acid (D), and dihydromyricetin (E), respectively, in the hydrophobic pocket of tyrosinase (c), which indicates the inhibition mechanism on the diphenolase activity of tyrosinase.

The combination mode and binding sites of tyrosinase and five typical compounds were studied by molecular simulation. The results showed that these compounds enter the hydrophobic activity cavity of tyrosinase, change the enzyme conformation, which in turn affect the catalytic activity. The hydrogen bonds between Met 280, Val 283, His 85 residues and compounds, the pi–pi bonds between Phe 264, His 244, His 259, or His 263 and compounds or pi–alkyl bonds between Val 283, Val 248 and compounds, may be related to the identification and fix the ligand and tyrosinase. Besides phenolic hydroxyls, the scaffold components of different compounds may also effect on their antityrosinase activities. Particularly, different hydrophobic groups may have significant contribution to binding with the hydrophobic cavity of the target proteins. The molecular docking results showed the detailed information and the visual evidence of the binding position

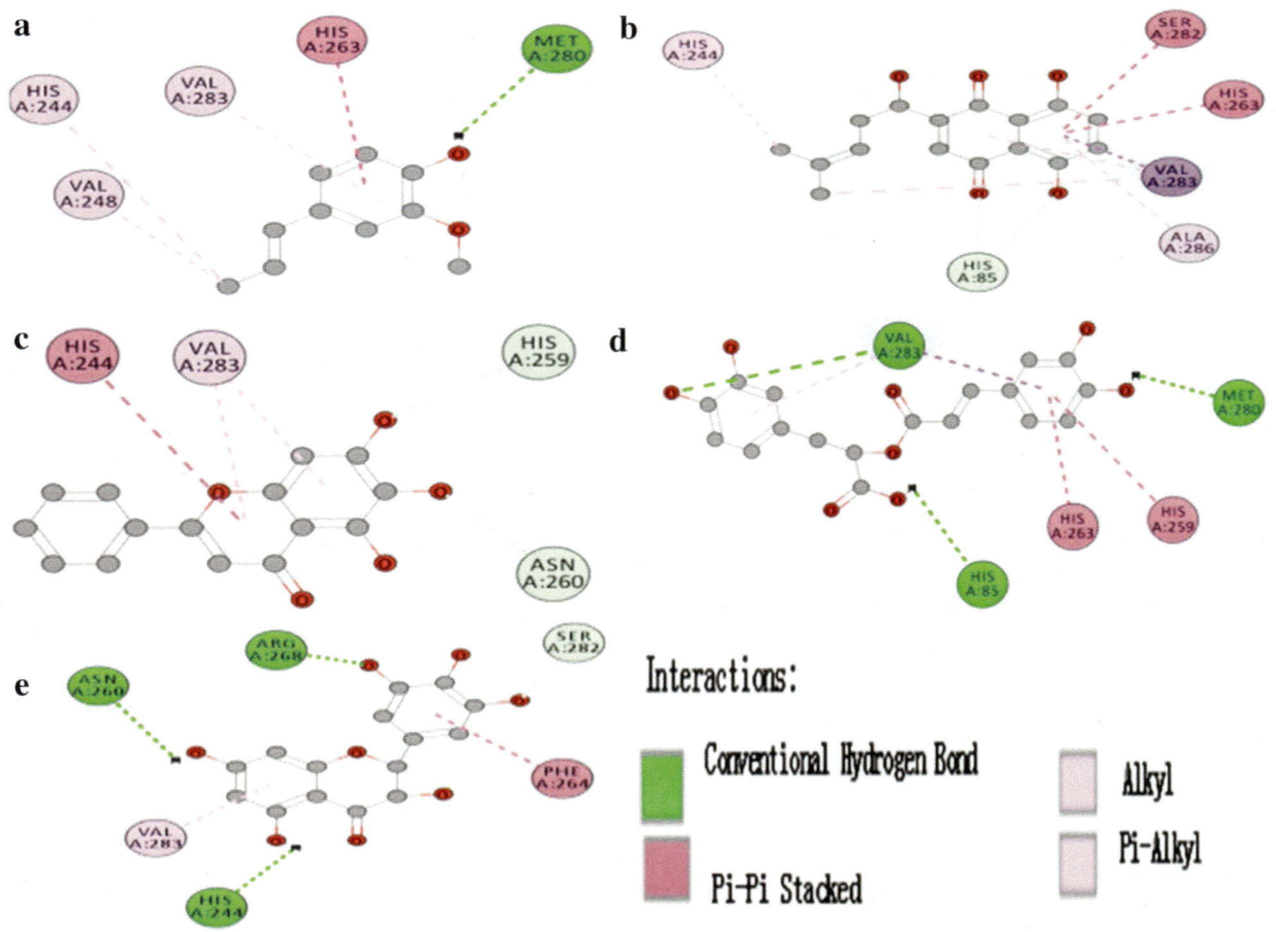

Fig. 4 Docking simulations 2D diagram of binding position and binding mode between tyrosinase and compound isoeugenol (**a**), shikonin (**b**), baicalein (**c**), rosmarinic acid (**d**), and dihydromyricetin (**e**), respectively

between the tyrosinase and inhibitors. The similar binding position and binding mode may be the similar inhibition mechanism. However, without any experimental evidence, the developed models will be too early to be applicable for antityrosinase activity of compounds. The result of Seo [29] indicated that CDOCKER and CDOCKER interaction energies of quercetin and its analogues were decreased by C151W mutation whereas benzoic acid and its analogues did not lower the energies. In particular, the results illustrated the blockage of pi–pi stacked or pi–alkyl interactions between quercetin and quercetin-4′-methyl ether and His154 or Val132. These results indicate that the influence of Cys 151 residue of Keap1 keeps on the interaction between compounds and Keap1 protein.

DPPH free radical scavenging activity

Figure 6 shows that isoeugenol, shikonin, baicalein, rosmarinic acid, and dihydromyricetin had obvious DPPH free radical scavenging activity. The IC_{50} values of DPPH free radical scavenging capacity of isoeugenol, shikonin, baicalein, rosmarinic acid, and dihydromyricetin were respectively 101.6 μmol/L, 83.2 μmol/L, 58.6 μmol/L, 28.5 μmol/L, and 12.4 μmol/L ($n=3$, $P<0.05$, Table 1). The order of activity was: isoeugenol < shikonin < baicalein < rosmarinic acid < dihydromyricetin.

The result of Zhu [17] indicated that IC_{50} of DPPH radical scavenging activity of rosmarinic acid extract was 5.5 ± 0.2 μg/mL, and IC_{50} of α-glucosidase inhibitory activity was 0.23 ± 0.01 mg/mL. The result of Liu [30] showed that IC_{50} of DPPH radical scavenging activity of the dihydromyricetin–lecithin complex was 22.60 μg/mL. The result of Xu [31] showed that the scavenging capacity of hydroxyl radical (·OH), superoxide radical (O_2·), and alkane radical (ROO·) for dihydromyricetin was 83.9%, 90.0%, and 63.9% respectively.

ABTS free radical scavenging activity

Figure 7 shows that isoeugenol, shikonin, baicalein, rosmarinic acid, and dihydromyricetin had obvious ABTS

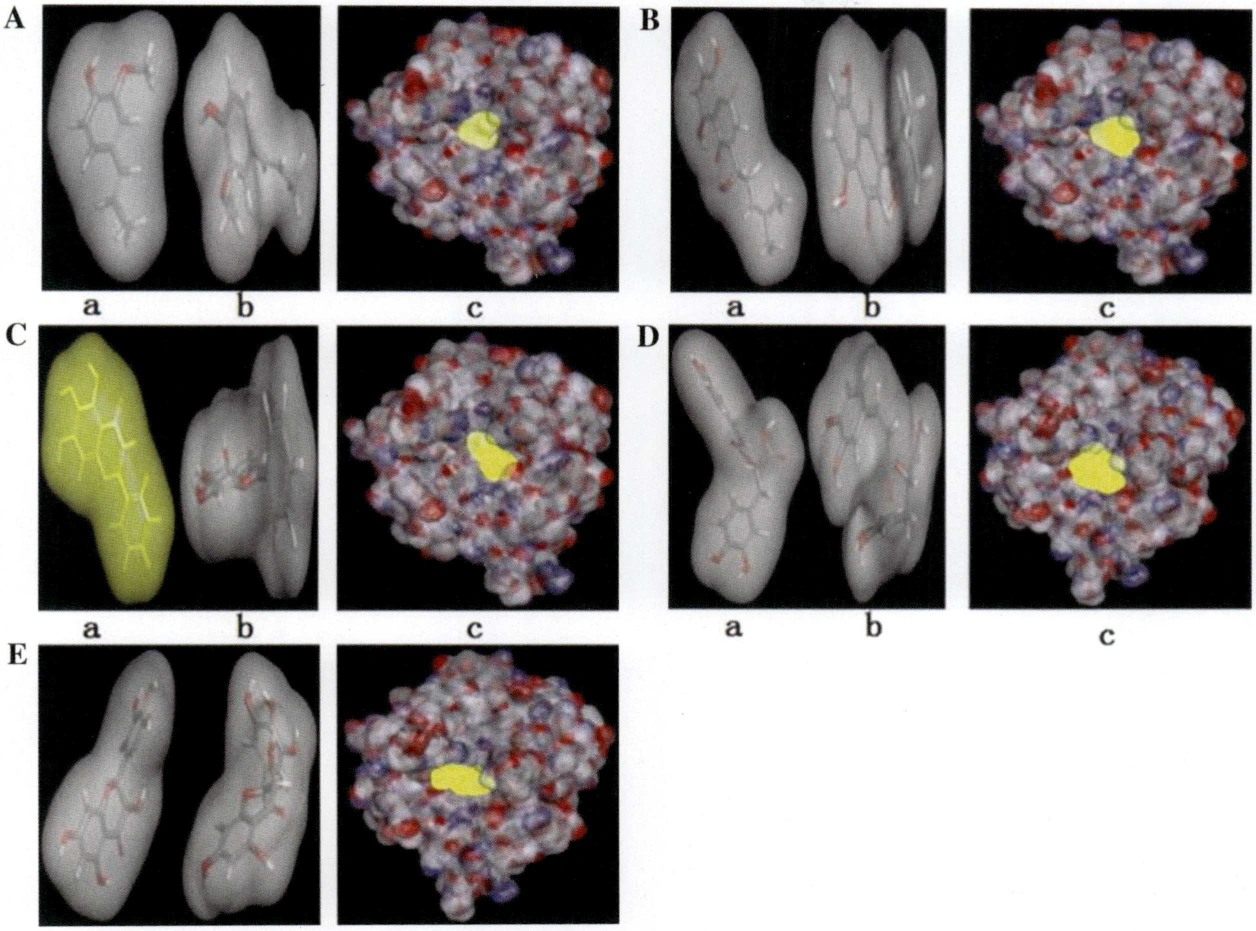

Fig. 5 Colored 3D-representations of the protein–ligand complex showed that surface and conformation changes of compounds before (a) and after (b) docking into tyrosinase, and docking simulation of compound isoeugenol (**A**), shikonin (**B**), baicalein (**C**), rosmarinic acid (**D**), and dihydromyricetin (**E**), respectively, in the hydrophobic pocket of tyrosinase (c)

free radical scavenging activity. The IC_{50} values of ABTS free radical scavenging capacity of isoeugenol, shikonin, baicalein, rosmarinic acid, and dihydromyricetin were respectively 36.36 μmol/L, 27.27 μmol/L, 9.09 μmol/L, 6.82 μmol/L, and 3.41 μmol/L ($n=3$, $P<0.05$, Table 1). The order of activity was: isoeugenol < shikonin < baicalein < rosmarinic acid < dihydromyricetin.

Hydroxyl free radical scavenging activity

Figure 8 shows that isoeugenol, shikonin, baicalein, rosmarinic acid, and dihydromyricetin had obvious hydroxyl free radical scavenging activity. The IC_{50} values of hydroxyl free radical scavenging capacity of isoeugenol, shikonin, baicalein, rosmarinic acid, and dihydromyricetin were respectively 32.5 μmol/L, 18.3 μmol/L, 11.6 μmol/L, 8.3 μmol/L, and 4.2 μmol/L ($n=3$, $P<0.05$, Table 1). The order of activity was: isoeugenol < shikonin < baicalein < rosmarinic acid < dihydromyricetin.

Superoxide free radical scavenging activity

Figure 9 shows that isoeugenol, shikonin, baicalein, rosmarinic acid, and dihydromyricetin had obvious superoxide free radical scavenging activity. The IC_{50} values of superoxide free radical scavenging capacity of isoeugenol, shikonin, baicalein, rosmarinic acid, and dihydromyricetin were respectively 38.2 μmol/L, 31.5 μmol/L, 16.1 μmol/L, 12.3 μmol/L, and 7.6 μmol/L ($n=3$, $P<0.05$, Table 1). The order of activity was: isoeugenol < shikonin < baicalein < rosmarinic acid < dihydromyricetin.

Lipid peroxidation assay in liver mitochondria in vitro

Figure 10 shows that isoeugenol, shikonin, baicalein, rosmarinic acid, and dihydromyricetin had obvious activity of inhibiting lipid peroxidation. The IC_{50} values of inhibiting lipid peroxidation of isoeugenol, shikonin, baicalein, rosmarinic acid, and dihydromyricetin were respectively 25.1 μmol/L, 16.67 μmol/L, 12.5 μmol/L, 8.33 μmol/L, and 6.25 μmol/L ($n=3$, $P<0.05$, Table 1). The order

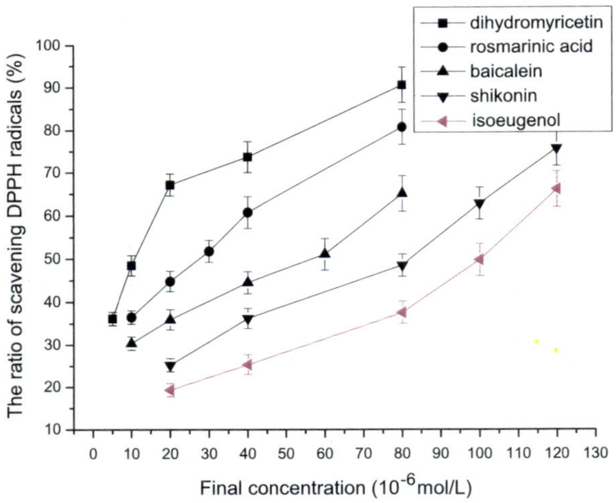

Fig. 6 The relationship between final concentration and the ratio of scavenging DPPH radicals. The IC_{50} values of DPPH free radical scavenging capacity of isoeugenol, shikonin, baicalein, rosmarinic acid, and dihydromyricetin were respectively 101.6 μmol/L, 83.2 μmol/L, 58.6 μmol/L, 28.5 μmol/L, and 12.4 μmol/L (n = 3, $P < 0.05$). *DPPH* 1,1-diphenyl-2-picrylhydrazyl

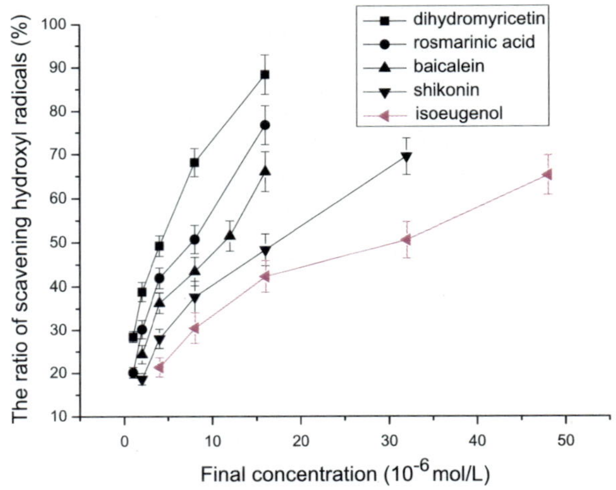

Fig. 8 The relationship between final concentration and the ratio of scavenging hydroxyl radicals. The IC_{50} values of hydroxyl free radical scavenging capacity of isoeugenol, shikonin, baicalein, rosmarinic acid, and dihydromyricetin were respectively 32.5 μmol/L, 18.3 μmol/L, 11.6 μmol/L, 8.3 μmol/L, and 4.2 μmol/L (n = 3, $P < 0.05$)

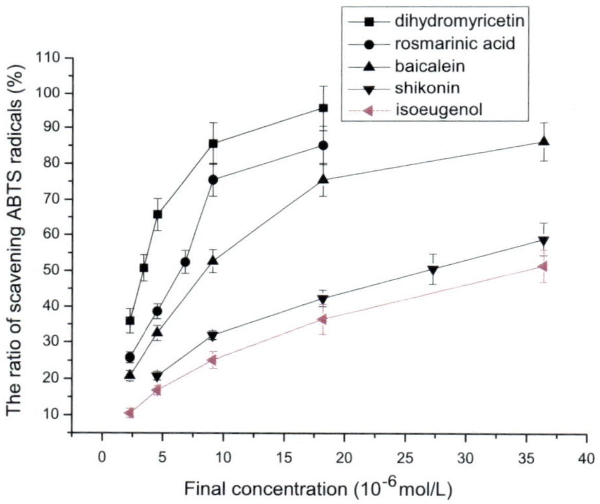

Fig. 7 The relationship between final concentration and the ratio of scavenging ABTS radicals. The IC_{50} values of ABTS free radical scavenging capacity of isoeugenol, shikonin, baicalein, rosmarinic acid, and dihydromyricetin were respectively 36.36 μmol/L, 27.27 μmol/L, 9.09 μmol/L, 6.82 μmol/L, and 3.41 μmol/L (n = 3, $P < 0.05$). ABTS = 2,2′-azino-bis-(3-ethylbenzothiazoline-6-sulphonic acid)

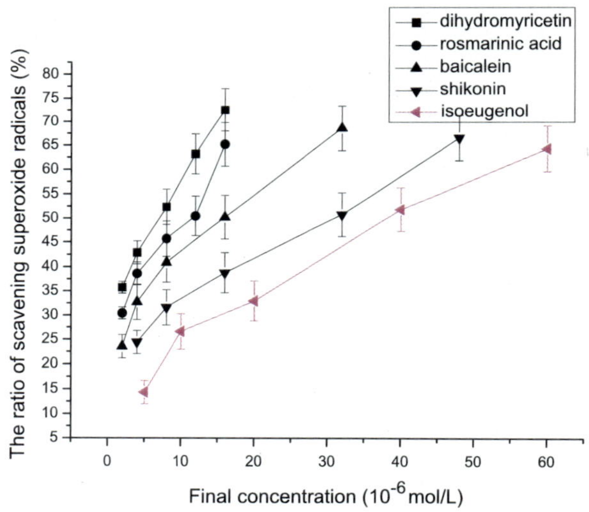

Fig. 9 The relationship between final concentration and the ratio of scavenging superoxide radicals. The IC_{50} values of superoxide free radical scavenging capacity of isoeugenol, shikonin, baicalein, rosmarinic acid, and dihydromyricetin were respectively 38.2 μmol/L, 31.5 μmol/L, 16.1 μmol/L, 12.3 μmol/L, and 7.6 μmol/L (n = 3, $P < 0.05$)

of activity was: isoeugenol < shikonin < baicalein < rosmarinic acid < dihydromyricetin.

Supercoiled pBR322 plasmid DNA assay

Figure 11a shows that in the absence of AAPH, the plasmid DNA was mainly supercoiled. The supercoiled form of plasmid DNA was changed into the linear forms and open circular with the addition of 10 mM AAPH. In the presence of 10 μM compounds, the amount of supercoiled form increased, but the amount of the linear and circular forms decreased. The amount of supercoiled plasmid DNA was quantified by the Bio-Rad Quantity One software. Figure 11b shows the observed values. Thus, these compounds exhibited

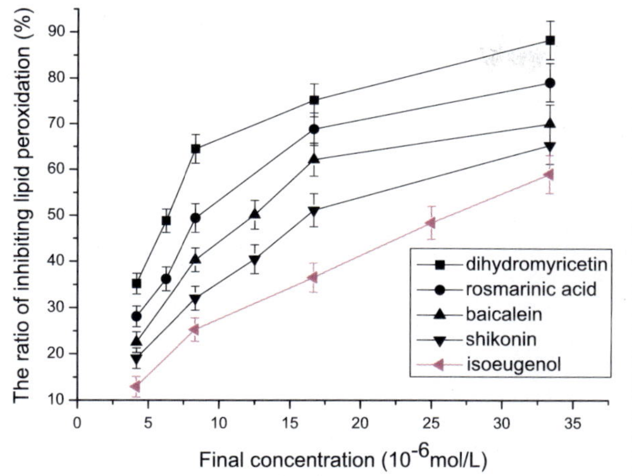

Fig. 10 The relationship between final concentration and the ratio of inhibiting lipid peroxidation. The IC_{50} values of inhibiting lipid peroxidation of isoeugenol, shikonin, baicalein, rosmarinic acid, and dihydromyricetin were respectively 25.1 μmol/L, 16.67 μmol/L, 12.5 μmol/L, 8.33 μmol/L, and 6.25 μmol/L ($n = 3$, $P < 0.05$)

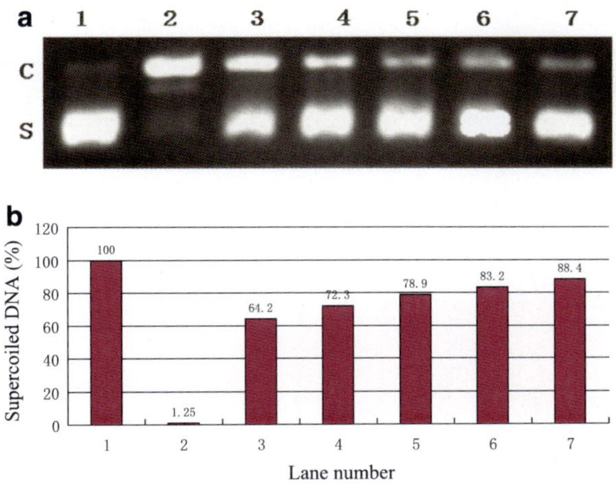

Fig. 11 **a** Agarose gel electrophoretic patterns of supercoiled pBR322 plasmid DNA converted into the open circular by AAPH in the presence or absence of samples (10 μM). **b** The effects of samples on supercoiled pBR322 plasmid DNAconverted into the open circular by AAPH in the presence or absence of samples(10 μM). Lane 1: control (native pBR322 DNA, without AAPH); Lane 2: AAPH; Lane 3: AAPH + isoeugenol; Lane 4: AAPH + shikonin; Lane 5: AAPH + baicalein; Lane 6: AAPH + rosmarinic acid; Lane 7: AAPH + dihydromyricetin. The density of the supercoiled DNA form was quantified by Quantity One (Bio-Rad). Data are the average of three determinations; *C* open circular, *S* supercoil, *AAPH* 2,2′-azobis(2-methylpropionamidine)dihydrochloride

protection against free radical injury induced by AAPH in a dose-dependent manner. The order of inhibition activity was: isoeugenol < shikonin < baicalein < rosmarinic acid < dihydromyricetin.

An index of DNA damage is used as the change of bacteriophage or plasmid DNA from the supercoiled form to the linear forms. Strand breaks in pBR322 DNA can be caused by the presence of AAPH [32].

Discussion

Isoeugenol is the major constituent of *E. caryophyllata* Thunb. The result of Hubungan [33] indicated that antioxidant activities in the following orders: butylated hydroxytoluene (BHT) > mannich product of isoeugenol > isoeugenol > mannich product of eugenol > eugenol. The result of Ko [34] indicated that demethyldi-isoeugenol inhibited Fe^{2+}-induced lipid peroxidation. It also scavenged superoxide anion generated by peroxyl radical (ROO.) derived from AAPH.

Shikonin is the major constituent of *Arnebia euchroma(Royle)Johnst.* The observed results revealed that shikonin demonstrated higher reducing ability (0.431%), and deoxy-shikonin showed maximum inhibition (0.440%) to DPPH-radical scavenging assay.

Baicalein is the major constituent of *Rheum officinale*. The results of Nishioka [35] revealed that baicalein can inhibit the express of human intestinal sucrase in the Caco-2 cells. The results of Tsai [36] revealed that baicalein can protect against the acute lung injury induced by lipopolysaccharide in rats. The results of Jeli [37] revealed that baicalein exhibit good inhibitory activities of both production of cytokine IL-6 and tyrosine kinase.

Rosmarinic acid can inhibit the enzymatic browning of fruits and vegetables. The result of Ha [38] showed that rosmarinic acid possess mushroom tyrosinase inhibitory activities (IC_{50} of 4.0 μM). The result of Ding [39] showed that rosmarinic acid methyl ester can inhibit tyrosinase, and reduce the melanin contents in B16 cells. The result of Fujimoto [40] showed that rosmarinic acid afforded a highly tyrosinase-inhibitory active product. Rosmarinic acid has antioxidant and prooxidant activities. The result of Sánchez-Campillo [41] indicated that rosmarinic acid can be used as a good photo-protective agent.

Zhao et al. [42] evaluated the antioxidant properties of Citri Exocarpium Rubrum based on its DPPH free radical scavenging activity, ferric ion reducing antioxidant power (FRAP) and trolox equivalent antioxidant capacity (TEAC) assays. Bivariate correlation analysis revealed correlations between the characteristic peaks and the antioxidant activities of the samples. *Sambucus williamsii* Hance (*Jiegumu*) is traditionally used in Chinese medicine to treat bone and joint diseases. The major phytochemicals are phenolic acids, lignans, and terpenoids. This compounds may have the antioxidant, anti-inflammatory, bone fracture healing, and anti-osteoporotic effects [43].

Tyrosinase (EC 1.14.18.1) play a key role in melanin biosynthesis [44]. Due to the over expression of tyrosinase, excessive melanin leads to melasma and age spots [45]. Tyrosinase is responsible for the browning of vegetables and fruits in the food industry, which results in reduced market value and shorter product shelf life [46]. Increased attention has also drawn to the applications of antioxidants and tyrosinase inhibitors as preservatives in skin-protective ingredients in cosmetics and in the food industry. On the other hand, ROS could induce oxidative damage of proteins and DNA, and peroxidation of membrane lipids. Lipid peroxidation will generate malondialdehyde (MDA), and do harm to cells [47]. It may be useful in diets to obtain properly antioxidants.

Conclusion

In conclusion, isoeugenol, shikonin, baicalein, rosmarinic acid, and dihydromyricetin exhibited good antityrosinase activities. These compounds also exhibited good antioxidant effects on lipid peroxidation, supercoiled pBR322 plasmid DNA, and DPPH, ABTS, hydroxyl, or superoxide free radical scavenging activity. The different molecular structures lead to the different antityrosinase and antioxidant activities. The activity order is isoeugenol < shikonin < baicalein < rosmarinic acid < dihydromyricetin. The results showed the compounds with more phenolic hydroxyls have more antioxidant and antityrosinase activities. This was the first study of molecular docking for modeling the antityrosinase activity of compounds. This was also the first study of the lipid peroxidation inhibition activity of compounds in liver mitochondria induced by Fe^{2+}/vitamin C(Vc) system in vitro, the protective effects on supercoiled pBR322 plasmid DNA. In a word, the results support the use of compounds as the new anti-aging candidate drugs, cosmetic materials and food additives.

Abbreviations

ROS: reactive oxygen species; L-DOPA: L-3,4-dihydroxyphenylalanine; DPPH: diphenyl-2-picrylhydrazyl; TBA: thiobarbituric acid; ABTS: 2, 2′-azino-bis (3-ethylbenzothiazoline-6-sulfonic acid); AAPH: 2,2′-azobis(2-methylpropionamidine)dihydrochloride; DMSO: dimethyl sulfoxide; IC50: inhibitory concentration 50.

Authors' contributions

ARZ, SWC, and QLS proposed and designed the experiment. HHD, YYY, LXZ, and XYY were involved in the experiment. SWC and QLS revised the manuscript and were responsible for the overall research. All authors read and approveed the final manuscript.

Author details

[1] State Key Laboratory of Food Science and Technology, Nanchang University, Nanchang 330047, Jiangxi, China. [2] Jiangxi University of Traditional Chinese Medicine, Nanchang, Jiangxi, China. [3] Department of Chemistry, Nanchang University, Nanchang, Jiangxi, China.

Acknowledgements

Not applicable.

Competing interests

The authors declare that they have no competing interests.

Consent for publication

Not applicable.

Funding

This project was supported by the National Natural Sciences Foundation of China (Nos. 20962014, 81473455, 31560038), the Traditional Chinese Medicine Sciences Foundation of Jiangxi (Nos. 2015A042, 2017A288), and the Sciences Foundation of Jiangxi University of Traditional Chinese Medicine (No. 201610412020).

References

1. Kim D, Park J, Kim J. Flavonoids as mushroom tyrosinase inhibitors: a fluorescence quenching study. J Agric Food Chem. 2006;54:935–41.
2. Khatib S, Nerya O, Musa R. Chalcones as potent tyrosinase inhibitors: the importance of a 2,4-substituted resorcinol moiety. Bioorg Med Chem. 2005;13:433–41.
3. Shimizu K, Kondo R, Sakai K. Inhibition of tyrosinase by flavonoids, stilbenes and related 4–substituted resorcinols: structure-activity investigations. Planta Med. 2000;66:11–5.
4. Nerya O, Musa R, Khatib S. Chalcones as potent tyrosinase inhibitors: the effect of hydroxyl positions and numbers. Phytochem. 2004;65:1389–95.
5. Shimizu K, Yasutake S, Kondo R. A new stilbene with tyrosinase inhibitory activity from Chlorophora excelsa. Chem Pharm Bull. 2003;51:318–9.
6. Kenji O, Toshiyuki T, Tetsuro I. Inhibitory effects of resveratrol derivatives from dipterocarpaceae plants on tyrosinase activity. Biosci Biotechnol Biochem. 2003;67:1587–9.
7. Ohguchi K, Tanaka T, Iliya I. Gnetol as a potent tyrosinase inhibitor from Genus Gnetum. Biosci Bio-technol Biochem. 2003;67:663–5.
8. Thomeby-andersson K, Sterner O, Hansson C. Tyrosi-nase-mediated formation of a reactive quinone from the depigmenting agents, 4-tert-butyphenol and 4-tert-butyl-catechol. Pigment Cell Res. 2000;13:33–8.
9. Seyoum A, Asres K, El-Fiky FK. Structure-radical scavenging activity relationships of flavonoids. Phytochem. 2006;67:2058–70.
10. Cai YZ, Sun M, Xing J. Structure-radical scavenging activity relationships of phenolic compounds from traditional Chinese medicinal plants. Life Sci. 2006;78:2872–88.
11. Ferro S, De Luca L, Germano MP, Buemi MR, Lelo L. Chemical exploration of 4-(4-fluorobenzyl) piperidine fragment for the development of new tyrosinase inhibitors. Eur J Med Chem. 2017;125:591–8.
12. Pillaiyar T, Manickam M, Namasivayam V. Skin whitening agents: medicinal chemistry perspective of tyrosinase inhibitors. J Enzyme Inhib Med Chem. 2017;32:403–25.
13. Wang JL, Cheng LP, Wang TC, Deng W, Wu FH. Molecular modeling study of CP-690550 derivatives as JAK3 kinase inhitors through combined 3D-QSAR, molecular docking, and dynamics simulation techbiques. J Mol Graph Model. 2017;72:178–86.
14. Jin T. Dehydrozingerone, chalcone, and isoeugenol analogues as in vitro anticancer agents. J Nat Prod. 2006;69:1445–9.
15. Chen CH. Involvement of reactive oxygen species, but not mitochondrial permeability transition in the apoptotic induction of human SK-Hep-1 hepatoma cells by shikonin. Planta Med. 2003;69:1119–24.
16. Li-Weber M. New therapeutic aspects of flavones: the anticancer properties of Scutellaria and its main active constituents Wogonin, Baicalein and Baicalin. Cancer Treat Rev. 2009;35:57–68.
17. Zhu F, Asada T, Sato A. Rosmarinic acid extract for antioxidant, antiallergic, and α-glucosidase inhibitory activities, isolated by supramolecular technique and solvent extraction from Perilla leaves. J Agric Food Chem. 2014;62:885–92.

18. Xin ML, Ma Y, Lin W, Xu K, Chen M. Use of dihydromyricetin as antioxidant for polypropylene stabilization. J Therm Anal Calori. 2015;120:1741–7.
19. Chen LH, Hu YH, Song W, Song KK, Liu X, Chen QX. Synthesis and antityrosinase mechanism of benzaldehyde thiosemicarbazones: novel tyrosinase inhibitors. J Agric Food Chem. 2012;60:1542–9.
20. Dong HH, Liu J, Liu XR, Yu YY, Cao SW. Molecular docking and QSAR analyses of aromatic heterocycle thiosemicarbazone analogues for finding novel tyrosinase inhibitors. Bioorg Chem. 2017;75:106–17.
21. Dong HH, Liu J, Liu XR, Yu YY, Cao SW. Combining molecular docking and QSAR studies for modeling the antityrosinase activity of aromatic heterocycle thiosemicarbazone analogues. J Mol Struct. 2018;1151:353–65.
22. Lee YL, Yang JH, Mau JL. Antioxidant properties of water extracts from Monascus fermented soybeans. Food Chem. 2008;106:1127–37.
23. Wan CP, Yu YY, Zhou SR, Liu W, Cao SW. Antioxidant activity and free radical-scavenging capacity of Gynura divaricata leaf extracts at different temperatures. Phcog Mag. 2011;7:40–5.
24. De Avellar IGJ, Magalhaas MMM, Silvan AB. Reevaluating the role of 1,10-phenanthroline in oxidative reactions involving ferrous ions and DNA damage. BBA-Gen Subjects. 2004;1675:46–53.
25. Shen J, Huang C, Jiang L, Gao F. Enhancement of cisplatin induced apoptosis by suberoylanilide hydroxamic acid in human oral squamous cell carcinoma cell lines. Biochem Pharmacol. 2007;73:1901–9.
26. Zuo AR, Yu YY, Li J, Xu BB, Yu XY, Qiu Y, Cao SW. Study on the relation of structure and antioxidant activity of isorhamnetin, quercetin, phloretin, silybin and phloretin isonicotinyl hydrazone. Free Rad Antiox. 2011;1:39–47.
27. Lin X, Yang DJ, Cai WQ, Zhao QY, Gao YF, Chen Q, Wang R. Endomorphins, endogenous opioid peptides, provide antioxidant defense in the brain against free radical-induced damage. BBA-Mol Basis Dis. 2003;195:1639–45.
28. Zuo AR, Yu YY, Shu QL, Zheng LX, Wang XM, Peng SH, Xie YF, Cao SW. Hepatoprotective effects and antioxidant, antityrosinase activities of phloretin and phloretin isonicotinyl hydrazone. J Chin Med Assoc. 2014;77:290–301.
29. Seo JY, Kim SK, Nguyen PH, Lee JY, Tung PHT, Sung SH, Oh WK. Chemical constituents from a *Gynostemma laxum* and their antioxidant and neuroprotective activities. Chin Med. 2017;12:15–27.
30. Liu BG, Du JQ, Zeng J, Chen CG, Niu SY. Characterization and antioxidant activity of dihydromyricetin–lecithin complex. Eur Food Res Technol. 2009;230:325–31.
31. Xu JJ, Yao MY, Xu G. Study on antioxidant activities of dihydromyricetin. Food Sci. 2007;28:43–5.
32. Zhang P, Omaye S. DNA strand breakage and oxygen tension: effects of β-carotene, α-tocopherol and ascorbic acid. Food Chem Toxicol. 2001;39:239–45.
33. Hubungan A, Antioksidan A, Isoeugenol D, Vanilin E, Dan T. Structure-antioxidant activities relationship. Indonesian J Chem. 2010;7:10–4.
34. Ko FN, Liao CH. KuoYH, LinYL. Antioxidant properties of demethyldiisoeugenol. Biochim Biophys Acta. 1995;1258:145–52.
35. Nishioka T, Kawabata J, Aoyama Y. Baicalein, an alpha-glucosidase inhibitor from Scutellaria baicalensis. J Nat Prod. 1998;61:1413–5.
36. Tsai CL, Lin YC, Wang HM. Baicalein, an active component of Scutellaria baicalensis, protects against lipopolysaccharide-induced acute lung injury in rats. J Ethnopharmacol. 2014;153:197–201.
37. Jeli D, Lower-Nedza AD, Brantner AH. Baicalin and Baicalein Inhibit Src Tyrosine Kinase and Production of IL-6. J Chem. 2016;8:1–6.
38. Ha TJ, Lee MH, Kwon HS. Oxidation of rosmarinic acid catalyzed by mushroom tyrosinase. J Korean Soc Appl Bio Chem. 2011;54:619–22.
39. Ding HY, Tzunghan C, Liang CH. Antioxidant and antimelanogenic properties of rosmarinic acid methyl ester from Origanum vulgare. Food Chem. 2010;123:254–62.
40. Fujimoto A, Shingai Y, Nakamura M, Maekawa T, Sone Y. Anovel ring-expanded product with enhanced tyrosinase inhibitory activity from classical Fe-catalyzed oxidation of rosmarinic acid, a potent antioxidative. Bioorg Med Chem Lett. 2011;42:7393–6.
41. Sánchez-Campillo M, Gabaldon JA, Castillo J, Benavente-García O. Rosmarinic acid, a photo-protective agent against UV and other ionizing radiations. Food Chem Toxicol. 2009;47:386–92.
42. Zhao Y, Kao CP, Liao CR, Wu KC, Zhou X, Ho YL, Chang YS. Chemical compositions, chromatographic fingerprints and antioxidant activities of Citri Exocarpium Rubrum (*Juhong*). Chin Med. 2017;12:6–20.
43. Xiao HH, Zhang Y, Cooper R, Yao XS, Wong MS. Phytochemicals and potential health effects of *Sambucus williamsii* Hance (*Jiegumu*). Chin Med. 2016;11:36–51.
44. Han YK, Park YJ, Ha YM, Park D, Lee JY, Lee N. Characterization of a novel tyrosinase inhibitor, (2RS,4R)-2-(2,4-dihydroxyphenyl) thiazolidine-4-carboxylic acid (MHY384). BBA-Gen Subjects. 2012;542:1820–6.
45. Fu B, Li H, Wang X, Lee FSC, Cui S. Isolation and identification of flavonoids in licorice and a study of their inhibitory effects on tyrosinase. J Agric Food Chem. 2005;53:7408–13.
46. Zhang JP, Chen QX, Song KK, Xie JJ. Inhibitory effects of salicylic acid family compounds on the diphenolase activity of mushroom tyrosinase. Food Chem. 2006;95:579–84.
47. Stangl V, Lorenz M, Ludwig A. The flavonoid phloretin suppresses stimulated expression of endothelial adhesion molecules and reduces activation of human platelets. J Nutr. 2005;135:172–8.

10

Authenticity analyses of Rhizoma Paridis using barcoding coupled with high resolution melting (Bar-HRM) analysis to control its quality for medicinal plant product

Bao-Zhong Duan[1,2,3], Ya-Ping Wang[4], Hai-Lan Fang[2,3], Chao Xiong[1,2], Xi-Wen Li[2*], Ping Wang[1] and Shi-Lin Chen[1,2*]

Abstract

Background: Rhizoma Paridis (Chonglou) is a commonly used and precious traditional Chinese medicine. *Paris polyphylla* Smith var. *yunnanensis* (Franch.) Hand. -Mazz. and *Paris polyphylla* Smith var. *chinensis* (Franch.) Hara are the two main sources of Chonglou under the monograph of Rhizoma Paridis in Chinese Pharmacopoeia. In the local marketplace, however, this medicine is prone to be accidentally contaminated, deliberately substituted or admixed with other species that are similar to Rhizoma Paridis in shape and color. Consequently, these adulterations might compromise quality control and result in considerable health concerns for consumers. This study aims to develop a rapid and sensitive method for accurate identification of Rhizoma Paridis and its common adulterants.

Methods: DNA barcoding coupled with high resolution melting analysis was applied in this research to distinguish Rhizoma Paridis from its adulteration. The internal transcribed spacer 2 (ITS2) barcode was selected for HRM analysis to produce standard melting profile of the selected species. DNA of the tested herbal medicines was isolated and their melting profiles were generated and compared with the standard melting profile of *P. polyphylla* var. *chinensis*.

Results: The results indicate that the ITS2 molecular regions coupled with HRM analysis can effectively differentiate nine herbal species, including two authentic origins of Chonglou and their seven common adulterants. Ten herbal medicines labeled "Chonglou" obtained from a local market were collected and identified with our methods, and their sequence information was analyzed to validate the accuracy of HRM analysis.

Conclusions: DNA barcoding coupled with HRM analysis is a accurate, reliable, rapid, cost-effective and robust tool, which could contribute to the quality control of Rhizoma Paridis in the supply chain of the natural health product industry (NHP).

Keywords: Authentication, Rhizoma Paridis, DNA barcoding, High resolution melting, Adulterations, Natural health products

Background

Rhizoma Paridis (Chonglou) is a precious traditional Chinese medicine. It originates from the dried rhizomes of both *Paris polyphylla* Smith var. *yunnanensis* (Franch.) Hand. -Mazz. and *P. polyphylla* Smith var. *chinensis* (Franch.) Hara, according to the Chinese Pharmacopoeia [1]. This medicine is most notably an ingredient of the hemostasis prescription 'Yunnan Baiyao' [2]. It plays an important clinical role in treating snake bites, fractures, parotitis, tumors, analgesia and traumatic bleeding. Recent pharmacological studies have indicated that Chonglou exhibits a variety of pharmacological activities, including anti-cancer, anti-inflammatory, antibacterial

*Correspondence: xwli@icmm.ac.cn; slchen@icmm.ac.cn
[2] Institute of Chinese Materia Medica, China Academy of Chinese Medical Sciences, Beijing 100700, China
Full list of author information is available at the end of the article

and immuno-regulatory activities [3]. Unfortunately, slow growth and over-harvesting for the past several years have led to a significant decline in Chonglou's population and caused it to be listed as a vulnerable species by the IUCN (International Union for Conservation of Nature and Natural Resources). The lack of supply and subsequent high price can result in adulteration of Chonglou, including accidentally contamination, deliberately substitution or admixture with other species [4]. More specifically, Chonglou is often contaminated with several common adulterants: *P. thibetica* Franch, *P. tengchongensis* Y.H. Ji, C.J. Yang & Y.L. Huang, *P. forrestii* (Takht.) H. Li, *P. mairei* H. Lév, *Tupistra* spp., *Trillium tschonoskii* Maxim. and *Polygonum paleaceum* Wall. These adulterants are usually of poor quality and some might even be toxic. Contaminated with these plants can pose considerable health threat for the consumers [5]. It was reported that several *Tupistra* species can induce headache and vomiting [6]. Thus, Chonglou authenticity is not only an issue of medicinal quality but also of safety. A fast, reliable and robust method is urgently needed to be established for the herbal industry and regulatory agencies to identify Chonglou species from their adulterants.

With rapid advances in sequencing technologies, Herbgenomics provides an effective platform to support biological analyses of complex herbal products [7, 8]. It is now being widely applied to DNA-based herbal identification through the establishment of an herbal gene bank. DNA-based methods have gained popularity for unequivocal plant species identification because DNA molecules can be found in all tissues and they cannot be affected by environment or physiological factors [9–13]. DNA barcoding, a method that use the sequence of a standard region of DNA for the purpose of species identification, has been recognized as a powerful tool for the identification of medicinal plants and their adulterants at the species level [4, 14–17]. However, DNA sequencing of each individual sample is expensive, time consuming and cannot easily be applied to studies of large samples because of financial constraints [18]. High resolution melting (HRM) analysis is a closed-tube post-PCR analysis that can differentiate between samples even with a single base change in DNA sequences. This technique permits the genotyping and the quantification of adulterants and has been proved to be fast, reliable, low-cost in terms of consumables [19, 20]. Very recently, the Bar-HRM analysis has been introduced for species identification and authentication. The use of just Bar-HRM for species authentication and detection of adulteration in commercial products has been reported [21, 22]. To date, it has not been applied as a tool for the species authentication of Chonglou.

The goal of this research is to develop a rapid, scientifically rigorous and accurate method to identify and authenticate two types of Chonglou, namely *P. polyphylla* var. *yunnanensis* and *P. polyphylla* var. *chinensis*, from their adulterants. For that purpose, Bar-HRM analysis using universal DNA barcoding ITS2 region was conducted. The proposed methodology was further applied to differentiate ten herbal medicines labeled as Chonglou bought in market place. This will provide the first evidence for the utility of Bar-HRM analysis to test the authenticity of Chonglou sold in the local market place.

Methods

Reference plant material and DNA extraction

Thirty two fresh rhizome samples from nine species were collected from the Yunnan Province, People's Republic of China, including *P. polyphylla* var. *yunnanensis*, *P. polyphylla* var. *chinensis*, *P. thibetica*, *P. tengchongensis*, *P. forrestii*, *P. mairei*, *Tupistra* spp., *T. tschonoskii* and *P. paleaceum* (Table 1). The rhizomes were gently washed and dried at 50 °C. All of the materials were authenticated by Professor Conglong Xia of the College of Pharmaceutical Science, Dali University. In addition, ten herbal medicines labeled "Chonglou" were purchased from a local market in the Yunnan Province. All voucher specimens and herbal medicines were deposited in the Herbarium of Dali University (DLU). Samples taken from dried rhizomes (30 mg) were rubbed for 2 min at a frequency of 30 r/s. Extraction proceeded by using the modified Plant Genomic DNA Extraction Kit (Tiangen Biotech Co., Ltd., Beijing, China). The DNA was diluted to 50 ng/μL and later stored at − 20 °C for further use.

HRM-PCR amplification

A conserved region of the ITS2 region of nuclear ribosomal DNA was used as the optimal region for the assay because of it has previously correctly identified the medicinal plants of the genus *Paris* [23]. DNA was amplified using the polymerase chain reaction (PCR). The real-time PCR mixture (25 μL) contained 50 ng of genomic DNA, 12.5 μL of 2 × HRM PCR master mix, 1 μL forward (5′-ATGCGATACTTGGTGTGAAT-3′) primer (10 μmol/L), and 1 μL reverse (5′-GACGCTTCTCCAGACTACAAT-3′) primer (10 μmol/L), and distilled water up to the final volume. Real-time PCR was performed in a Rotor-Gene Q MDx cycler (Qiagen, Hilden, Germany) under the following conditions: 94 °C for 3 min followed by 40 cycles of 94 °C for 30 s, 56 °C for 30 s and 72 °C for 45 s. The fluorescent data were acquired at the end of each extension step of the PCR cycle. HRM was performed as follows: pre-melt at 95 °C

Table 1 The origin of the plant species used in the study and their GenBank accession numbers

No.	Family	Botanical name	Voucher number	Genbank accessions number
1	*Liliaceae*	*Paris polyphylla* var. *yunnanensis* (Franch.) Hand. -Mazz.	YN0001MT01, YN0001MT02, YN0001MT03, YN0001MT04, YN0001MT05, YN0001MT06	KX458130, KX458131, KX458132, KX458133, KX458134, KX458135
2		*Paris polyphylla* var. *chinensis* (Franch.) H. Hara	YN0011MT01, YN0011MT02, YN0011MT03	KX458140, KX458141, KX458142
3		*Paris thibetica* Franch.	YN0012MT01, YN0012MT02, YN0012MT03	KX458136, KX458137, KX458138, KX458139
4		*Paris tengchongensis* Y.H. Ji, C.J. Yang & Y.L. Huang	YN0007MT01, YN0007MT02, YN0007MT03, YN0007MT04, YN0007MT05, YN0007MT06	KX458121, KX458122, KX458123, KX458124, KX458125, KX458126
5		*Paris forrestii* (Takht.) H. Li	YN0009MT01, YN0009MT02, YN0009MT03	KX458127, KX458128, KX458129
6		*Paris mairei* H. Lév	YN0005MT01, YN0005MT02, YN0005MT03	KX458118, KX458119, KX458120
7		*Tupistra* spp. (not define)	YN0016MT03, YN0016MT04, YN0016MT05	/
8		*Trillium tschonoskii* Maxim.	YN0016MT10, YN0016MT11, YN0016MT12	KX458143, KX458144, KX458145
9	*Polygonaceae*	*Polygonum paleaceum* Wall.	YN0016MT01, YN0016MT02	KX458146, KX458147

for 1.5 min, followed by a temperature raise from 65 to 95 °C with 0.1 °C degree increments and a 2 s hold time for each acquisition step.

The Rotor-Gene Q software (Qiagen, Hilden, Germany) was used to genotype the different varieties and the herbal products. The negative derivative of the fluorescence (F) over temperature (T) (dF/dT) curve displayed the melting temperature (Tm), and the normalized raw curve depicted the decreasing fluorescence against increasing temperature. Pre- and post-melt normalization regions were set to define the temperature boundaries of the normalized and difference plots and to generate normalized melting curves of the normalized and difference plots [24]. *P. polyphylla* var. *chinensis* was also used as reference species. To assess the discriminative power of Bar-HRM analysis, samples from both the fresh plants and dry tissue were used for PCR amplification and HRM analysis.

Sequencing and data analysis

To verify the HRM analysis results, all the PCR products were directly sequenced in two directions using the automated ABI 3730 XL sequencer (Applied Biosystems, Foster City, CA, USA). Sequence results were submitted to the GenBank database (accession numbers were listed in Table 1), assembled with CodonCode Aligner 5.1.5 (CodonCode Co., USA) and aligned using Clustal W. The neighbor-joining (NJ) trees were calculated and constructed using the MEGA 5.05 software with the Bootstrap method (1000 resembling) and the K2P model [25].

The Minimum Standards of Reporting Checklist contains details of the experimental design, and statistics, and resources used in this study (Additional file 1).

Results

Barcoding of PCR products by HRM analysis

The amplicons of ITS2 were analyzed with HRM to define their Tms. There exist some differences in ITS2 region among Chonglou and their adulterate species reflected by their Tm values (Table 2). Although the Tms value of *Paris* genus were close to each other, each species still could be clearly discerned by the plots of the normalized melting curves (Fig. 1). Average genotype confidence percentages (GCPs) were also calculated and a cut-off value of 90% was used to assign a genotype for each region. The GCPs from the HRM analyses of the ITS2 region of nine species are listed in Table 3. As shown in Table 3, all species were sufficiently and confidently identified with a value of 100%. The highest GCP (81.28%) was found between the *P. mairei* and *P. polyphylla* var. *chinensis*

Table 2 The values of the melting temperatures of nine species measured by HRM analysis using ITS2 as marker

No.	Botanical name	Examin	Tm (°C)
1	*Paris polyphylla* var. *yunnanensis* (Franch.) Hand. -Mazz.	6	87.31 ± 0.07
2	*Paris polyphylla* var. *chinensis* (Franch.) H. Hara	3	86.88 ± 0.02
3	*Paris thibetica* Franch.	3	86.84 ± 0.02
4	*Paris tengchongensis* Y.H. Ji, C.J. Yang & Y.L. Huang	6	87.55 ± 0.04
5	*Paris forrestii* (Takht.) H. Li	3	86.68 ± 0.04
6	*Paris mairei* H. Lév	3	87.37 ± 0.03
7	*Tupistra* spp. (not define)	3	92.66 ± 0.08
8	*Trillium tschonoskii* Maxim.	3	88.91 ± 0.17
9	*Polygonum paleaceum* Wall.	2	91.02 ± 0.02

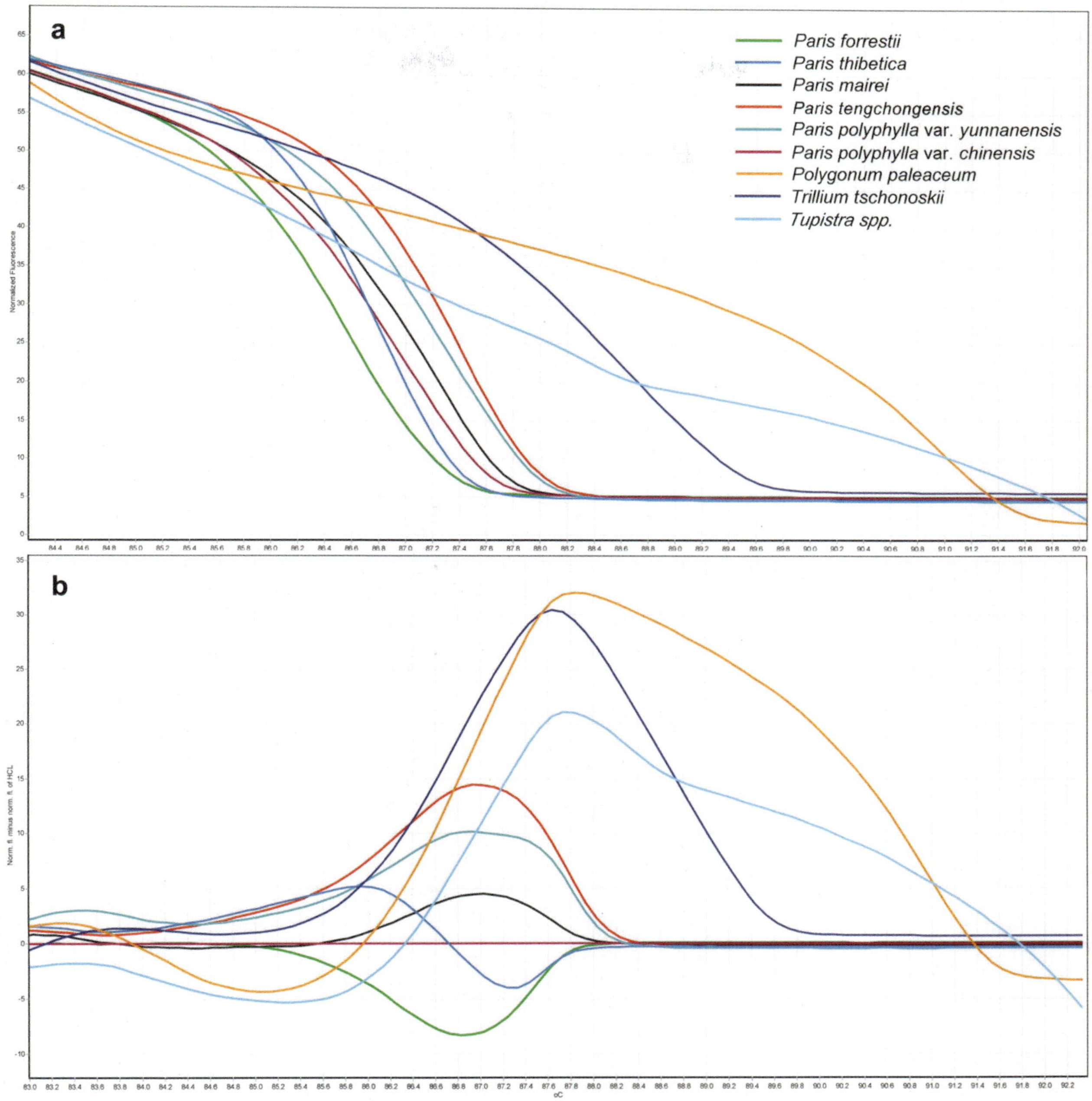

Fig. 1 **a** The normalized melting profiles of nine plant species obtained by HRM analysis with ITS2 as the universal marker. **b** The difference graphs of nine species using *Paris polyphylla* var. *chinensis* as a reference genotype. A color-code table listing the species was used

species, while the lowest (0.0) was between *Paris* and the other genera. The melting profiles of the ITS2 amplicons from the nine species were assessed by plotting two different curves: the derivate melt curve (Fig. 1a) and the difference plot melt curve (Fig. 1b). The normalized HRM curves with the barcode marker ITS2 showed that all the nine species could be easily and visually distinguished.

Species authentication using DNA sequencing

To validate the results of HRM analysis, amplicon sequences of all samples from the nine reference plant species were sequenced. Twenty-seven ITS2 sequences from eight species were successfully obtained, except for *Tupistra* spp. These sequences were used to construct phylogenetic tree [neighbor-joining (NJ)]. Eight

Table 3 The results of average genotype confidence percentages from the HRM analysis of nine species

Taxon	*P. forrestii*	*P. tengchongensis*	*P. mairei*	*P. polyphylla* var. *chinensis*	*P. polyphylla* var. *yunnanensis*	*P. thibetica*	*Trillium tschonoskii*	*Polygonum paleaceum*	*Tupistra* spp.
P. forrestii	100								
P. tengchongensis	0.13	100							
P. mairei	19.11	16.85	100						
P. polyphylla var. *chinensis*	48.71	4.55	*81.28*	100					
P. polyphylla var. *yunnanensis*	1.24	72.1	44.33	18.75	100				
P. thibetica	28.57	3.32	47.6	63.51	16.66	100			
Trillium tschonoskii	0	0.06	0	0	0.01	0	100		
Polygonum paleaceum	0	0	0	0	0	0	0.04	100	
Tupistra spp.	0	0.02	0.02	0.01	0.02	0	0.94	0.6	100

The highest GCP was found between the P. mairei and P. polyphylla var. chinensis, which are presented in italics

species can be clearly distinguished by the NJ tree (Fig. 2), namely *P. polyphylla* (var. *yunnanensis* and var. *chinensis*), *P. thibetica, P. tengchongensis, P. forrestii, P. mairei, T. tschonoskii* and *P. paleaceum.* The genetic relationships reflected by the NJ tree were in good agreement with the Bar-HRM results. The sequence of each amplicon and the alignment among eight species are shown in Fig. 3. Sequencing results revealed that the differences in the melting curves maybe caused by deletions, insertions and a number of SNPs in the ITS2 region. In brief, the variations of the eight species in ITS2 region are capable to produce differences in the HRM analysis profile.

Application of Bar-HRM to commercial herbal medicine

As mentioned previously, Chonglou sold in the local market places can be confused with certain other species that are similar in shape and color with the authentic Chonglou. To evaluate the accuracy of Bar-HRM method and to assure the quality of Chonglou in local market, the proposed methodology was further applied to authenticate ten batches of samples labelled as "Chonglou". The HRM curves of nine reference plant species and ten samples are shown in Fig. 4. *T*m values and GCPs of ten samples obtained from the HRM analysis are shown in Tables 4 and 5. As shown in Fig. 4 and Tables 4 and 5, the *T*ms of five Chonglou samples (Com-1, Com-2, Com-3, Com-8, and Com-10) ranged from 87.29 to 87.33 °C, which agreed with the *T*m of *P. polyphylla* var. *yunnanensis*, and the curves overlapped completely. These results demonstrated that all these five samples were *P. polyphylla* var. *yunnanensis.* Among them, three samples (Com-4, Com-5, and Com-6) were identified as *P. tengchongensis.* Com-7 sharing a similar plot with *T. tschonoskii*. Com-9 was identified as *P. mairei.* These results indicate that Bar-HRM analysis can be effectively used to differentiate Chonglou from its adulterants.

Discussion

Species identification is critical to ensuring the quality of herbal medicine. HRM analysis is a method that measures the dissociation rates of double-stranded DNA into single-stranded DNA in increasing temperatures [26]. Minute difference in amplicon size or composition, even a simple nucleotide, can be detected. In general, different genotypes have their own unique transitions, including changes in curve shape and in the plots of their melting curves, which can be shown in their HRM profiles [24].

At present, several methods, such as high performance liquid chromatography (HPLC) and near infrared spectroscopy (NIR), have been introduced to discriminate the controversial *Paris* species [27, 28]. However, the HPLC method is relatively expensive and NIR spectroscopy suffers from low precision and tedious calibration, which is not ideal for the rapid screening of large numbers of samples. For these reasons, molecular biology-based analysis is becoming increasingly popular for the differentiation

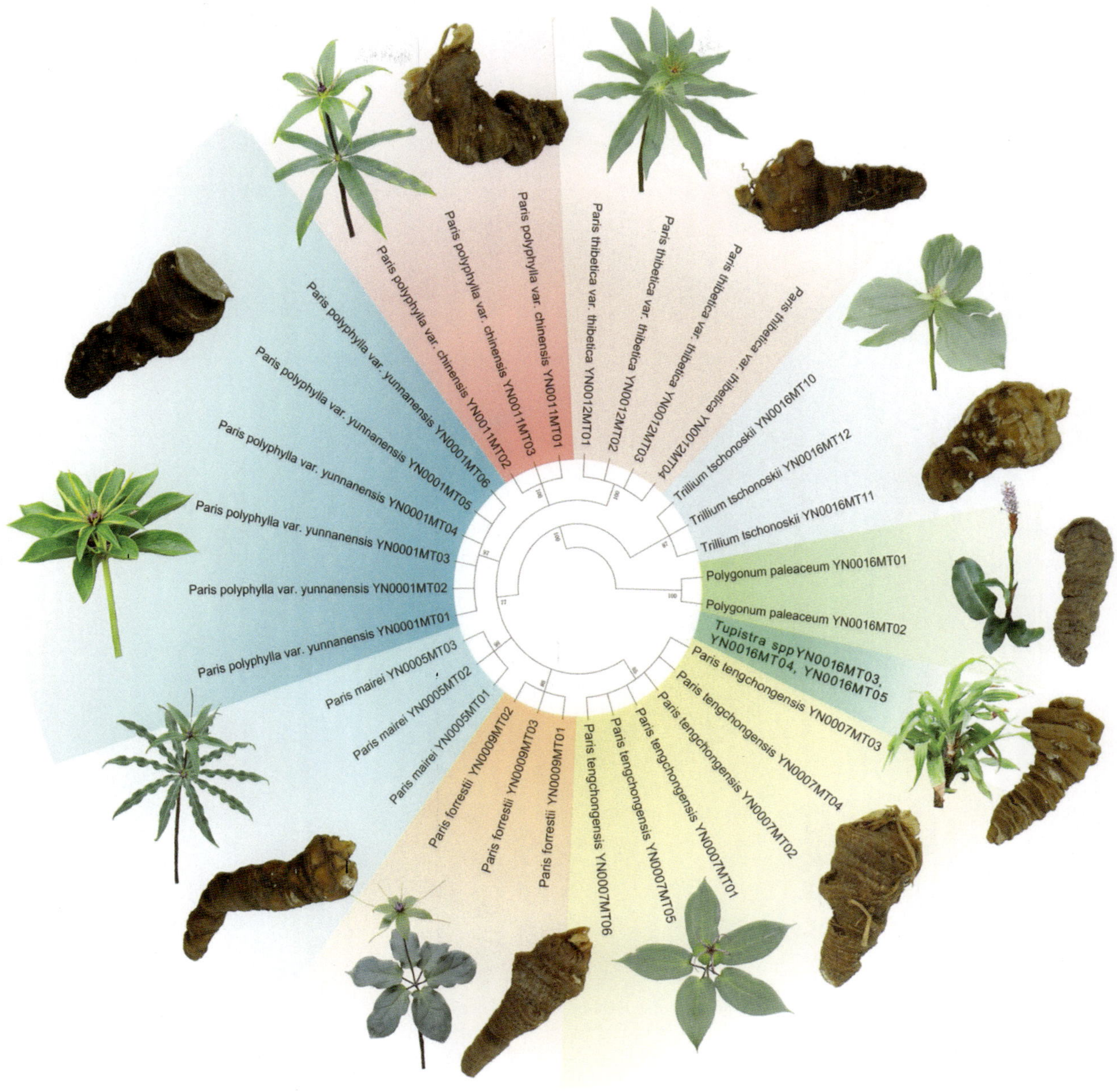

Fig. 2 The phylogenetic tree of Rhizoma Paridis and its adulterants constructed from the ITS2 sequences using the N-J method (Bootstrap scores ≥ 50%). Representatives of the species illustrate the morphological variation in *Paris* and related species

and identification of species in several scientific fields [29]. Among the various molecular biology techniques, DNA barcoding, ITS2, has been successfully applied to distinguish *Paris* species [23]. However, DNA sequencing technology is relatively expensive and time-consuming since the sequencing process is about 1–2 days. The use of Bar-HRM can overcome the cost and time issues (the whole process only takes 4 h). Moreover, this new approach has its own advantage compared with previously employed methods. The Bar-HRM analysis is performed in one completely "closed" tube and the results are available for analysis at the end of the run.

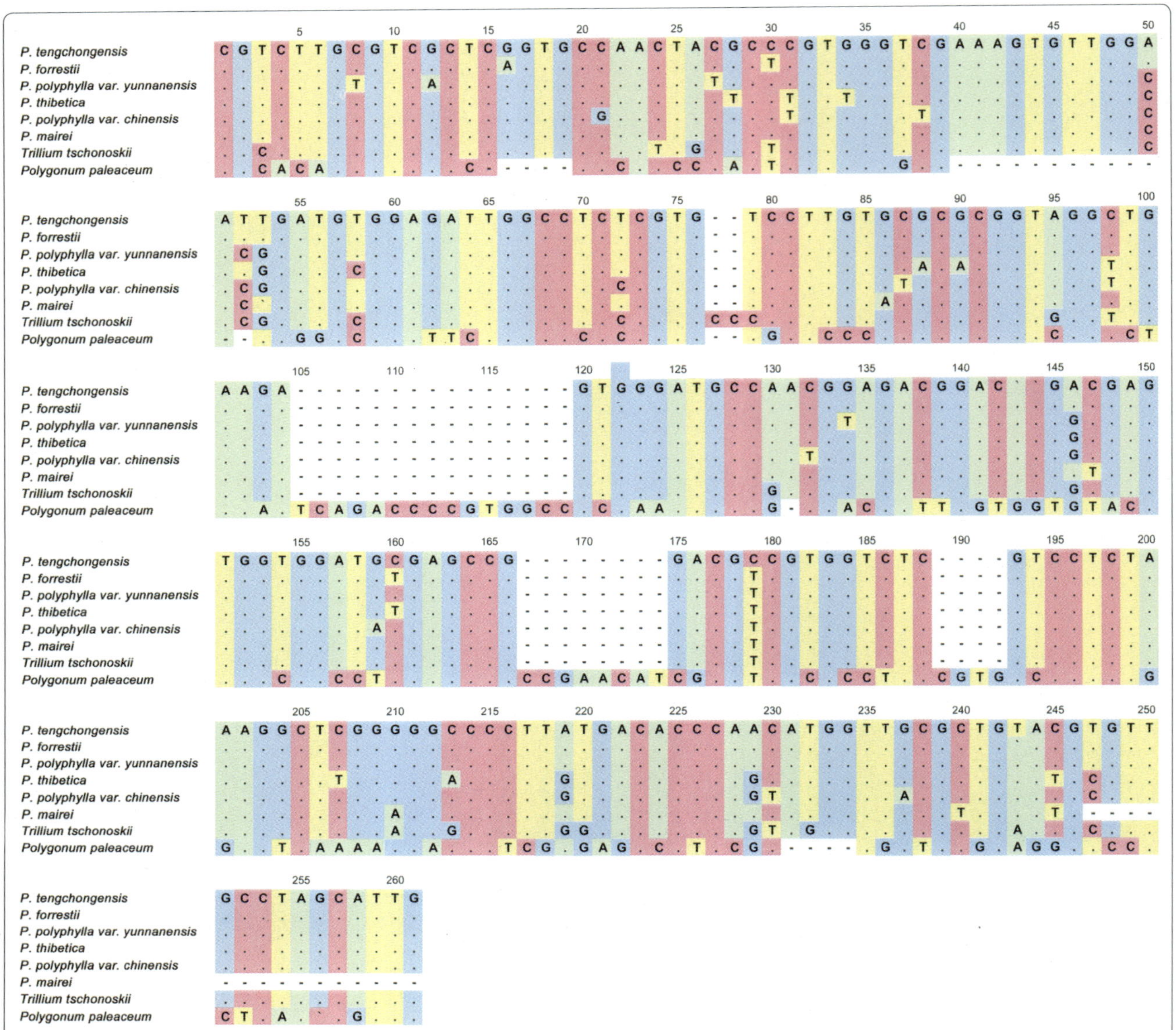

Fig. 3 The DNA sequence alignment analysis of nine plant species showing differences in the DNA level alignment confirmed the Bar-HRM results

In this study, we have successfully applied Bar-HRM analysis for the rapid detection and identification of two major *Paris* species and their seven adulterants. The results indicated that Bar-HRM is a sensitive, fast, cheap, and reliable method for identifying and tracking herbal medicines. To validate the accuracy of polymorphisms detected by HRM analysis, the sequences of the reference plant specie were analyzed. Each PCR product was amplified and both strands were sequenced in opposite directions. Although the PCR products of *Tupistra* spp. were clearly visible as a single band on agarose gel, the sequence information of *Tupistra* spp. was not obtained, and there are no documented reports on its ITS2 sequences information in the GeneBank. The multi-copy of ITS2 region may lead to the failure of sequence. However, the HRM melting curves could be used to distinguish Chonglou from its adulterants clearly, included *Tupistra* spp. Considering these features, Bar-HRM can be a useful tool for quality control of herbal medicines in the supply chain of the natural health product industry (NHP) and medicine supervisory institutions. In conclusion, this study substantially contributes to the protection of public health worldwide.

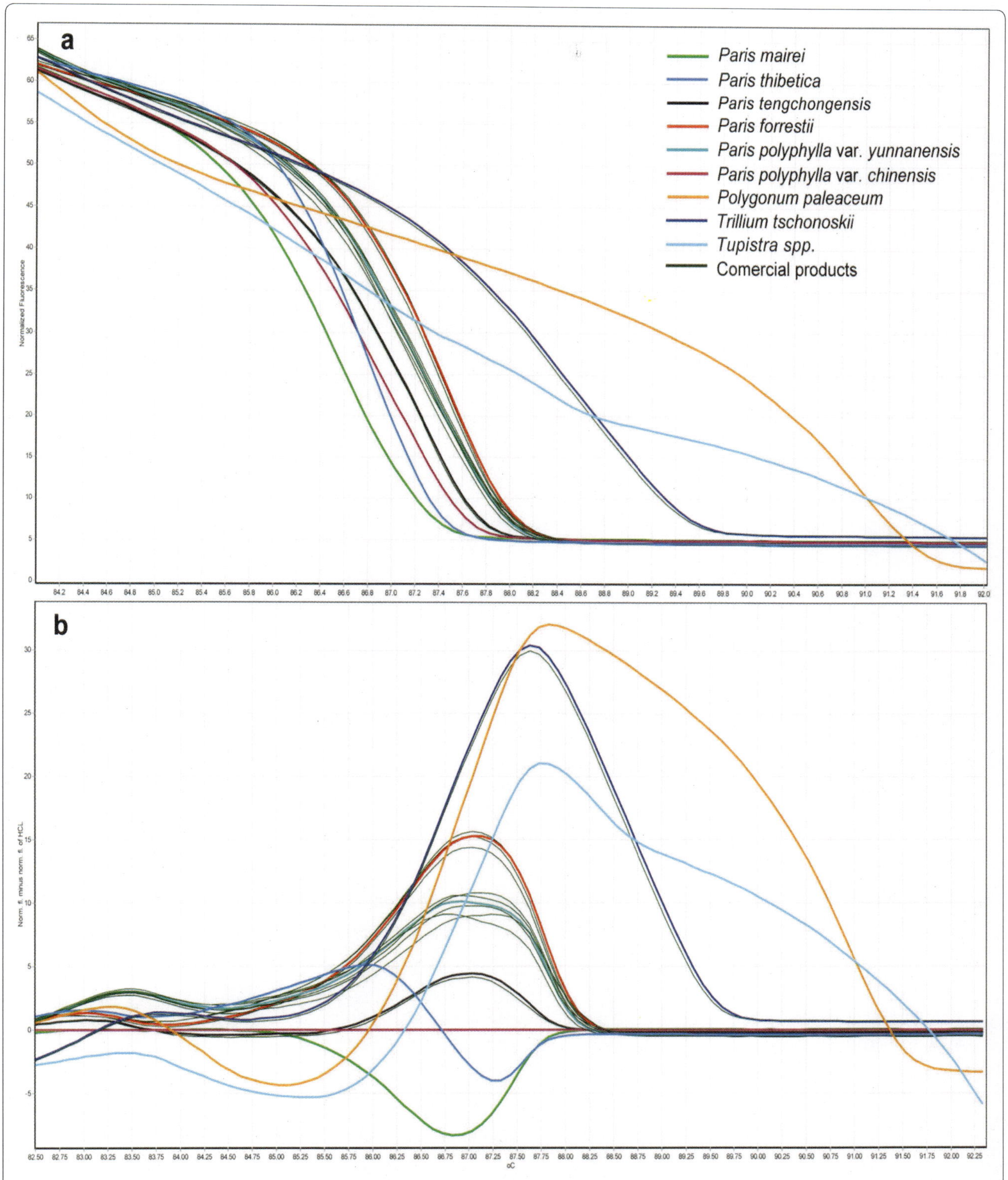

Fig. 4 The Bar-HRM analysis of nine plant species and ten commercial Chonglou products using HRM analysis with the ITS2 marker. **a** Normalized melting curves. **b** Difference curves, with the mean *Paris polyphylla* var. *chinensis* curve used as a reference genotype. A color-code table listing the species was used

Table 4 The list of ten commercial "Chonglou" products that were identified using ITS2 sequencing coupled with high resolution melting temperature values

Code	Asserted species	Tm (°C)	HRM
Com-1	Chong-Lou (not define)	87.30	*Paris polyphylla* var. *yunnanensis*
Com-2	Chong-Lou (not define)	87.29	*Paris polyphylla* var. *yunnanensis*
Com-3	Chong-Lou (not define)	87.32	*Paris polyphylla* var. *yunnanensis*
Com-4	Chong-Lou (not define)	87.57	*Paris tengchongensis*
Com-5	Chong-Lou (not define)	87.55	*Paris tengchongensis*
Com-6	Chong-Lou (not define)	87.52	*Paris tengchongensis*
Com-7	Chong-Lou (not define)	88.40	*Trillium tschonoskii* Maxim.
Com-8	Chong-Lou (not define)	87.31	*Paris polyphylla* var. *yunnanensis*
Com-9	Chong-Lou (not define)	87.39	*Paris mairei*
Com-10	Chong-Lou (not define)	87.33	*Paris polyphylla* var. *yunnanensis*

Com Commercial

Conclusions

The Bar-HRM analysis has been used in this study to differentiate Chonglou, namely *P. polyphylla* var. *yunnanensis* and *P. polyphylla* var. *chinensis*, from their adulterate species. Species-specific PCR amplification of the ITS2 region was performed to validate the results of HRM analysis. The difference between Chonglou species and their adulterants can be observed from their sequencing information. The proposed method has been proved to be accurate, reliable, rapid, cost-effective and robust for identifying Chonglou from its adulterants. Bar-HRM analysis is also feasible for high-throughput assays, and could be well applied to other herbal species in the future, ensuring the perceived value and quality of herbal medicines.

Abbreviations

Bar-HRM: barcoding coupled with high resolution melting; HRM: high resolution melting; ITS2: internal transcribed spacer 2; IUCN: International Union for Conservation of Nature; GCPs: genotype confidence percentages; PCR: polymerase chain reaction; *Tm*: melting temperature; HPLC: high performance liquid chromatography; NIR: near infrared spectroscopy; NHP: natural health product industry.

Authors' contributions

BZD and HLF carried out the molecular experiments, analyzed the data and wrote the manuscript. YPW wrote the manuscript, CX carried out the data analyses, PW thoroughly revised the manuscript. XWL and SLC conceived of the study, contributed to the design and interpretation of the research. All authors read and approved the final manuscript.

Author details

[1] College of Pharmaceutical Science, Hubei University of Chinese Medicine, Wuhan 430065, China. [2] Institute of Chinese Materia Medica, China Academy of Chinese Medical Sciences, Beijing 100700, China. [3] College of Pharmaceutical Science, Dali University, Dali 671000, China. [4] Centre for Cancer and Inflammation Research, School of Chinese Medicine, Hong Kong Baptist University, Hong Kong, China.

Acknowledgements

We acknowledge the help of Conglong Xia and Zhigang Duan (Dali University) for their help in the collection of plant samples and the identification of species.

Competing interests

The authors declare that they have no competing interests.

Table 5 The results of genotype confidence percentages from the HRM analysis of ten commercial "Chonglou" products

Taxon	COM-1	COM-2	COM-3	COM-4	COM-5	COM-6	COM-7	COM-8	COM-9	COM-10
P. forrestii	0.95	2.38	1.62	0.19	0.1	0.22	0	1.05	21	1.84
P. tengchongensis	75.04	61.77	68.07	*97.66**	*99.39**	*98.64**	0.09	76.7	14.91	61.04
P. mairei	39.09	57.09	49.88	19.82	14.73	21.98	0	41.96	*99.73**	49.81
P. polyphylla var. *chinensis*	15.75	27.23	22.04	5.84	3.87	6.49	0	16.9	83.79	23.51
P. polyphylla var. *yunnanensis*	*99.47**	*95.99**	*99.22**	79.11	69.88	78.62	0.02	*99.21**	40.64	*97.72**
P. thibetica	14.48	20.85	18.49	4.93	3.02	4.81	0	13.77	48.15	23.46
Trillium tschonoskii	0.01	0.01	0.01	0.04	0.06	0.04	*98.93*	0.02	0	0.01
Polygonum paleaceum	0	0	0	0	0	0	0.03	0	0	0
Tupistra spp.	0.02	0.03	0.02	0.02	0.02	0.02	1.12	0.02	0.02	0.01

*Over the 90% confidence percentage threshold are presented in italics

Consent for publication

Not applicable.

Funding

This study was supported by Grants from The National Natural Science Foundation of China (31460084), the National Key Technology Support Program (2015BAI05B02), the Science and Technology Cooperation Project of Hong Kong, Macao and Taiwan (2015DFM30030), the Training Scheme of reserve Talents for Young and Middle-aged Academic and Technical Leaders of the Yunnan Province (2015HB058), and the Doctoral Science Foundation of Dali University (KYBS201737).

References

1. Commission CP. Pharmacopoeia of the People's Republic of China. Peking: Chin Med Science Press; 2015.
2. Wu S, Gao W, Duan H, Jia W. Advances in studies on chemical constituents and pharmacological activities of Rhizoma Paridis. Chin Tradit Herb Drug. 2004;35(3):344–6.
3. Li H. The genus *Paris* (*Trilliaceae*). Beijing: Science Press; 1998.
4. Newmaster SG, Grguric M, Shanmughanandhan D, Ramalingam S, Ragupathy S. DNA barcoding detects contamination and substitution in North American herbal products. BMC Med. 2013;11(1):1–13.
5. Ekor M. The growing use of herbal medicines: issues relating to adverse reactions and challenges in monitoring safety. Front Pharmacol. 2013;4(4):177.
6. Xia LY. Handbook of toxicity of traditional Chinese medicine. Hohhot: Inner Mongolia Science Technology Press; 2006.
7. Chen SL, Song JY, Sun C, Xu J, Zhu YJ, Verpoorte R, Fan TP. Herbal genomics: examining the biology of traditional medicines. Science. 2015;347(6219):S27–9.
8. Chen SL, Song JY. Herbgenomics. China J Chin Mater Med. 2016;41(21):3881–9.
9. Cabral P, Soares T, Lima A, De Miranda FD, Souza FB, Gonçalves L. Genetic diversity in local and commercial dry bean (*Phaseolus vulgaris*) accessions based on microsatellite markers. Gen Mol Res. 2011;10(1):140–9.
10. Chen SL, Pang XH, Song JY, Shi LC, Yao H, Han JP, Leon C. A renaissance in herbal medicine identification: from morphology to DNA. Biotechnol Adv. 2014;32(7):1237–44.
11. Gad HA, El-Ahmady SH, Abou-Shoer MI, Al-Azizi MM. Application of chemometrics in authentication of herbal medicines: a review. Phytochem Anal. 2013;24(1):1–24.
12. Al SSRE. Authentication methods for drugs used in Ayurveda, Siddha and Unani Systems of medicine: an overview. Int J Pharm Sci Res. 2012;3(8):2352.
13. Fu JG, Dai L, Lin Z, Lu HM. Houttuynia cordata Thunb: a review of phytochemistry and pharmacology and quality control. Chin Med. 2013;4(3):101–23.
14. Chen SL, Yao H, Han JP, Liu C, Song JY, Shi LC, Zhu YJ, Ma XY, Gao T, Pang XH. Validation of the ITS2 region as a novel DNA barcode for identifying medicinal plant species. PLoS ONE. 2010;5(1):e8613.
15. Techen N, Parveen I, Pan Z, Khan IA. DNA barcoding of medicinal plant material for identification. Curr Opin Biotechnol. 2014;25(2):103–10.
16. Chen JJ, Zhao QS, Liu YL, Zha SH, Bing Z. Identification of maca (*Lepidium meyenii* Walp.) and its adulterants by a DNA-barcoding approach based on the ITS sequence. Chin J Nat Med. 2015;13(9):653–9.
17. Han JP, Pang XH, Liao BS, Hui Y, Song JY, Chen SL. An authenticity survey of herbal medicines from markets in China using DNA barcoding. Sci Rep. 2016;6:1–9.
18. Osathanunkul M, Madesis P, de Boer H. Bar-HRM for authentication of plant-based medicines: evaluation of three medicinal products derived from *Acanthaceae* species. PLoS ONE. 2015;10(5):e128476.
19. Wu S, Wirthensohn MG, Hunt P, Gibson JP, Sedgley M. High resolution melting analysis of almond SNPs derived from ESTs. Theor Appl Genet. 2008;118(1):1–14.
20. Ganopoulos I, Argiriou A, Tsaftaris A. Adulterations in Basmati rice detected quantitatively by combined use of microsatellite and fragrance typing with high resolution melting (HRM) analysis. Food Chem. 2011;129(2):652–9.
21. Osathanunkul M, Suwannapoom C, Osathanunkul K, Madesis P, de Boer H. Evaluation of DNA barcoding coupled high resolution melting for discrimination of closely related species in phytopharmaceuticals. Phytomedicine. 2016;23(2):156–65.
22. Li JJ, Song M, Xiong C, Zhao B, Sun W. Application of barcode high-resolution melting for rapid authentication of the medicinal plant *Psammosilene tunicoides*. Biotechnol Biotechnol Equip. 2016;30(4):790–6.
23. Zhu YJ, Chen SL, Yao H, Tan R, Song JY, Luo K, Lu J. DNA barcoding the medicinal plants of the genus *Paris*. Acta Pharm Sin. 2010;45(3):376–82.
24. Wittwer CT, Reed GH, Gundry CN, Vandersteen JG, Pryor RJ. High-resolution genotyping by amplicon melting analysis using LCGreen. Clin Chem. 2003;49(6):853–60.
25. Tamura K, Peterson D, Peterson N, Stecher G, Nei M, Kumar S. MEGA5: molecular evolutionary genetics analysis using maximum likelihood, evolutionary distance, and maximum parsimony methods. Mol Biol Evol. 2011;28(10):2731–9.
26. Reed GH, Wittwer CT. Sensitivity and specificity of single-nucleotide polymorphism scanning by high-resolution melting analysis. Clin Chem. 2004;50(10):1748–54.
27. Zhang T, Liu H, Liu XT, Xu DR, Chen XQ, Wang Q. Qualitative and quantitative analysis of steroidal saponins in crude extracts from *Paris polyphylla* var. *yunnanensis* and *P. polyphylla* var. *chinensis* by high performance liquid chromatography coupled with mass spectrometry. J Pharm Biomed Anal. 2010;51(1):114–24.
28. Zhao YL, Zhang J, Yuan TJ, Shen T, Li W, Yang SH, Hou Y, Wang YZ, Jin H. Discrimination of wild *Paris* based on near infrared spectroscopy and high performance liquid chromatography combined with multivariate analysis. PLoS ONE. 2014;9(2):e89100.
29. Li XW, Yang Y, Henry RJ, Rossetto M, Wang YT, Chen SL. Plant DNA barcoding: from gene to genome. Biol Rev. 2015;90(1):157–66.

11

Chemical constituents from a *Gynostemma laxum* and their antioxidant and neuroprotective activities

Ji Yeon Seo[1], Sang Kyum Kim[2], Phi Hung Nguyen[3], Ju Yong Lee[1], Pham Ha Thanh Tung[1], Sang Hyun Sung[1] and Won Keun Oh[1*]

Abstract

Background: A few bioactivities of constituents from *Gynostemma laxum*, which has been collected in Vietnam, have been reported until now. There is no report about the effects of constituents from *G. laxum* although the nuclear factor (erythroid-derived 2)-like 2 (Nrf2)-mediated heme oxygenase-1 (HO-1) antioxidant defense system is involved in neuroprotection in the brain. Therefore, we investigated whether quercetin (**2**), benzoic acid (**10**) and their analogues (**1**, **3**–**9** and **11**) from *G. laxum* have the antioxidant and neuroprotective activities and also their underlying mechanism.

Methods: To examine their neuroprotective and antioxidant activities, oxytosis, total oxidant scavenging capacity (TOSC), 2,7-dichlorofluorescein (DCFDA), dihydroethidium (DHE), antioxidant response element (ARE)-luciferase reporter gene assays, Western blot analysis, real time-PCR, immunocytochemistry and in silico 3D molecular docking simulation were performed.

Results: The study of constituents using chromatographic techniques and spectroscopic analysis showed that *G. laxum* contained an abundance of quercetin (**2**), benzoic acid (**10**) and their analogues (**1**, **3**–**9** and **11**). Our data demonstrated that quercetin (**2**) and its analogue (**4**) among the constituents from *G. laxum* showed the strongest neuroprotective effect against oxytosis triggered by the excessive amount of glutamate. Compounds **2**, **4**, **6** and **11** exhibited reactive oxygen species (ROS) inhibitory and ARE transcriptional activities in immortalized hippocampal HT22 cell line. Among them, compound **4**, a second active compound, induced Nrf2/HO-1 activation. They were also fit stable onto the Tramtrack and Bric-à-Brac (BTB) domain of Kelch-like ECH-associated protein 1 (Keap1), a known Nrf2 inhibitor protein, based on the results of docking and interaction energies. Overall, these data suggest that –OH and –OCH_3 groups of quercetin and its analogues are responsible for their neuroprotective effect.

Conclusions: In summary, the major constituents of *G. laxum* had strong antioxidant and neuroprotective activities so that they could consider as a natural antioxidant supplement. Furthermore, *G. laxum* might be used beneficially in reducing oxidative complications with the further deep investigation in vivo.

Keywords: *Gynostemma laxum*, Quercetin analogues, Antioxidant, Neuroprotection, Keap1

*Correspondence: wkoh1@snu.ac.kr
[1] Korea Bioactive Natural Material Bank, Research Institute of Pharmaceutical Sciences, College of Pharmacy, Seoul National University, Seoul 08826, Republic of Korea
Full list of author information is available at the end of the article

Background

Oxidative stress can be defined as an imbalance between oxidants and the antioxidant system leading to oxidative damage at critical sites in tissues and cells [1]. The homeostasis between oxidants and antioxidants in the human body is maintained consistently under normal condition, and it is important for sustaining optimal physiology [2]. Recently, much interest has focused on the antioxidant activities of dietary components with the expectation that they may supplement the human natural defenses against various oxidant challenges [3].

Reactive oxygen species (ROS) such as the O_2^-, HO^- and other non-radicals oxygen analogues, e.g., H_2O_2 and $^1O_2$ are generated by an integral part of metabolism [4]. Thus, antioxidants have been interested in biologists and clinicians as they may help to protect the human body against damage due to ROS [5, 6]. Antioxidants have also been used to preserve food quality mainly by prevention of oxidative deterioration of lipid constituent. When antioxidants added to lipids and lipid-containing foods, their shelf-life can increase retarding the process of lipid peroxidation. At present, the most commonly used antioxidants are butylated hydroxyanisole, butylated hydroxytoluene, propyl gallate, and *tert*-butylhydroquinone [7]. However, they have suspected to be responsible for their harmful effects on various organs such as brain [8] and liver [9]. Specifically, ROS has been regarded as one of the major reasons to occur the neurological diseases including Alzheimer's [10], Parkinson's [11] and Huntington's diseases [12]. Therefore, development of more safer natural antioxidants from plant materials that can replace synthetic antioxidants has been of interest [13] as well as attenuation of ROS-mediated damages can be strategies to prevent or alleviate to neurodegenerative diseases [10, 14].

In the brain, nuclear factor (erythroid-derived 2)-like 2 (Nrf2)-mediated antioxidant enzymes including heme oxygenase-1 (HO-1) eliminate the intracellular ROS through the catabolism [15]. The recent many reports suggest that Kelch-like ECH-associated protein 1 (Keap1), which is an inhibitor protein of Nrf2, acts as a central regulator of the Nrf2-mediated cytoprotection and anti-inflammation. In this case, the N-terminal Broad complex, Tramtrack and Bric-à-Brac (BTB) domain of Keap1 plays important roles in sensing electrophilic antioxidants and interaction with the cullin 3 (Cul3)/E3 ubiquitin-protein ligase system which is an initial signal for proteasome degradation of Keap1 and Nrf2 complex. The C151 among the other cysteines in Keap1 has been considered as a responsible residue for interaction with electrophiles [16]. Thus, investigations of antagonists or interacting compounds into the active site of BTB domain in Keap1, particularly in C151, are also valuable approach for understanding the function of natural antioxidants.

The genus *Gynostemma*, which belongs to the Cucurbitaceae family, is comprised of about 21 species including *G. pentaphyllum*, *G. laxum*, and *G. pubescens*. These plants distribute over large areas in Japan, China, and also Vietnam [17]. Of the genus *Gynostemma*, many studies have been focused on the *G. pentaphyllum* with dammarane-type saponins as the discovery of new activities for treatment of metabolic disease [18–20], anti-cancer activity through the inhibition of proliferation [17], and learning and memory disorder [21]. However, the scientific study of chemical constituents and biological activities against neuroprotection with the *G. laxum* has not reported so far.

During the purpose of screening for antioxidants from natural plants, we found that an EtOAc fraction partitioned from 70% ethanolic extract of *G. laxum* exhibited significant antioxidant activities. Thus, we report for the first time on the characterization of the chemical constituents of *G. laxum* and their neuroprotective and antioxidant properties in vitro radical scavenging systems and neuronal cell models.

Methods

Plant material

The dried aerial parts of *G. laxum* were collected at Bac Kan province, Northern Vietnam in spring, 2013. A voucher specimen was deposited in the Medicinal Herbarium of Hanoi University of Pharmacy (HUP) with the accession number HNIP: 18500/16. Plant material was identified as *G. laxum* based on morphological characteristics. For DNA authentification of *G. Laxum*, total DNA was extracted from 200 mg of fresh plant leave using a Dneasy Plant Mini Kit (QIAGEN, Germany) with some modifications. PCR amplification and sequencing were conducted by Macrogen Inc. (Seoul, Korea) using a pair of primers: ITS1-F (5′-TCCGTAGGTGAACCTGCGG-3′), ITS4-R (5′-TCCTCCGCTTATTGATATGC-3′). The sequence of ITS region of sample and reference sequence of *G. laxum* (KF269126) from Genebank NCBI was aligned by Geneious Alignment (65% similarity). The combined length of the entire ITS region (ITS1, 5.8S and ITS2) from taxa was analyzed with a 535 nucleotides. As ITS region of *G. laxum* are highly matched with the sequence over 99.4% from Genebank (KF269126), the plant material was finally identified as *G. laxum* based on morphological characteristics and DNA barcoding methods (Additional file 2).

Total oxidant scavenging capacity (TOSC) assay

A slight modification of the method developed by Regoli and Winston was used to determine the TOSC of the quercetin and its analogues [22]. Peroxy radicals were produced by thermal homolysis of 60 mM 2,2′-azobis-amidinopropane (ABAP) in 200 mM potassium phosphate buffer, pH 7.4, at 35 °C. Reactions with 0.4 mM α-keto-γ-methiobutyric acid (KMBA) were carried out in 10 mL rubber septa-sealed vials in a final reaction volume of 1 mL. Ethylene production was measured by gas chromatographic analysis of 200 μL aliquots taken from the headspace of vials at indicated intervals during the reaction. Total ethylene formation was quantified from the area under the kinetic curve. Samples were monitored in sequence at 15 min intervals over a time course of 60 min. Analyses were performed with a Shimadzu-2010 (Shimadzu Corp., Tokyo, Japan) gas chromatograph equipped with a SPB-1 capillary column (30 m × 0.32 mm × 0.25 μm) and a flame ionizing detector (FID). The oven, injection, and FID temperatures were 60, 180, and 180 °C, respectively. Helium, at a flow rate of 30 mL/min, was used as the carrier gas.

Quantification of TOSC

The TOSC value for each concentration of the sample was calculated as following:

$$\mathrm{TOSC} = 100 - (\textstyle\int \mathrm{SA}/\int \mathrm{CA} \times 100). \quad (1)$$

Here, $\int$SA and $\int$CA are the integrated areas from the sample reaction and control reaction, respectively. Thus, a sample with no oxy-radical scavenging capacity would give an area equal to the control ($\int \mathrm{SA}/\int \mathrm{CA} = 1$) and a resulting TOSC value of 0. However, as the $\int$SA approaches 0, the hypothetical TOSC value approaches 100. sTOSC values were obtained from the slope of the linear regression lines for the TOSC curves and rTOSC values were quantified by dividing the sTOSC value of the sample by that obtained of trolox, as shown below:

$$\mathrm{rTOSC} = \mathrm{sTOSC(sample)}/\mathrm{sTOSC(trolox)} \quad (2)$$

Molecular docking simulation

Possible docking modes between the ligands and active site 1 of BTB domain of Keap1 (PDB code: 4CXT) or its mutant at C151W were monitored by CDOCKER protocol in CHARMm force fields. CDOCKER energy indicates the ligand–protein docking energy. Ligand interacting affinity was expressed as CDOCKER interaction energy and interacting bonds such as hydrogen bond, pi–alkyl, pi–sulfur and Van der Waals using Discovery Studio 4.0 (Accelrys, San Diego, CA).

2,7-Dichlorofluorescein (DCFDA) and dihydroethidium (DHE) assays

Oxidative stress was quantified in cells by DCFDA [23] or DHE [24] (Invitrogen Thermo Fisher Scientific, Rockford, IL) assays according to the previously reported methods with slight modifications.

Antioxidant response element (ARE)-reporter gene assay

HT22-ARE or SH-SY5Y-ARE cells [25] were plated onto 12-well plates at a density of 3 × 10^5 cells/well for 6 h, and then the cells were incubated in DMEM containing 1% FBS for another 6 h. After sample treatment, the cells were incubated for 16 h, and the collected cell lysates were used for measuring the luciferase activity according to the protocol guided by the manufacturer (Promega Corp., WI).

Western blot analysis

Thirty μg of proteins were loaded onto the SDS-PAGE gel, the gel was run at 200 V for 1–2 h, and then the proteins were transferred to Immobilion®-P 0.45 μm PVDF transfer membrane (Millipore, Billerica, MA). After blocking the non-specific proteins on the membrane, the primary antibodies for Nrf2 (H-300, Santa Cruz), HO-1 (sc-1797, Santa Cruz), Lamin B (sc-474, Santa Cruz) and β-actin (ab6276, Abcam) were loaded and were incubated for more than 18 h at 4 °C. After washing the membranes, secondary antibodies such as horseradish peroxidase-conjugated anti-rabbit, anti-goat or anti-mouse-immunoglobulin G were loaded and were incubated for 2 h at room temperature. The protein bands were visualized through the reaction with chemiluminescent substrates from Thermo Scientific (Rockford, IL) using Image Quant™ LAS4000 imaging system from GE Healthcare Life Sciences (Little Chalfont, UK). The relative protein expressions were calculated by using ImageJ software (National Institutes of Health, Bethesda, MD).

Immunocytochemistry

HT22 cells were seeded onto a 35 mm cell culture plates and the cells were treated with DMEM with 1% FBS, PS and 20 μM of compound 4 for 12 h. After fixation and permeabilization steps, the cells were incubated with 1% BSA solution. The cells were reacted with primary antibodies (1:200 ratio, 4 °C), and were sequentially incubated with secondary antibodies conjugated with FITC or Texas red (1:500 ratio) for 2 h. The nucleus was stained with 1 μg/mL DAPI for 1 min. After washing the cells, the cells were mounted by using the Vectashield mounting medium (Vector Laboratories, Burlingame, CA). The confocal immunofluorescence images were taken by Confocal microscopy TCS SP8 (Leica, Wetzlar, Germany).

Real-time PCR

The mRNA extraction was performed by the Trizol method and then the mRNA was immediately synthesized to cDNA using Maxim RT PreMix (random primer) manufactured from iNtRON Biotechnology (Seongnam, Korea). The cDNA was subjected to do the real time-PCR. Primers were used to amplify HO-1 (forward: CAGCCCCACCAAGTT and reverse: GGCGGTCTTAGCCTCTTCTGT) and 18S (forward: GCTTAATTTGACTCAACACGGGA and reverse: AGCTATCAATCTGTCAATCCTGTC). The real time-PCR was done using StepOne Real-Time PCR System provided by Thermo Fisher Scientific (Waltham, MA) at this time condition: 10 min incubation at 95 °C and 40 cycles of 15 s at 95 °C and 1 min at 60 °C. 2X SYBR green and ROX dye (Bioneer, Daejeon, Korea) were used to measure the relative mRNA expression level.

Statistical analysis

The significance of results was analyzed by the one-way analysis of variance (ANOVA) using Tukey's post hoc or the Newman–Keuls multiple range tests using SPSS statistics 23 (SPSS, Inc., Chicago, IL, USA).

Information of experimental design and resources

Details of our experimental design, statistics, and all resources used in this study were included in the Minimum Standards of Reporting Checklist (Additional file 1).

Results

Isolation and structure determination of chemical constituents from *G. laxum*

The EtOAc fr. of *G. laxum* was subjected to a succession of chromatographic procedures including silica gel, Shephadex LH-20, RP-C18, and HPLC to afford 11 compounds (**1**–**11**). Chemical structures of isolated compounds were identified by ^{1}H, ^{13}C, and HMBC NMR analyses, and comparing their physicochemical and spectroscopic data with those published in the literature (Additional file 2). Compound **2** was obtained as a yellow powder and gave a positive ferric chloride reaction. The UV displayed two maximum bands at 260 and 381 nm, characteristic of a flavon-3-ol. In addition, the ^{1}H and ^{13}C NMR spectra showed a typical ABX aromatic spin system for ring B [δ_H 7.81 (1H, d, 2.0, H-2′), 6.98 (1H, dd, 2.0, 8.5, H-5′), and 7.68 (1H, d, 8.5, H-6′)], with corresponding carbons at δ_C 120.2, 117.3, and 112.1, respectively. Two oxygenated quaternary carbons at δ_C 148.5 (C-3′) and 147.7 (C-4′) supported this observation. Therefore, compound **2** was determined to be quercetin [26]. In comparison, the ^{1}H and ^{13}C NMR spectroscopic patterns of compounds **2**, **3**, and **4** were identical except only for the signals assignable for a methoxy group in **3** and **4** [δ_H 3.93 (3H, s), δ_C 56.4–56.5]. The methoxy group was found to be attached at C-3′ in compound **3** and at C-4′ in compound **4** by an HMBC experimental analyses. Thus, compounds **3** and **4** were characterized as quercetin-3′-methyl ether and quercetin-4′-methyl ether, respectively. As compounds **5** and **6** possessed two methoxy moieties in the structure, one methoxy group was attached to C-3, and the other one was substituted at C-3′ in **5** and C-4′ in **6**, respectively. Ermanin (**7**) and kaempferol-3-methyl ether (**9**) were also similar with **5** and **6** bearing a methoxy group at C-3 (δ_C 131.3–132.6). The significant differences in the ^{1}H NMR spectra of **7** and **9**, as compared to **5** and **6**, were the pattern of substitution in the B-ring at δ_H 8.05–8.25 (2H, br, d, 9.0) and 6.90–7.12 (2H, br, d, 9.0), indicative of H-2′/6′ and H-3′/5, respectively. Therefore, compound **9** was characterized as kaempferol-3-methyl ether, and compound **7** as to be ermanin, respectively.

Phytochemical study suggests that the aerial part of *G. laxum* is an abundant source of natural phenolics, which were identified as quercetin (**2**), quercetin analogues (**3**–**9**), benzoic acid (**10**) and benzoic acid analogues (**1**, **11**). It is well known that phenolics have a wide impact on the living system and that the most interested property of phenolics is antioxidant property [27]. Isolated compounds were determined as 3,4-dihydroxybenzoic acid (**1**), quercetin (**2**), quercetin-3′-methyl ether (**3**), quercetin-4′-methyl ether (**4**), quercetin-3,4′-dimethyl ether (**5**), quercetin-3,3′-dimethyl ether (**6**), ermanin (**7**), quercetin-3′,4′-dimethyl ether (**8**), kaempferol-3-methyl ether (**9**), benzoic acid (**10**), and 3-ethoxy-4-hydroxybenzoic acid (**11**) (Fig. 1).

Quercetin (**2**): Yellow powder; m.p. (uncorrected) 312–318 °C, $FeCl_3$ test: positive; UV (MeOH) λ_{max} nm: 260, 381; ^{13}C NMR (125 MHz, acetone-d_6): δ_C 178.2, 165.3, 164.1, 158.9, 153.3, 148.5, 147.7, 132.8, 123.9, 120.2, 117.3, 112.1, 104.6, 95.8, 94.9; ^{1}H NMR.

Quercetin-4′-methyl ether (**4**): Yellowish powder; $FeCl_3$ test: positive; ^{13}C NMR (125 MHz, acetone-d_6): δ_C 178.1, 164.5, 163.1, 158.8, 154.5, 147.4, 147.0, 132.3, 124.1, 120.7, 117.8, 112.9, 105.6, 96.7, 95.6, 56.4.

Oxytosis inhibitory activities of isolated compounds from *G. laxum*

The neuroprotective effects of the isolated compounds **1**–**11** were evaluated by an oxytosis assay which is a type of cytotoxicity assays with the extremely high concentration of glutamate treatment on the HT22 cells. Quercetin (**2**), quercetin analogues (**4**–**6**) and compound **11** at 20 μM exerted significant cytoprotective effect against cell death induced by 10 mM glutamate. Among them, compounds **2**, **4**, **6** and **11** had shown the protective effects at treatment concentrations at a range of 1, 5, 10, and 20 μM. The cells did not get damage at the treatment of compounds **2**, **4**, **6** and **11** whereas condensed and shrunk cells were observed at a single glutamate treatment (Fig. 2).

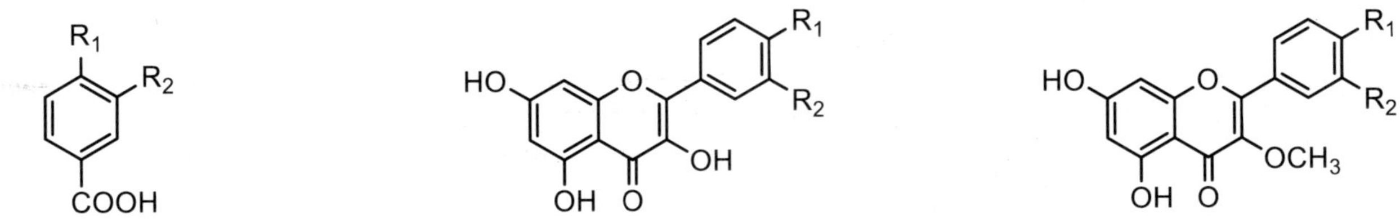

(**1**) $R_1 = R_2 = OH$
(**10**) $R_1 = R_2 = H$
(**11**) $R_1 = OH, R_2 = OCH_2CH_3$

(**2**) $R_1 = R_2 = OH$
(**3**) $R_1 = OH, R_2 = OCH_3$
(**4**) $R_1 = OCH_3, R_2 = OH$
(**8**) $R_1 = R_2 = OCH_3$

(**5**) $R_1 = OCH_3, R_2 = OH$
(**6**) $R_1 = OH, R_2 = OCH_3$
(**7**) $R_1 = OCH_3, R_2 = H$
(**9**) $R_1 = OH, R_2 = H$

Fig. 1 Chemical structures of isolated compounds

ROS inhibitory activities of isolated compounds from *G. laxum*

To understand responsible mechanism for the neuroprotective effect of compounds **2**, **4**, **6** and **11**, intracellular ROS and superoxide anion were measured by staining with molecular probes such as DCFDA for total ROS or DHE for superoxide anion. Intracellular ROS and superoxide anion produced by glutamate were effectively eliminated by compounds **2**, **4** and **11**. Interestingly the ROS-removing effect of compounds **2** and **4** was higher than compound **6** (Fig. 3a).

ARE transcriptional activities of isolated compounds from *G. laxum*

To elucidate whether quercetin (**2**) or its analogues (**4** or **6**) attenuate an intracellular ROS production and whether these effects are involved in ARE transcriptional activity, ARE reporter gene assay was performed using HT22-ARE and SH-SY5Y-ARE cells which contain ARE-luciferase reporter gene. The results demonstrated that compounds **2–4**, **6** and **11** induced ARE transcriptional activity over 2.5 times of relative value compared to the control at 20 μM in HT22-ARE and SH-SY5Y cells (Fig. 3b, c; Additional file 2).

Nrf2-mediated HO-1 induction by compound 4

The Nrf2/HO-1 related study about compound **4** (quercetin-4′-methyl ether), which was shown the excellent neuroprotective and ARE gene transcriptional activities, has not been elucidated so far. As shown in Fig. 4, compound **4** enhanced the Nrf2 accumulation in nucleus and translocation of Nrf2 from cytoplasm to nucleus at 20 μM. It also increased mRNA and protein expressions of HO-1 in hippocampal neuroblastoma HT22 cells by concentrations in a range of 5–20 μM (Fig. 4). These data indicate that compound **4** have HO-1 inducing effects mediated by Nrf2 activation.

TOSC activities of quercetin and its analogues (2–9) from *G. laxum*

In the present study, when quercetin (**2**) and quercetin analogues (**3–9**) reduced ethylene production in the presence of each sample in a concentration-dependent manner. The slopes of the regression lines were calculated from the linear portion of TOSC vs. concentration of the quercetin and quercetin analogues used, and the sTOSC and rTOSC values against peroxy radicals are listed in Table 1. Ethylene generation from KMBA oxidation upon thermal homolysis of ABAP was markedly inhibited by the quercetin and quercetin analogues. Quercetin (**2**) showed the greatest sTOSC value against peroxy radicals followed in decreasing order by compounds **4**, **3**, **8**, **6**, **9**, **5**, and **7**. Quercetin with two hydroxy groups in B ring displayed the highest sTOSC value of 11.76 ± 1.27 TOSC/μM, and compound **4** with a methoxy moiety substituted at C-4′ of the B ring (5.54 ± 0.40 TOSC/μM) showed significantly greater antioxidant capacities against peroxy radicals than Trolox, a positive antioxidant (2.88 ± 0.14 TOSC/μM), respectively. Compound **3** with a methoxy group at C-3′ and **8** with two methoxy groups in B ring (3.39 and 3.32 TOSC/μM, respectively) showed slightly lower activity than compounds **2** and **4**. Both methoxy substitutions at the 3-hydroxy group in C ring and 3′-hydroxy group of catechol in B ring (compound **5**) were significantly decreased the sTOSC values. In addition, compound **6** showed more strong scavenging capacity than compound **5** (significantly different by Student's *t* test, $p < 0.05$), with the same skeleton compound **9** also showed stronger effect than **7** (Table 1). Thus, the

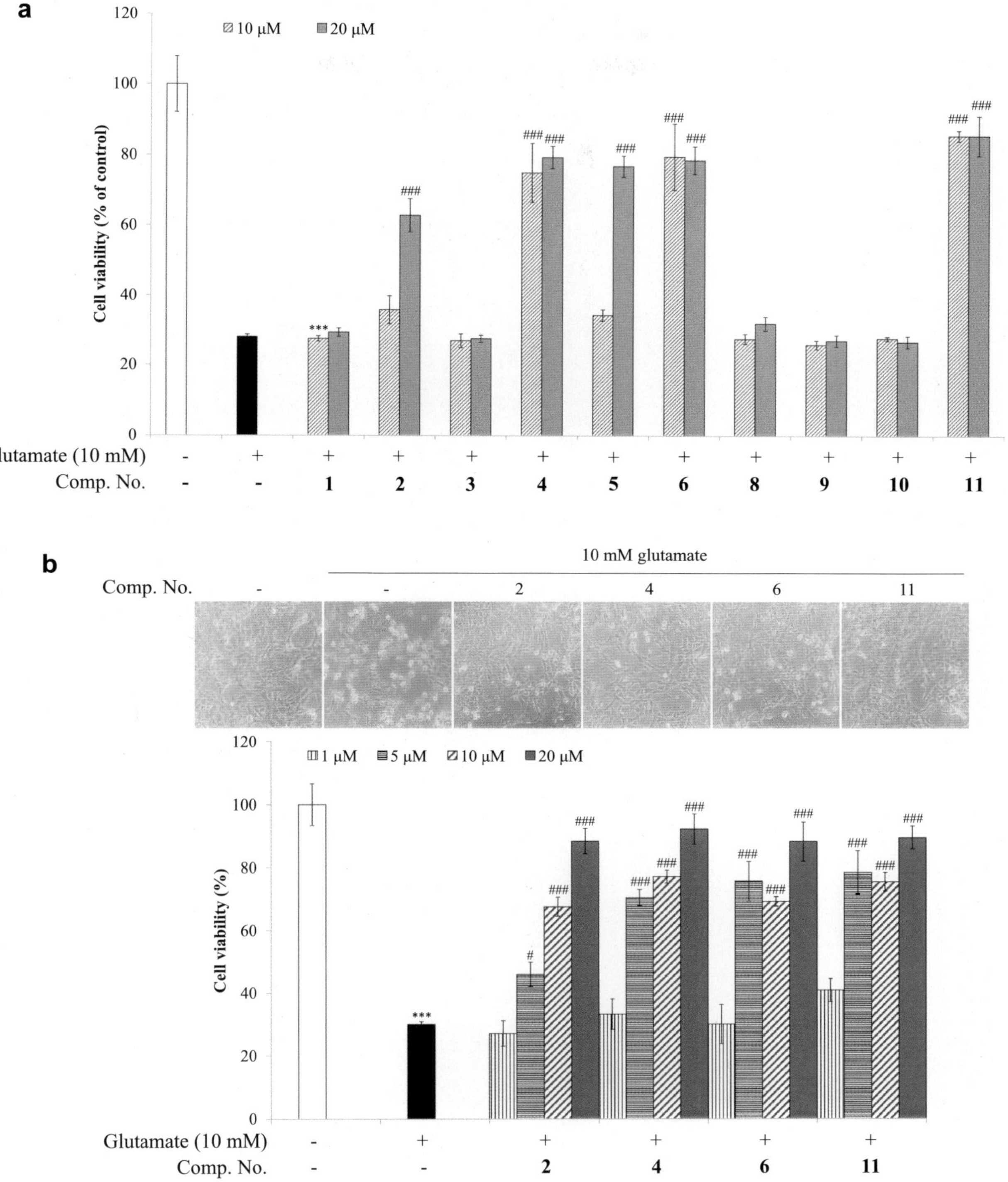

Fig. 2 Neuroprotective effects of isolated compounds from *G. laxum* in HT22 cells. **a** Cells were treated with each isolated compound from *G. laxum* at 10 or 20 μM in the presence or absence of 10 mM glutamate for 12 h. Values expressed to AV ± SD. N = 3, the significance was presented as ***$p < 0.001$ compared to the control, ###$p < 0.001$ compared to the glutamate-treated cell group. **b** Cells were treated with compounds **2**, **4**, **6**, and **11** at 1, 5, 10, and 20 μM in the presence of 10 mM glutamate for 12 h. Values expressed to AV ± SD. N = 3, the significance was presented as ***$p < 0.001$ compared to the control, #$p < 0.05$ and ###$p < 0.001$ compared to the glutamate-treated cell group

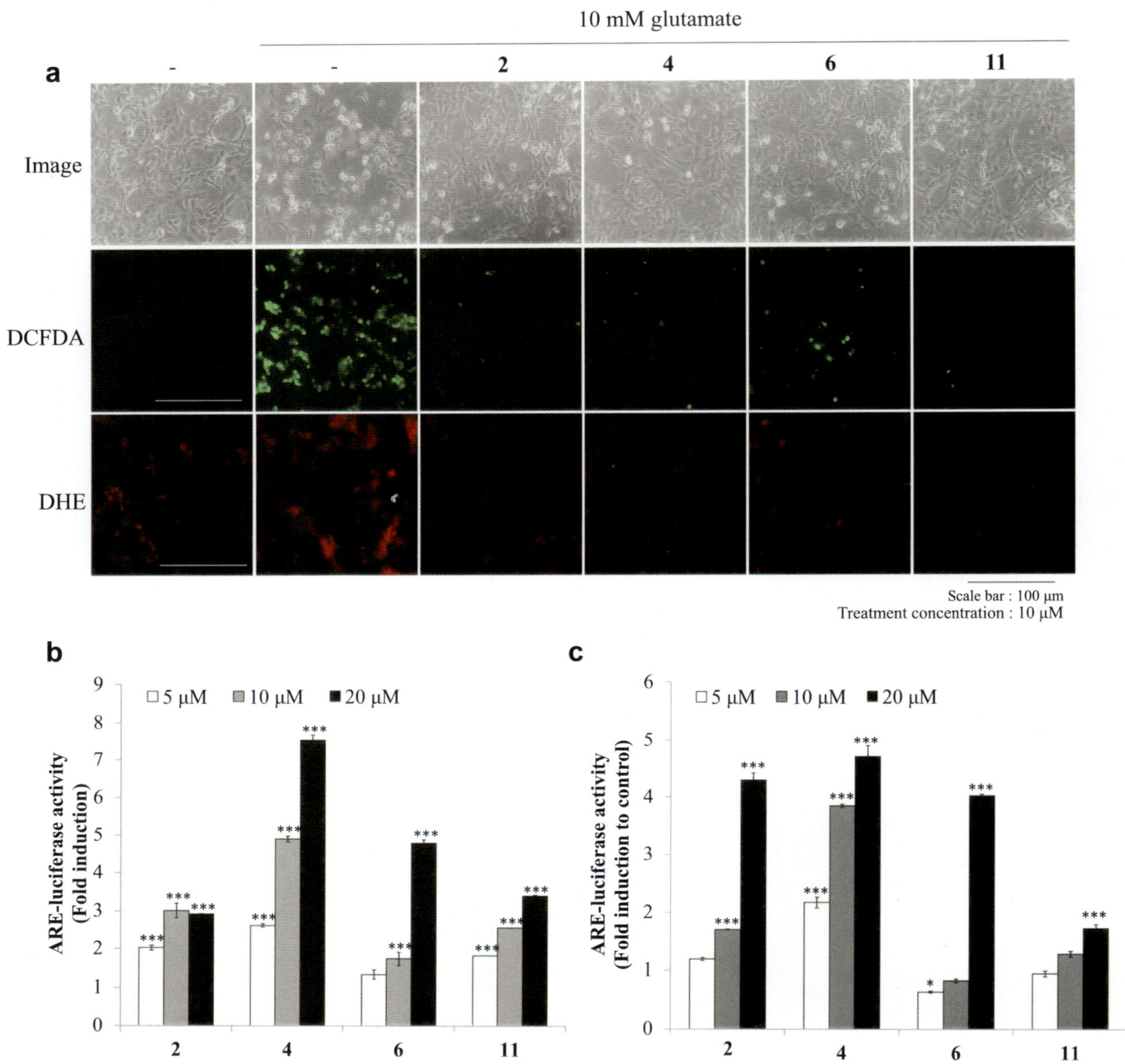

Fig. 3 Effects of compounds **2**, **4**, **6**, and **11** on ROS inhibitory and ARE transcription inducing activities. **a** DCFDA and DHE assays were visualized as the bright field cell images, intracellular ROS and superoxide anion levels by compounds **2**, **4**, **6**, and **11** at 10 μM for 10 h plus 10 mM glutamate. The magnification is ×200. **b** ARE-luciferase reporter gene assay was performed using HT22-ARE cells. Cells were treated with compounds **2**, **4**, **6**, and **11** at 5, 10, and 20 μM for 16 h. The specific methods are described in "Methods" section. Values expressed to AV ± SD. N = 3, the significance was presented as *$p < 0.05$ and ***$p < 0.001$ compared to the control

methoxy group may play a role in decreasing activity when attached to C-4′ position of the catechol.

Molecular docking simulation of isolated compounds to BTB domain of Keap1

We investigated whether isolated compounds from *G. laxum* can be docked in BTB domain of Keap1 and also can interact with amino acids positioned at BTB domain including the C151 residue by comparing with the docking and docking interaction energies of sulforaphane (SFN) as the positive control (Table 2). As results, quercetin had the lowest CDOCKER and CDOCKER interaction energies which indicate the binding affinity to Keap1. Consequently, the compounds fit stably onto the BTB domain and it was ordered by compounds **2**, **3**, **4**, and **8** at CDOCKER and **5**, **6**, **9**, and **7** at CDOCKER

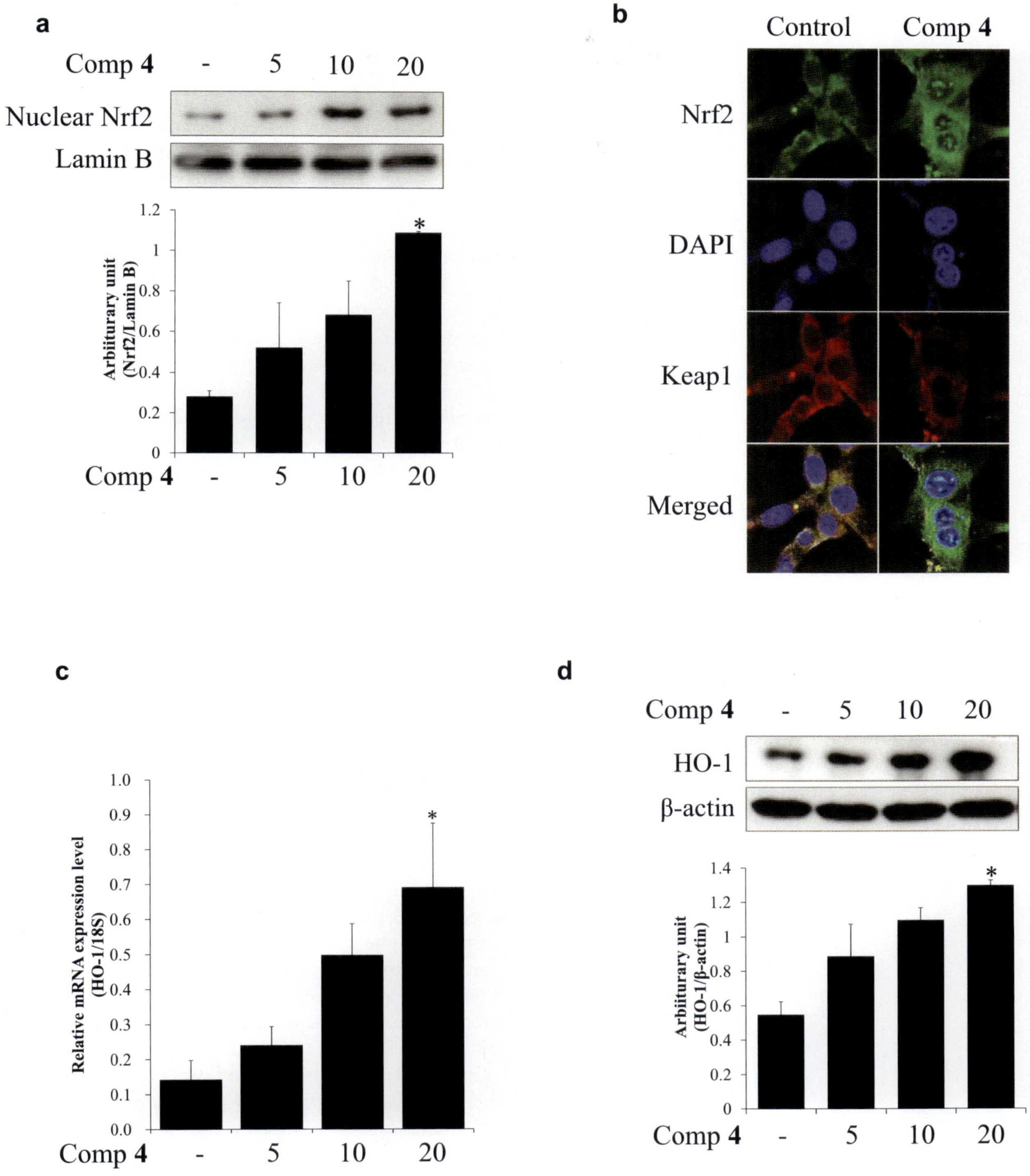

Fig. 4 Nrf2-mediated HO-1 induction by compound **4** in HT22 cells. **a** Nuclear Nrf2 accumulation by compound **4** at 5, 10, and 20 μM was analyzed by Western blotting. **b** Translocation of Nrf2 into nucleus by compound **4** at 20 μM was determined by the immunocytochemistry procedure using confocal fluorescence microscope. **c** Real-time PCR evaluated the mRNA expression of HO-1 by treatment of compound **4** at 5, 10, and 20 μM for 24 h. Values expressed to AV ± SD. N = 3, the significance was presented as $*p < 0.05$ compared to the control. **d** HO-1 expression pattern by treatment of compound **4** at 5, 10, and 20 μM for 24 h. Values expressed to AV ± SD. N = 2, the significance was presented as $*p < 0.05$ compared to the control

Table 1 TOSC values of quercetin and quercetin analogues against peroxyl radicals

Compound	Concentration (μM)	TOSC value	sTOSC value (TOSC/μM)	rTOSC value
2	0.625	3.2	11.76 ± 1.27[a]	4.08
	1.25	11.5	($R^2 = 0.9772$)	
	2.5	28.4		
	5	41.7		
	10	71.8		
	20	94.4		
3	2.5	7.7	3.39 ± 0.34[c]	1.18
	5	27.3	($R^2 = 0.9717$)	
	10	38.1		
	20	68.6		
	40	92.0		
4	1.25	8.0	5.54 ± 0.40[b]	1.92
	2.5	12.1	($R^2 = 0.9894$)	
	5	28.2		
	10	72.0		
	20	93.6		
	40	97.4		
5	10	−0.8	0.44 ± 0.05[d]	0.15
	20	7.1	($R^2 = 0.9781$)	
	40	12.9		
	80	35.4		
6	5	4.2	1.04 ± 0.03[d]	0.36
	10	11.5	($R^2 = 0.9977$)	
	20	21.2		
	40	41.2		
	80	69.8		
7	10	0.5	0.12 ± 0.02[d]	0.04
	20	−0.1	($R^2 = 0.9268$)	
	40	2.8		
	80	9.0		
8	1.25	0.4	3.22 ± 0.15[c]	1.12
	2.5	8.3	($R^2 = 0.9957$)	
	5	14.5		
	10	32.5		
	20	54.5		
	40	88.6		
	80	95.8		
9	5	4.4	0.53 ± 0.07[d]	0.18
	10	6.65	($R^2 = 0.9686$)	
	20	11		
	40	13.2		
	80	27.2		

The TOSC values of each concentration are mean from three independent measurements. The sTOSC values were obtained from the slope of the linear regression line for the TOSC curves, and the rTOSC values were determined by dividing the sTOSC value of the sample by that of Trolox. The specific TOSC values of Trolox against peroxyl radicals were 2.88 ± 0.14 TOSC/μM. Values with different letters are significantly different from each other (ANOVA followed by Newman–Keuls multiple range test, $p < 0.05$)

interaction energies respectively. The compounds **2**, **3**, and **4** docked to the BTB domain better than SFN and the quercetin (**2**) and its analogues (**3**–**9**) interacted with the BTB domain better than SFN. The C151 interacted with rings A and C of compounds **2** and **4**, the most active compounds, by pi–alkyl bonds in the contrast of other quercetin analogues. To investigate the involvement of C151 in docking of quercetin and its analogues to BTB domain of Keap1, C151 was mutated to W151. As results, CDOCKER and CDOCKER interaction energies of quercetin and its analogues were decreased by C151W mutation whereas benzoic acid and its analogues did not lower the CDOCKER and CDOCKER interaction energies. Interestingly, C151W mutation changed the space of active site of BTB domain in Keap1 so that the binding heads of compounds **2** and **4** against binding site also changed by opposite site. The changes in binding style lead to the interaction characteristics of compounds **2** and **4** in BTB domain of Keap1. In particular, the results illustrated the blockage of pi–pi stacked or pi–alkyl interactions between active compounds (**2**, **4**) and H154 or V132 (Table 2; Fig. 5). In summary, when C151 was mutated to W151 in Keap1, compounds **2**–**9** had shown higher energy differences than those of SFN at both CDOCKER and CDOCKER interaction energies. These results indicate that the influence of C151 residue of Keap1 keeps on the interaction between compounds and Keap1 protein.

Discussion

The phytochemical study suggests that the aerial part of *G. laxum* is an abundant source of natural phenolics, which were identified as quercetin (**2**), quercetin analogues (**3**–**9**), benzoic acid (**10**) and benzoic acid analogues (**1**, **11**). It is well known that phenolics have a wide impact on the living system and that the most interested property of phenolics is antioxidant property [27].

In this study, we used oxidative glutamate toxicity model for determination of neuroprotective effects by quercetin, benzoic acid and their analogues. Oxidative glutamate toxicity is categorized by oxytosis which is a unique oxidative stress-induced programmed cell death, and also it is accompanied by glutathione depletion due to the inhibition of cystine uptake via the cystine/glutamate antiporter [28]. Compound **2**, **4**, **6** and **11** exerted strong protective effects against the oxidative glutamate toxicity.

The Nrf2/Keap1-mediated HO-1 pathway is a possible mechanism for understanding the protective effects of quercetin, benzoic acid and their analogues. It has been well known that Nrf2 regulates the antioxidant enzymes including HO-1 through binding to ARE. Under the

Table 2 Molecular docking and interaction energies of isolated compounds from *G. laxum*

	CDOCKER energy		CDOCKER interaction energy	
	Wild type	C151W mutation	Wild type	C151W mutation
SFN	-20.7 ± 0.5^{c}	$-19.1 \pm 1.0^{e,*}$	-19.1 ± 0.4^{bc}	-17.8 ± 0.9^{a}
1	-19.3 ± 0.7^{c}	$-22.5 \pm 0.4^{g,**}$	-18.1 ± 0.6^{b}	$-21.1 \pm 0.4^{b,\#\#}$
2	-26.6 ± 0.2^{e}	$-21.4 \pm 0.4^{fg,**}$	-28.9 ± 0.1^{de}	$-23.8 \pm 0.4^{c,\#\#}$
3	-23.8 ± 0.5^{d}	$-18.2 \pm 0.7^{de,**}$	-29.2 ± 1.2^{de}	$-24.1 \pm 0.8^{c,\#}$
4	-24.7 ± 0.4^{de}	$-20.8 \pm 0.1^{f,**}$	-30.8 ± 0.5^{e}	$-26.5 \pm 0.3^{e,\#}$
5	-16.2 ± 0.4^{b}	$-11.0 \pm 1.1^{b,**}$	-30.1 ± 0.6^{de}	$-26.1 \pm 1.1^{de,\#}$
6	-15.3 ± 0.4^{ab}	$-9.3 \pm 0.6^{a,***}$	-29.4 ± 0.5^{de}	$-24.0 \pm 1.0^{c,\#\#}$
7	-14.0 ± 0.3^{a}	$-9.0 \pm 0.2^{a,***}$	-29.7 ± 0.9^{de}	$-24.5 \pm 0.1^{cd,\#}$
8	-19.9 ± 0.1^{c}	$-14.1 \pm 0.2^{c,***}$	-31.3 ± 0.4^{e}	$-25.0 \pm 0.3^{cde,\#\#\#}$
9	-14.8 ± 0.5^{ab}	$-9.8 \pm 0.4^{ab,**}$	-27.7 ± 0.4^{d}	$-23.3 \pm 1.0^{c,\#}$
10	-13.6 ± 1.0^{a}	$-17.4 \pm 0.2^{d,*}$	-14.7 ± 1.1^{a}	$-18.6 \pm 0.1^{a,\#}$
11	-21.0 ± 1.7^{c}	-22.4 ± 0.4^{g}	-21.4 ± 1.8^{c}	-23.2 ± 0.2^{c}

Values with different letters are significantly different from each other (ANOVA followed by Tukey's post hoc multiple range test, $p < 0.05$). The triple best fits were selected by CDOCER analysis using discovery studio 4.0. SFN, a representative antioxidant, and a C151 residue modifier, was used as a positive control. The significance was analyzed by the post hoc Turkey method (* $p < 0.05$, ** $p < 0.01$, *** $p < 0.001$ compared to the wild type of Keap1 in CDOCKER energy, # $p < 0.05$, ## $p < 0.01$, ### $p < 0.001$ compared to the wild type of Keap1 in CDOCKER interaction energy)

condition of oxidative stress, Nrf2 detaches from Keap1 due to the conformation change of Nrf2-Keap1 complex and then released Nrf2 moves to the nucleus, binds to the promoter region of ARE site [29]. Previously, many studies have reported that quercetin and its analogues are effectively scavenged oxy-radicals responsible for the pathogenesis of many diseases, including cancer, neurodegenerative, and cardiovascular diseases, and ageing [30–32]. The neuroprotective and Nrf2-mediated HO-1-inducing activities by quercetin were reported on HT22 cells [33] and its hippocampus effects on hippocampus-dependent learning and memory in mice fed with different diets related with oxidative stress [34].

Quercetin is a typical flavonol and is abundant in many commonly consumed fruits and vegetables, particularly apples, cranberries, blueberries, and onions. A number of studies suggested that antioxidant properties may be responsible for pharmacological activities of quercetin [22]. This observation in the result of a TOSC assay reveals that substitution of methoxy moiety in B ring may be responsible for the decrease of antioxidant activity against peroxyl radicals. Moreover, this is interesting that the presence of a hydroxy group at the 3′ position of B ring is more important than the 4′ position for antioxidant activities.

The cysteine residues in the BTB domain of Keap1, which play the key role in dimerization of Keap1, are covalently modified by oxidative or electrophilic molecules. The modification of disulfide bonds in cysteine residues of the BTB domain in Keap1 leads to dissociation of Cul3, and additionally releases Nrf2. Moreover, the stability of Nrf2 gets robust by decreasing ubiquitination-mediated protein degradation in proteasome [16]. The previous report suggested that C151 is essential for the biological action of sulforaphane (SFN), a representative antioxidant enriched in broccoli, as well as SFN reacts with four cysteine residues in Keap1 including C151 and thereby it modifies the C151 residue in Keap1 [35]. The results of in silico 3D molecular docking simulation indicate that the hydroxy and methoxy groups are important for Keap1 stability by influencing on docking to BTB domain. Compound **3** was stably fit than compound **4** which means that a hydroxy group in B ring also has critical role in docking to BTB domain. On the contrast, the CDOCKER interaction energy had shown in compound **8** < **4** < **3** < **2** and **5** < **7** < **6** < **9** in ascending power. When it compared to compounds **3** and **6**, docking energy of compound **3** was much lower than compound **6** while interaction energy of compound **3** was similar to compound **6**. Overall, hydroxy group in quercetin and its analogues involves in the Keap1 stability by improving to the docking of compounds in BTB domain, and methoxy group enhances the interaction of compounds with BTB domain of Keap1 (Table 2).

Conclusions

Taken together, the investigation of the structure-active relationship between quercetin and its analogues and antioxidant and neuroprotective activities related to Keap1 showed that the essential role of hydroxy and methoxy groups in B ring of flavonol-type compounds. This study investigated for the first time the significant

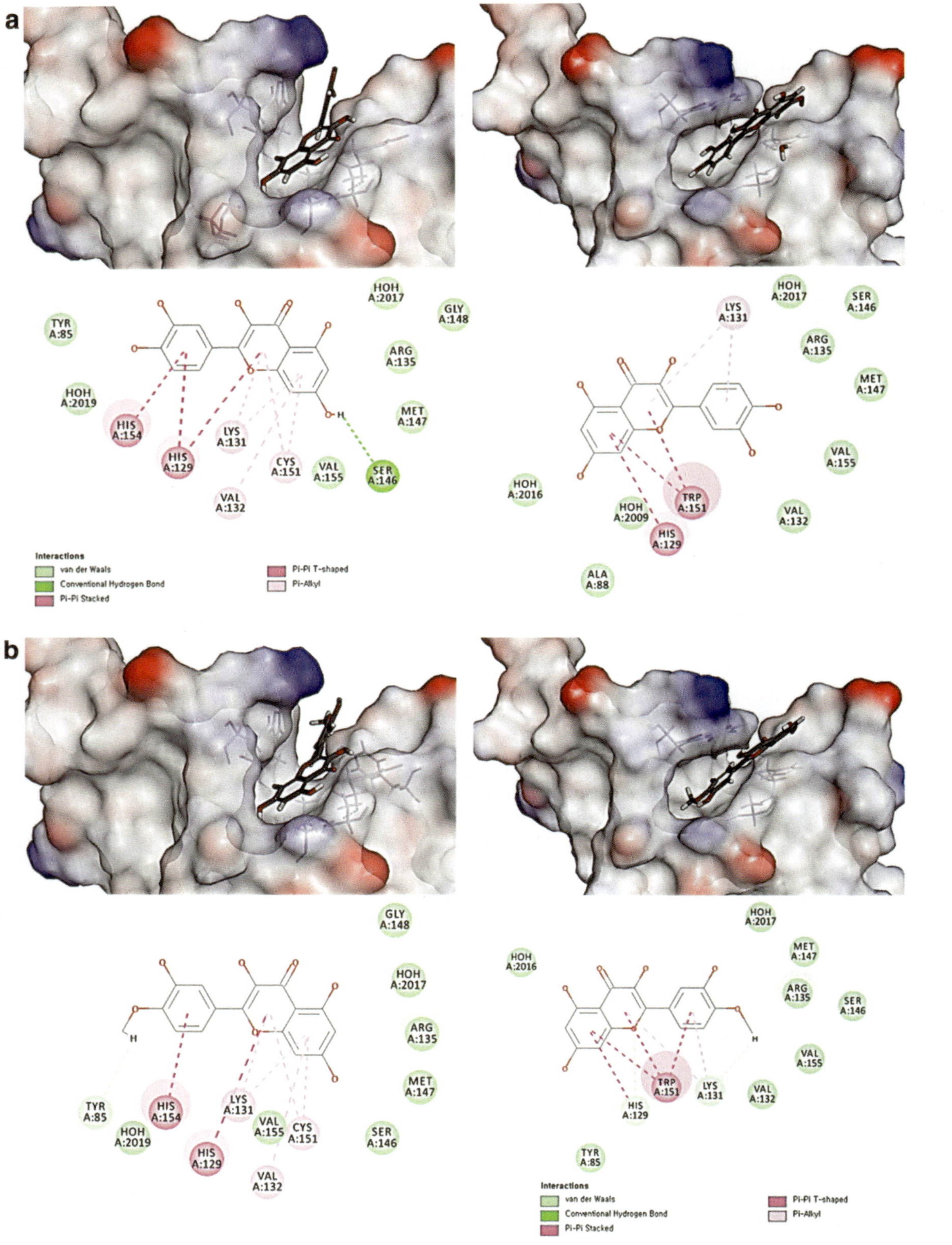

Fig. 5 Molecular docking and interaction images of compounds **2** and **4** with Keap1. **a** Quercetin docked in BTB domain of Keap1 (*left-up side*) and mutant BTB domain at C151W of Keap1 (*right-up side*). The interpolated structures were shown in this figure. The 2D diagram of ligand interactions was illustrated at *down side*. **b** Quercetin-4′-methyl ether docked in BTB domain of Keap1 (*left-up side*) and mutant BTB domain at C151W of Keap1 (*right-up side*). The interpolated structures were shown in this figure. The 2D diagram of ligand interactions was illustrated at *down side*

antioxidant and neuroprotective properties as well as the principles of the aerial part of *G. laxum*. The finding demonstrates that the *G. laxum* can be considered as an abundant natural antioxidant source so that it could be used beneficially in reducing oxidative stress complications.

Abbreviations

G. laxum: *Gynostemma laxum*; ROS: reactive oxygen species; ARE: antioxidant response element; Nrf2: nuclear factor (erythroid-derived 2)-like 2; HO-1: heme oxygenase-1; BTB: N-terminal broad complex, tramtrack and bric-a-brac; Keap1: Kelch-like ECH-associated protein 1; Cul3: cullin 3; TOSC: total oxidant scavenging capacity; ABAP: 2,2′-azobis-amidinopropane; KMBA: α-keto-γ-methiobutyric acid; FID: flame ionizing detector; PDB: protein data bank; DCFDA: 2,7-dichlorofluorescein; DHE: dihydroethidium.

Authors' contributions

JYS provided to experimental ideas and design partially, performed the experiments for neuroprotective effects, wrote the manuscript and contributed to biological and in silico data. SKK and PHN performed TOSC and antioxidant assays and analyzed the data. JYL and TPHT analyzed the content of quercetin in *G. laxum* and plant authentication. SHS provided many ideas and MS identification at results and discussion. WKO contributed to supervision, discussion and reviewed/edited the manuscript. WKO is guarantors of this work and had full access to all the data in this study and take responsibility for the data. All authors read and approved the final manuscript.

Author details

[1] Korea Bioactive Natural Material Bank, Research Institute of Pharmaceutical Sciences, College of Pharmacy, Seoul National University, Seoul 08826, Republic of Korea. [2] College of Pharmacy, Chungnam National University, Daejeon 34134, Republic of Korea. [3] College of Pharmacy, Chosun University, Gwangju 61452, Republic of Korea.

Acknowledgements

We would like to express our acknowledgements to Prof. Jong-Sang Kim from Kyungpook National University, Prof. Tran Van On, and Prof. Msc Nghiem Duc Trong, Department of Botany, at Hanoi University of Pharmacy, Vietnam.

Competing interests

The authors declare that they have no competing interests.

Funding

This work was financially supported in part by grants from the KBNMB (NRF-2012M3A9B8021570) and from the Bio & Technology Development (2016M3A9A5919548) of the National Research Foundation of Korea (NRF), which is funded by the Ministry of Science, information & communication technology (ICT) & Future Planning.

References

1. Droge W. Free radicals in the physiological control of cell function. Physiol Rev. 2002;82:47–95.
2. Ray PD, Huang BW, Tsuji Y. Reactive oxygen species (ROS) homeostasis and redox regulation in cellular signaling. Cell Signal. 2012;24:981–90.
3. Panza VS, Wazlawik E, Schutz GR, Comin L, Hecht KC, da Silva EL. Consumption of green tea favorably affects oxidative stress markers in weight-trained men. Nutrition. 2008;24:433–42.
4. Halliwell B. Antioxidants in human health and disease. Annu Rev Nutr. 1996;16:33–50.
5. Halliwell B. Establishing the significance and optimal intake of dietary antioxidants: the biomarker concept. Nutr Rev. 1999;57:104–13.
6. Prior RL, Cao G. In vivo total antioxidant capacity: comparison of different analytical methods. Free Radic Biol Med. 1999;27:1173–81.
7. Shahidi F. Antioxidants in food and food antioxidants food additives. Nahrung. 2000;44:158–63.
8. Wang Q, Sun AY, Simonyi A, Kalogeris TJ, Miller DK, Sun GY, Korthuis RJ. Ethanol preconditioning protects against ischemia/reperfusion-induced brain damage: role of NADPH oxidase-derived ROS. Free Radic Biol Med. 2007;43:1048–60.
9. Witschi HP. Enhanced tumour development by butylated hydroxytoluene (BHT) in the liver, lung and gastro-intestinal tract. Food Chem Toxicol. 1986;24:1127–30.
10. Dumont M, Beal MF. Neuroprotective strategies involving ROS in Alzheimer disease. Free Radic Biol Med. 2011;51:1014–26.
11. Drechsel DA, Patel M. Role of reactive oxygen species in the neurotoxicity of environmental agents implicated in Parkinson's disease. Free Radic Biol Med. 2008;44:1873–86.
12. Lim JL, Wilhelmus MM, de Vries HE, Drukarch B, Hoozemans JJ, van Horssen J. Antioxidative defense mechanisms controlled by Nrf2: state-of-the-art and clinical perspectives in neurodegenerative diseases. Arch Toxicol. 2014;88:1773–86.
13. Bonilla J, Atares L, Chiralt A, Vargas M. Recent patents on the use of antioxidant agents in food. Recent Pat Food Nutr Agric. 2011;3:123–32.
14. Kim HG, Ju MS, Kim DH, Hong J, Cho SH, Cho KH, Park W, Lee EH, Kim SY, Oh MS. Protective effects of Chunghyuldan against ROS-mediated neuronal cell death in models of Parkinson's disease. Basic Clin Pharmacol Toxicol. 2010;107:958–64.
15. Gao Y, Xu X, Chang S, Wang Y, Xu Y, Ran S, Huang Z, Li P, Li J, Zhang L, et al. Totarol prevents neuronal injury in vitro and ameliorates brain ischemic stroke: potential roles of Akt activation and HO-1 induction. Toxicol Appl Pharmacol. 2015;289:142–54.
16. Cleasby A, Yon J, Day PJ, Richardson C, Tickle IJ, Williams PA, Callahan JF, Carr R, Concha N, Kerns JK, et al. Structure of the BTB domain of Keap1 and its interaction with the triterpenoid antagonist CDDO. PLoS ONE. 2014;9:e98896.
17. Zhu H, Liu Z, Tang L, Liu J, Zhou M, Xie F, Wang Z, Wang Y, Shen S, Hu L, et al. Reversal of P-gp and MRP1-mediated multidrug resistance by H6, a gypenoside aglycon from *Gynostemma pentaphyllum*, in vincristine-resistant human oral cancer (KB/VCR) cells. Eur J Pharmacol. 2012;696:43–53.
18. Niu Y, Yan W, Lv J, Yao W, Yu LL. Characterization of a novel polysaccharide from tetraploid *Gynostemma pentaphyllum* makino. J Agric Food Chem. 2013;61:4882–9.
19. Nguyen PH, Gauhar R, Hwang SL, Dao TT, Park DC, Kim JE, Song H, Huh TL, Oh WK. New dammarane-type glucosides as potential activators of AMP-activated protein kinase (AMPK) from *Gynostemma pentaphyllum*. Bioorg Med Chem. 2011;19:6254–60.
20. Norberg A, Hoa NK, Liepinsh E, Van Phan D, Thuan ND, Jornvall H, Sillard R, Ostenson CG. A novel insulin-releasing substance, phanoside, from the plant *Gynostemma pentaphyllum*. J Biol Chem. 2004;279(40):41361–7.
21. Hong SW, Yang JH, Joh EH, Kim HJ, Kim DH. Gypenoside TN-2 ameliorates scopolamine-induced learning deficit in mice. J Ethnopharmacol. 2011;134:1010–3.
22. Cao G, Sofic E, Prior RL. Antioxidant and prooxidant behavior of flavonoids: structure–activity relationships. Free Radic Biol Med. 1997;22:749–60.
23. Wang H, Joseph JA. Quantifying cellular oxidative stress by dichlorofluorescein assay using microplate reader. Free Radic Biol Med. 1999;27:612–6.
24. Zielonka J, Vasquez-Vivar J, Kalyanaraman B. Detection of 2-hydroxyethidium in cellular systems: a unique marker product of superoxide and hydroethidine. Nat Protoc. 2008;3:8–21.
25. Seo JY, Ju SH, Oh J, Lee SK, Kim JS. Neuroprotective and cognition-enhancing effects of compound K isolated from red ginseng. J Agric Food Chem. 2016;64:2855–64.
26. Halabalaki M, Urbain A, Paschali A, Mitakou S, Tillequin F, Skaltsounis AL. Quercetin and kaempferol 3-*O*-[alpha-L-rhamnopyranosyl-(1→2)-alpha-L-arabinopyranoside]-7-*O*-alpha-L-rhamnopyranosides from *Anthyllis hermanniae*: structure determination and conformational studies. J Nat Prod. 2011;74:1939–45.
27. Karakaya S. Bioavailability of phenolic compounds. Crit Rev Food Sci Nutr. 2004;44:453–64.

28. Tan S, Schubert D, Maher P. Oxytosis: a novel form of programmed cell death. Curr Top Med Chem. 2001;1:497–506.
29. Nguyen T, Nioi P, Pickett CB. The Nrf2-antioxidant response element signaling pathway and its activation by oxidative stress. J Biol Chem. 2009;284:13291–5.
30. Russo M, Spagnuolo C, Tedesco I, Bilotto S, Russo GL. The flavonoid quercetin in disease prevention and therapy: facts and fancies. Biochem Pharmacol. 2012;83:6–15.
31. Boots AW, Haenen GR, Bast A. Health effects of quercetin: from antioxidant to nutraceutical. Eur J Pharmacol. 2008;585:325–37.
32. Kashyap D, Mittal S, Sak K, Singhal P, Tuli HS. Molecular mechanisms of action of quercetin in cancer: recent advances. Tumour Biol. 2016;37:12927–39.
33. Yang EJ, Kim GS, Kim JA, Song KS. Protective effects of onion-derived quercetin on glutamate-mediated hippocampal neuronal cell death. Pharmacogn Mag. 2013;9:302–8.
34. Xia SF, Xie ZX, Qiao Y, Li LR, Cheng XR, Tang X, Shi YH, Le GW. Differential effects of quercetin on hippocampus-dependent learning and memory in mice fed with different diets related with oxidative stress. Physiol Behav. 2015;138:325–31.
35. Hu CQ, Eggler AL, Mesecar AD, van Breemen RB. Modification of Keap1 cysteine residues by sulforaphane. Chem Res Toxicol. 2011;24:515–21.

12

Rapid screening and identification of bioactive compounds specifically binding to beta 2-adrenoceptor from San-ao decoction using affinity magnetic fine particles coupled with high-performance liquid chromatography–mass spectrometry

Fuhuan Fei, Huanmei Sun, Xixi Cheng, Jiajun Liu, Jing Wang, Qian Li and Yajun Zhang*

Abstract

Background: San-ao decoction (SAD) has been widely used in Chinese medicine against respiratory diseases, such as asthma and rhinallergosis. The bioactive compounds for such pharmacological action remain unknown.

Methods: We developed a methodology to isolate the bioactive compounds of SAD. The assay involved the immobilization of beta 2-adrenoceptor (β_2-AR) onto magnetic fine particles, the capture of target compounds by the immobilized receptor, the identification of the receptor bound compounds by reversed-phase high-performance liquid chromatography coupled with tandem mass spectrometry.

Results: Vicenin, shaftoside, isoshaftoside, liquiritin apioside and isoliquiritin apioside were identified as β_2-AR ligands in SAD extract. The binding of these compounds to β_2-AR occurred on serine^{169}, serine^{170} and phenylalanine^{256} of the receptor.

Conclusions: The developed methodology has high stability and specificity for recognizing and isolating target compounds. It is an alternative method for rapidly screening bioactive compounds of immobilized receptor from Chinese prescriptions.

Keywords: Affinity selection methods, Beta 2-adrenoceptor, Bioactive compounds, Magnetic fine particles, San-ao decoction

Background

Drug discovery involves identifying compounds that prevent or control diseases and play an important role in maintaining human health [1–3]. Despite increased investments in manpower, materials and financial resources for pharmaceutical research, the number of innovative drugs approved has declined during the last few decades [4, 5]. This is mainly due to the incompatibility between the increasing difficulties in drug discovery and the relatively low efficiency of the current lead screening methods. Efforts to create new, more efficient methodologies are urgently needed.

Natural products are the main source of virtually all medicinal preparations, and between 1981 and 2010, 34% of approved small molecule drugs were from natural products [6]. The impressive contribution of natural products to medicine, including traditional Chinese medicine, has promoted their use in driving drug discovery [7–9]. The classic approaches depend on the

*Correspondence: zhangyj@nwu.edu.cn
Key Laboratory of Resource Biology and Biotechnology in Western China, Ministry of Education, College of Life Sciences, Northwest University, Xi'an 710069, China

bioassay-guided screening of natural products, such as animal- and cell-based methods, have been continuously improved to utilize technological advances and achieve high throughput [10]. More recently, developed functional assays and phenotypic screens, such as cellular membrane affinity chromatography and computer-aided virtual screening technologies have received increasing attention [11–15]. In our previous work, beta 2-adrenoceptor (β_2-AR) chromatography was established for the identification of bioactive compounds of the receptor [16]. This strategy has limitations of time-intensity and labor-intensity in preparation of chromatographic columns. The structure of β_2-AR may misfold during the high pressure environment. Here, we established a bio-affinity technique by the utilization of magnetic material to remove the isolation and identification bottlenecks in identifying procedures [17–21]. Magnetic fine particle (MFP)-based ligand isolation methods are highly desirable because they utilize the unique properties of MFPs, such as convenient solid–liquid separation, high surface area and good biocompatibility [22–24]. Subsequently, with the molecular docking technology, we predicted the potential activity of bioactive compounds obtained from ligand capture [25].

San-ao decoction (SAD) is a basic prescription for treating respiratory diseases in Chinese practice. The formula is indexed in the Pharmacopoeia of the People's Republic of China 2015, and consists of three herbs: *Herba Ephedrae, Semen Armeniacae Amarum* and *Radix Glycyrrhizae*. Pharmacologically, respiratory ailments are mainly mediated by the β_2-AR, which belongs to the G-protein coupled receptor (GPCRs) superfamily [26, 27]. We hypothesized that SAD contains bioactive compounds that bind to β_2-AR. In this work, we immobilized β_2-AR onto MFPs to construct a new biologically relevant isolation material. The immobilized β_2-AR MFPs were used to rapidly screen bioactive compounds of the receptor from SAD. The compounds of interest were subsequently isolated and identified by high-performance liquid chromatography–tandem mass spectrometry (HPLC–MS/MS). Molecular docking confirmed the binding between the bioactive compounds and β_2-AR. The receptor-functionalized MFPs provide a convenient and effective strategy for isolating ligands from traditional Chinese medicines.

Methods

The Minimum Standards of Reporting Checklist contains details of the experimental design, and statistics, and resources used in this study (Additional file 1).

Chemicals and instruments

Ferric chloride hexahydrate ($FeCl_3 \cdot 6H_2O$) (99%) and ferrous chloride tetrahydrate ($FeCl_2 \cdot 4H_2O$) (99%) were purchased from Tianjin Tianli Chemical Reagents Ltd (Tianjin, China). Analytical-grade sodium hydroxide, trisodium citrate, ethanol and aqueous ammonia (25 wt%) were acquired from Shanghai Chem. Reagent Co. (shanghai, China). Reference standards of salbutamol (batch no. 100328–200703), terbutaline (batch no. 100273–201202) and shaftoside (batch no. 111912–201703) were purchased from the National Institutes for Food and Drug Control (Beijing, China). Vicenin (batch no. B21399), isoshaftoside (batch no. B21563), liquiritin apioside (batch no. B25831) and isoliquiritin apioside (batch no. B20987) were purchased from Shanghai yuanye Bio-Technology Co., Ltd (Shanghai, China). *Herba Ephedra, Semen Armeniacae Amarum* and *Radix Glycyrrhizae* were obtained at a local medicinal market and identified by Professor Xiao Chaoni in the College of Life Sciences of Northwest University.

An AKTA10 low-pressure chromatographic system from GE Healthcare Life Sciences (Uppsala, Sweden) was utilized for β_2-AR purification. Chromatographic analysis of the drugs were performed on an EClassical 3100 series apparatus (Dalian Elite Analytical Instruments Company, Dalian, China) equipped with an isocratic pump, a column oven and an ultraviolet–visible detector. Separation and identification of the bioactive compounds were carried out on an Agilent 1100 series of high-performance liquid chromatography (Santa Clara, CA, USA) coupled with an SL trap mass spectrometer (Waldbronn, Germany). The size distribution of MFPs was determined by dynamic light scattering (DLS) using a Malvern ZS ZEN 3600 system (Malvern, Worcestershire, UK).

Preparation of SAD

SAD was extracted by heat reflux [28]. Briefly, nine grams of each herb (*Herba Ephedrae, Semen Armeniacae Amarum* and *Radix Glycyrrhizae*) were weighed according to the Pharmacopoeia formula dosages. The mixture was decocted three times with 8 volumes of water (v/w) and 1.0 h for each time. The three filtrates were combined and concentrated to a certain volume via evaporation. Appropriate volumes of ethanol were added to the concentrated solution to give a final ethanol concentration of 80%. The mixture was stored for 12.0 h under an ambient atmosphere and was collected by filtration. The filtrate was concentrated to 1.0 g/mL under vacuum at 40 °C and stored at 4 °C for further experiments.

Synthesis of magnetic fine particles

Magnetic fine particles were synthesized by chemical coprecipitation based on the reaction of $Fe^{3+} + Fe^{2+} + OH^- \rightarrow Fe_3O_4$ [29]. We dissolved $FeCl_3{\cdot}6H_2O$ (10.812 g, 40 mM) and $FeCl_2{\cdot}4H_2O$ (3.9742 g, 20 mM) in 150 mL of distilled water. Oxygen was removed by a nitrogen stream for 1.0 h. An aliquot of 20 mL aqueous NaOH solution (8.0 g, 10 mM) was added to the mixture slowly and uniformly using a drop funnel. The solution was mechanically stirred for 1.0 h until the color turned black. The black solution was heated to 90 °C and then maintained at 90 °C for 1.0 h to ripen the particles. Decreasing the temperature to 25 °C, we collected the magnetic material using a magnet. The collected material was dispersed in 200 mL of 0.3 M sodium citrate solution and heated for 1.0 h at 80 °C. The solvent was removed after collecting the magnetic Fe_3O_4 FPs using a magnet. The Fe_3O_4 FPs were thoroughly rinsed with acetone and kept at 30 °C until all the solvent was removed. The dried Fe_3O_4 FPs were modified with aminopropyltriethoxysilane (APTES) to synthesize $Fe_3O_4@NH_2$ FPs [30].

Preparation and purification of β_2-AR

His-tagged β_2-AR was prepared and purified according to the methods in our previous work [31]. Briefly, genetically engineered bacteria (*E. coli* BL21 (DE3)-pET32a-β_2-AR) were incubated in 50 mL of Luria–Bertani medium containing 100 μg/mL penicillin. When the OD value reached 0.4–0.6, isopropyl β-D-thiogalactopyranoside was added to the medium at a final concentration of 2.0 mM to induce the expression of the receptor. Ni-chelated Sepharose high-performance affinity column and Quaternary Sepharose Fast Flow column were utilized to purify β_2-AR by sequential. The fraction of interest was collected by eluting the Ni-chelated Sepharose high-performance affinity column using 50% phosphate buffer (20 mM, containing 0.5 M NaCl and 0.5 M imidazole, pH 7.4). The purification of the collected fraction was performed on the Quaternary Sepharose Fast Flow column. The elution containing β_2-AR was collected from the column by 20 mM phosphate buffer (containing 0.8 M NaCl, pH 7.4) with gradient elution ranging from 18 to 50%. The purity of β_2-AR was measured by sodium dodecyl sulfate-polyacrylamide gel electrophoresis (SDS-PAGE). The fraction with greater than 90% purity was used for further investigation (Fig. 1).

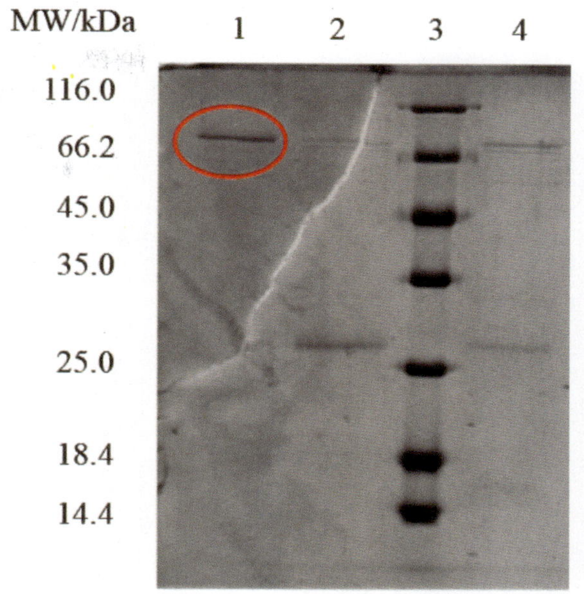

Fig. 1 SDS-PAGE analysis of β_2-AR. Lane 1, collection from Quaternary Sepharose Fast Flow column gradiently eluted by 18–26% phosphate buffer; Lane 2, collection from Quaternary Sepharose Fast Flow column gradiently eluted by 26–40% phosphate buffer; Lane 3, protein molecular weight marker (the molecular weights from top to bottom were 116.0, 66.2, 45.0, 35.0, 25.0, 18.4 and 14.4 kDa, respectively); Lane 4, collection from Quaternary Sepharose Fast Flow column gradiently eluted by 40–50% phosphate buffer. The concentration of phosphate buffer was 20 mM with the presence of 0.8 M NaCl

Immobilization of β_2-AR

As illustrated in Fig. 2, the purified β_2-AR was immobilized on the surface of $Fe_3O_4@NH_2$ FPs. In this case, we suspended 0.5 g of $Fe_3O_4@NH_2$ FPs in 50 mL acetonitrile containing 0.5 g N,N′-carbonyldiimidazole. The mixture was stirred for 6.0 h to activate the fine particles. After the removal of acetonitrile, the activated $Fe_3O_4@NH_2$ FPs were resuspended in 20 mM phosphate buffer and mixed with 10 mL of 0.24 mg/mL purified β_2-AR. The solution was mechanically stirred for 3.0 h at 4 °C to accomplish the reaction between the receptor and the imidazole residue on the $Fe_3O_4@NH_2$ FPs. The modified $Fe_3O_4@\beta_2$-AR FPs were collected using a magnet, while the unbound β_2-AR was removed. The obtained $Fe_3O_4@\beta_2$-AR FPs were suspended in 1% glycine solution and stirred for 30 min to quench the unreacted imidazole groups. The final $Fe_3O_4@\beta_2$-AR FPs were collected and washed three times with phosphate buffer. DLS was used to determine the size distribution of the $Fe_3O_4@\beta_2$-AR FPs.

Bioactivity of the immobilized β_2-AR

Salbutamol and terbutaline are both specific agonists of β_2-AR. They have similar structures such as meta-hydroxyl group, phenyl ring and N-terminus. Because of the same binding sites, salbutamol can be

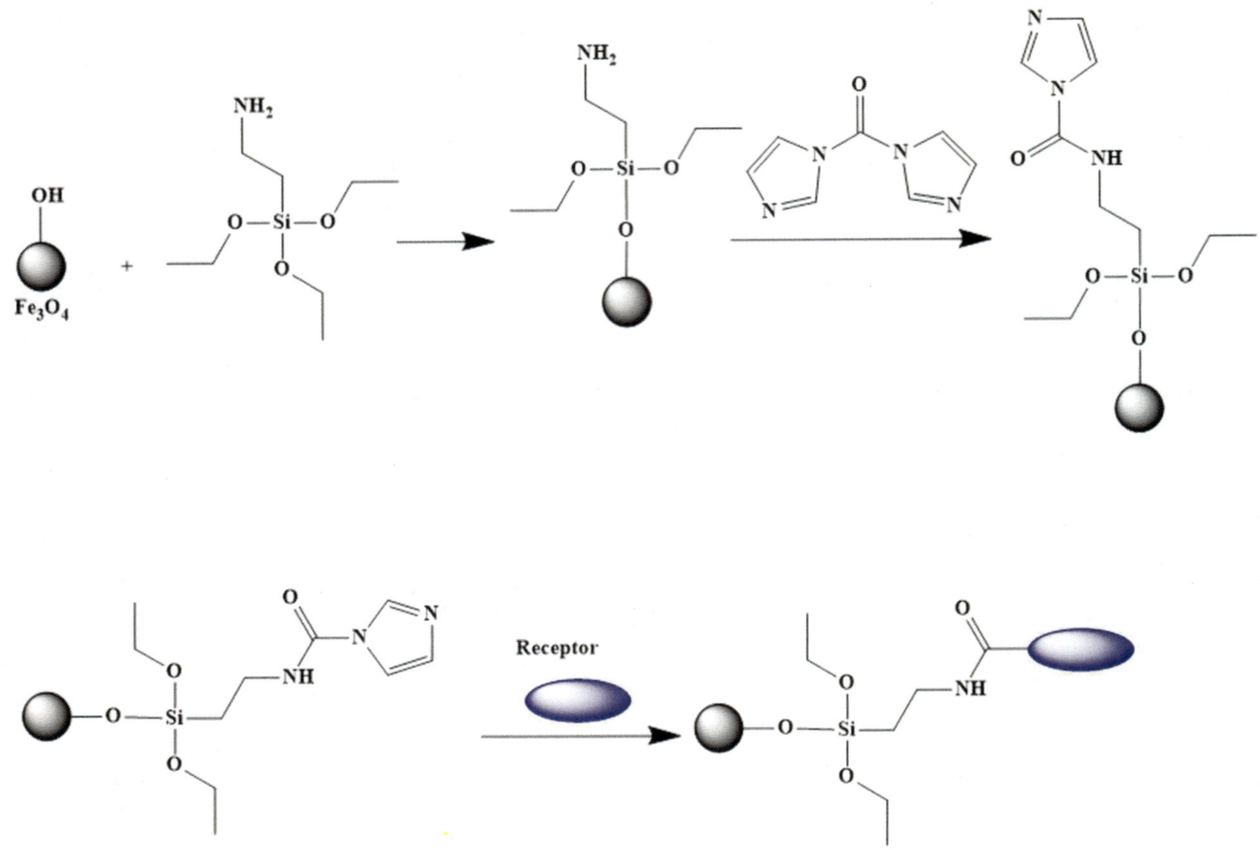

Fig. 2 The scheme for the immobilization of β_2-AR on the surface of Fe_3O_4 FPs. The structure of the compound was created using Chemdraw software. The blue ellipsoid represented β_2-AR

competitively displaced by terbutaline without any influence on the protein structure. Using the selective β_2-AR agonists salbutamol and terbutaline as probes, the bioactivity of $Fe_3O_4@\beta_2$-AR FPs was investigated by displacement experiments. Fifty milligrams of $Fe_3O_4@\beta_2$-AR FPs were incubated in 200 μL of salbutamol (10 μg/mL) and gently shaken for 30 min. The unbound salbutamol was discarded after collecting the fine particles using a magnet. The result $Fe_3O_4@\beta_2$-AR/salbutamol FPs were rinsed twice with 1.0 mL ammonium acetate buffer (10 mM, pH 7.4) and incubated with 100 μL competitive agent (terbutaline, 2.0 μg/mL) for 30 min to release the bound salbutamol [32]. The supernatant was collected after the fine particles were sequestered by a magnet. A similar procedure was performed with a control group of $Fe_3O_4@NH_2$ FPs, The drug concentration in the collected solution was determined by HPLC using an Agilent C_8 column (5 μm, 4.6 × 150 mm) with a mobile phase of 10% (v/v) methanol/water containing 0.1% (v/v) formic acid, a flow rate of 0.6 mL/min and a detection wavelength of 276 nm.

Screening of bioactive compounds in SAD

An aliquot of 50 mg $Fe_3O_4@\beta_2$-AR FPs was suspended in 200 μL of 0.2 g/mL SAD extract. This suspension was gently shaken for 30 min at room temperature. Following the removal of solvent, we washed the fine particles twice using 1.0 mL of 10 mM ammonium acetate. Bioactive compounds bound to the immobilized receptor were collected by treating the cleaned fine particles with 100 μL terbutaline (0.01 mg/mL) as a competitor. Terbutaline, a strong β_2-AR binder, has capacity to target all the three types of binding sites of β_2-AR [33]. As a result of competitive interaction, terbutaline can fully displace the potential ligands from the receptor. Simultaneously, this strategy is capable of probing the exact binding sites of the bound ligands inspired by the competitive displacement.

The released bioactive compounds were further separated and identified by HPLC–MS/MS with electrospray ionization (HPLC–ESI–MS/MS). An Agilent TC-C_{18} column (5 μm, 4.6 × 250 mm) was used with 40% (v/v) methanol/0.1% (v/v) formic acid as mobile phase. The flow rate was 0.6 mL/min and the column temperature was 30 °C. The nebulizing gas pressure was set at 50 psi. The flow rate and temperature of the dry gas were 10.0 L/min and 350 °C, respectively. Mass spectra were acquired in negative mode with scan range of 50–1000 amu.

Molecular docking

The crystal structure of β_2-AR was constructed by homologous modeling according to a previous work that utilized the methylated β_2-AR–Fab complex (PDB ID: 3KJ6) as the template. The structures of vicenin, shaftoside, isoshaftoside, liquiritin apioside and isoliquiritin apioside were created by ChemDraw Ultra 8.0 software (PerkinElmer Inc., Waltham, MA, USA), and was converted to pdbqt format using Chem3D Ultra 8.0 software (PerkinElmer Inc., Waltham, MA, USA) followed by MM2 energy minimization. Diverse receptor–ligand complexations were generated by AutoDock 4.2 which was downloaded from the Scripps Research Institute website (La Jolla, CA, USA). A grid box size of 62 × 56 × 50 points in the x, y and z directions was built to locate the receptor ligand binding domain. The grid center was set at x = 0.644, y = − 2.121 and z = − 7.094, which was large enough to accommodate the three known types of binding sites in β_2-AR.

Results

Morphological characterization of immobilized β_2-AR

The sizes of control Fe_3O_4@NH_2 FPs and Fe_3O_4@β_2-AR FPs were analyzed by DLS with intensity-weighted size distributions (Fig. 3). Both the two types of particles displayed a relatively uniform size distribution, with average sizes of 236.7 nm and 278.3 nm, respectively.

To determine whether the immobilization of β_2-AR on Fe_3O_4 FPs covalent bonds, we analyzed the Fe_3O_4@β_2-AR FPs by Fourier transform infrared spectroscopy (FT-IR) after complete rinse of the particles. Figure 4 depicted the representative spectra of Fe_3O_4, sodium citrate solution-modified Fe_3O_4, APTES-modified Fe_3O_4 and Fe_3O_4@β_2-AR FPs. The FT-IR adsorption band at 575 cm^{-1} corresponded to Fe–O bond vibrations in iron oxide. The strong absorption band at 3417 cm^{-1} was produced by O–H bond stretching on the Fe_3O_4 surface. The absorption peak at 1396 cm^{-1} was the typical absorption peak of carboxylate, providing an evidence

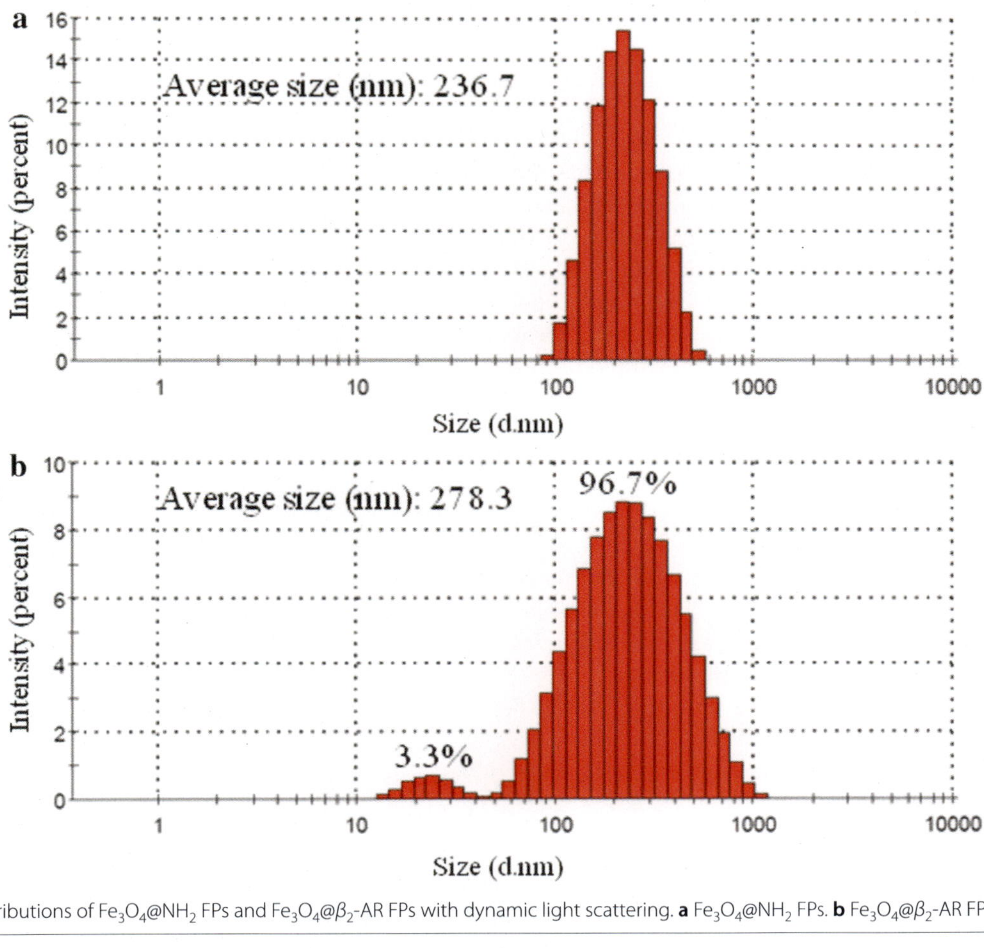

Fig. 3 Size distributions of Fe_3O_4@NH_2 FPs and Fe_3O_4@β_2-AR FPs with dynamic light scattering. **a** Fe_3O_4@NH_2 FPs. **b** Fe_3O_4@β_2-AR FPs

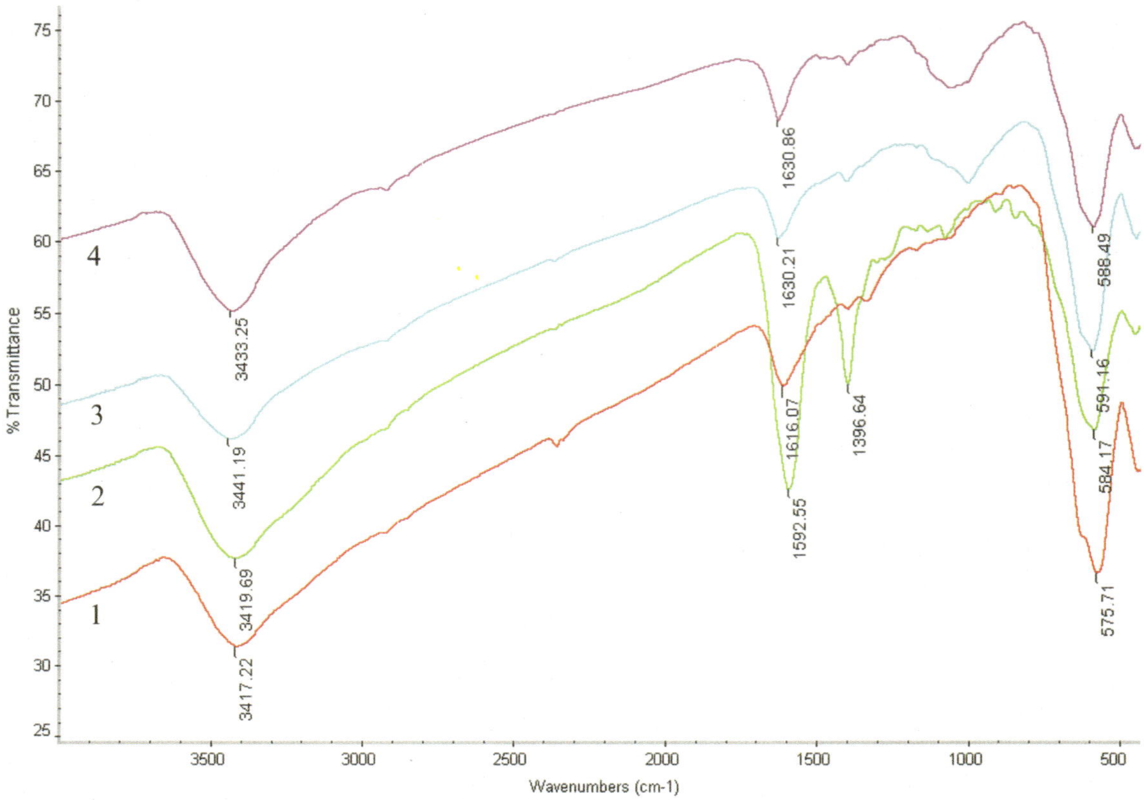

Fig. 4 FT-IR spectra of FPs. (1) Fe_3O_4 FPs. (2) Sodium citrate solution-modified Fe_3O_4 FPs. (3) APTES-modified Fe_3O_4 FPs. (4) $Fe_3O_4@\beta_2$-AR FPs

for the presence of –COOH on the Fe_3O_4 surface. Taking together, the citrate modification of Fe_3O_4 was occurred through chemical reaction rather than physical interactions. The spectrum of Fe_3O_4-APTES FPs displayed two broad bands at 3441 cm^{-1} and 1630 cm^{-1} due to N–H stretching and NH_2 bending modes of free NH_2 group. The strong absorbance observed at 3441 cm^{-1} was attributed to hydrogen bond formation. These results demonstrated that the immobilization of β_2-AR was accomplished by covalent reaction rather than physical absorption.

Bioactivity of immobilized β_2-AR

The bioactivity of $Fe_3O_4@\beta_2$-AR FPs was evaluated using salbutamol as a probe. A denaturing buffer solution (10 mM glycine–HCl, pH 2.0) was used to release the bound drug from the particles. The amounts of salbutamol adsorbed on the control and $Fe_3O_4@\beta_2$-AR NPs surfaces were determined to be 3 ± 1 and 52 ± 2 ng, respectively. The adsorption of metoprolol and prazosin (selective antagonists of β_1-AR and α_1-AR, respectively) on $Fe_3O_4@\beta_2$-AR FPs was examined under the same conditions. The amounts of the two antagonists on the $Fe_3O_4@\beta_2$-AR were 2 ± 1 and 3 ± 1 ng. On the basis of the pharmacological properties of the drugs, we concluded that the $Fe_3O_4@\beta_2$-AR FPs have the bioactivity of recognizing specific ligands of the immobilized receptor. The stability of the immobilized β_2-AR was investigated by measuring the amount of adsorbed salbutamol over 2 weeks. The relative standard deviation (RSD) of the content of the absorbed salbutamol was 2.1% (Table 1), indicating that immobilized β_2-AR was stable for at least 2 weeks.

Table 1 Stability investigation of the immobilized β_2-AR MFPs

Times (day)	Salbutamol binding contents (ng)	Relative standard deviation (RSD)
1	58	2.1%
3	56	
7	57	
10	54	
14	53	

The binding contents of salbutamol were determined by denaturing the receptor using 10 mM glycine–HCl (pH 2.0) and releasing the drug into solution

Competitive displacement of ligands bound on immobilized β_2-AR

Competitive experiments were performed to prevent false positives which were generated by non-specific binding. Salbutamol was used as a ligand while terbutaline served as a competitive agent. The competitive displacement procedure consisted of three steps: loading, washing, and displacing. In the loading step, we added 200 μL salbutamol (10 μg/mL) to the suspension of $Fe_3O_4@\beta_2$-AR FPs. Incubating the result suspension for 30 min, we collected the $Fe_3O_4@\beta_2$-AR FPs with bound salbutamol by a magnet while discarded the free drug in the supernatant. In the second step, we rinsed the $Fe_3O_4@\beta_2$-AR FPs by ammonium acetate (10 mM, pH 7.4) to remove non-specific binders on the immobilized receptor. In the final step, we incubated the suspension of the clean particles with 2.0 μg/mL terbutaline for 30 min. This aimed to release the bound ligand from the receptor by competitive displacement. Figure 5a showed the chromatograms of salbutamol and terbutaline reference standards. Under the desired conditions, the two drugs were totally separated without any inference. This condition was subsequently utilized to content of the two drugs during the displacement procedure. Figure 5b displayed the chromatograms of salbutamol in the solution post-incubation with control and $Fe_3O_4@\beta_2$-AR FPs. Compared with the original solution, a clear loss of salbutamol was observed in the supernatant after the incubation with $Fe_3O_4@\beta_2$-AR FPs. This loss raised from the specific binding of potential ligand onto the immobilized receptor. Figure 5c exhibited the chromatograms of salbutamol in the solution that was utilized to rinse control and $Fe_3O_4@\beta_2$-AR FPs. The control particles gave no peaks on the chromatograms, while the $Fe_3O_4@\beta_2$-AR

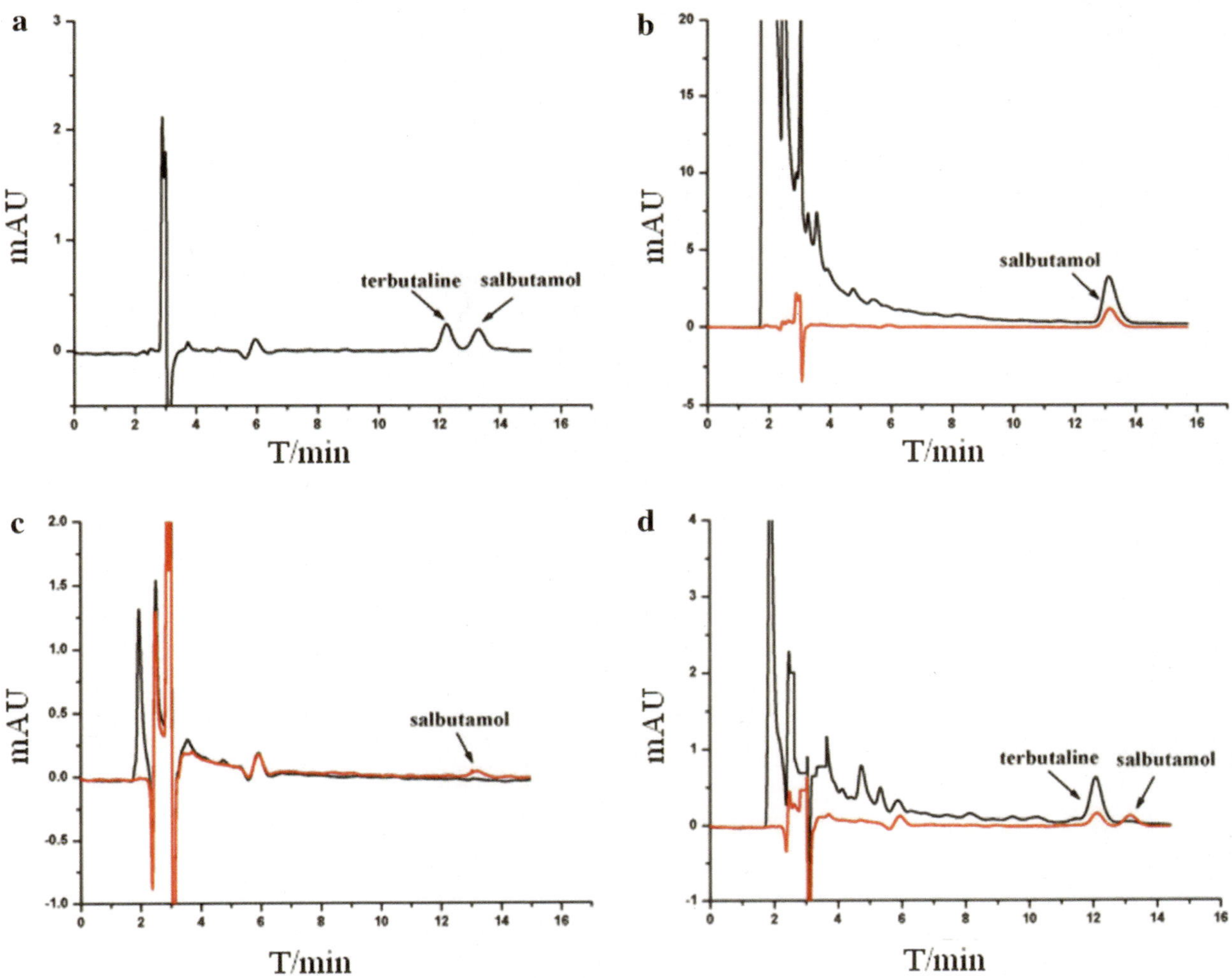

Fig. 5 Chromatograms of terbutaline and salbutamol in the collected supernatant from $Fe_3O_4@NH_2$ FPs (black curve) and $Fe_3O_4@\beta_2$-AR FPs (red curve) of the competitive displacement. **a** Terbutaline and salbutamol standards. **b** Loading salbutamol to $Fe_3O_4@\beta_2$-AR FPs. **c** Washing unbound salbutamol by ammonium acetate. **d** Displacing the bound salbutamol from $Fe_3O_4@\beta_2$-AR FPs by terbutaline

FPs resulted in a weak peak after the same rinsing treatment to control particles. The presence of this peak is expected because there will be a continuous ligand-dissociation/ligand-association from/with the ligand–protein complex at equilibrium [17]. As anticipated, this weak peak disappeared when we rinsed the particles for five times. Considering the speed of the whole methodology, we intended to use two times rinsing for further experiment since the weak peak had little influence on the determination of salbutamol in displacement procedure and was easy to be subtracted. Figure 5d depicted the chromatograms of salbutamol after incubating the Fe_3O_4@β_2-AR FPs with terbutaline (competitive agent) solution. Two intensive peaks were observed at 12.2 min and 13.1 min in the chromatogram. Using the reference standards, we identified the two peaks as salbutamol and terbutaline. This result indicated that terbutaline has the capacity to competitively displace the bound salbutamol on the particles. The method is feasible to be utilized for screening potential ligand and simultaneously probing the exact binding sites of the ligand on the receptor.

Screening bioactive compounds of β_2-AR from SAD

The total ion current chromatogram of the SAD extract and the eluted bioactive compounds specifically bound to β_2-AR were illustrated in Fig. 6a, b. Compared with the chromatogram of SAD extract, we observed five intensive peaks after treating the Fe_3O_4@β_2-AR FPs with SAD extract. No other peaks in SAD extract were detected in the same sample. These results demonstrated the

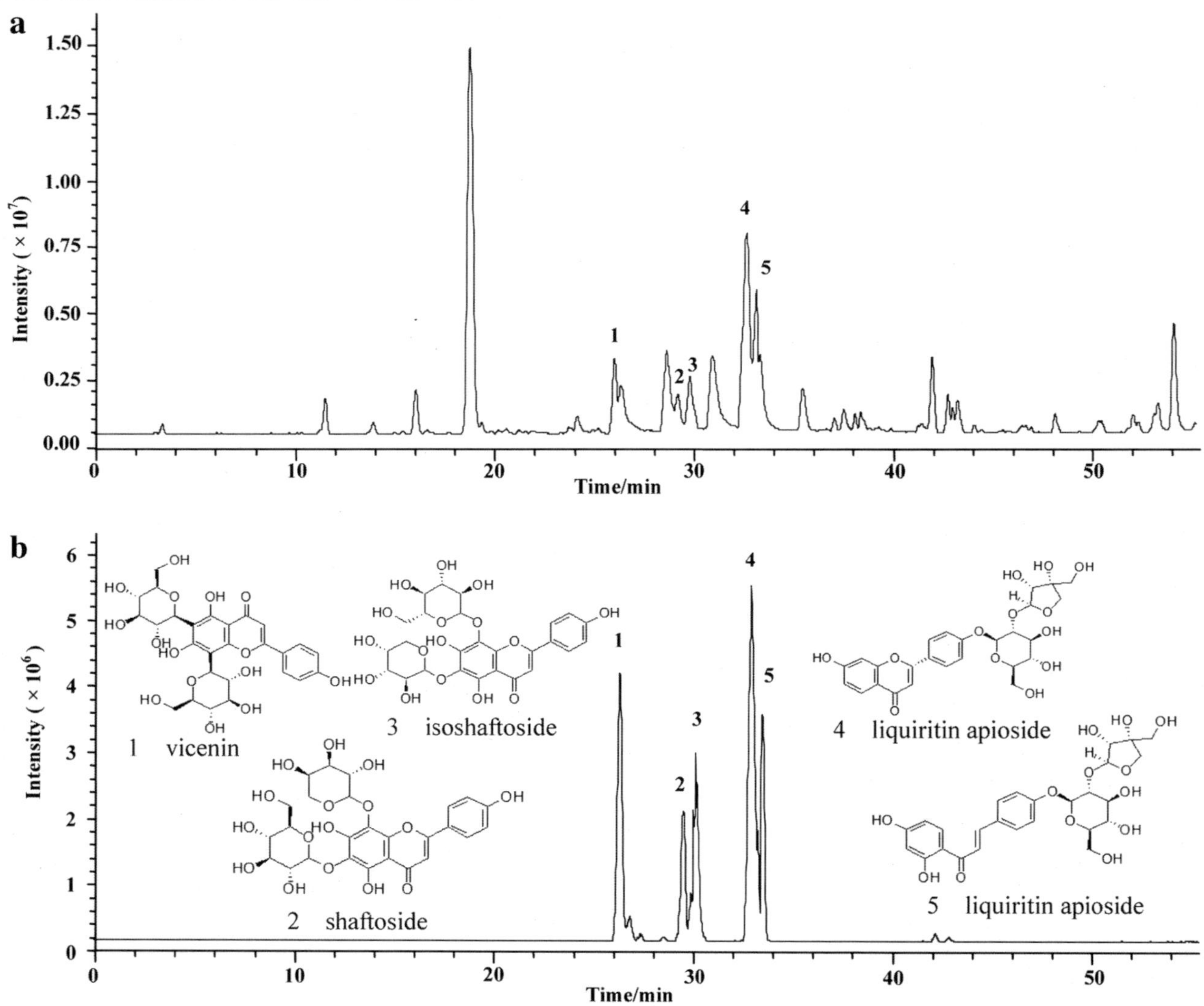

Fig. 6 Total ion current chromatograms of SAD extract and the bioactive compounds screened from the prescription. **a** SAD extract. **b** Bioactive compounds screened from SAD

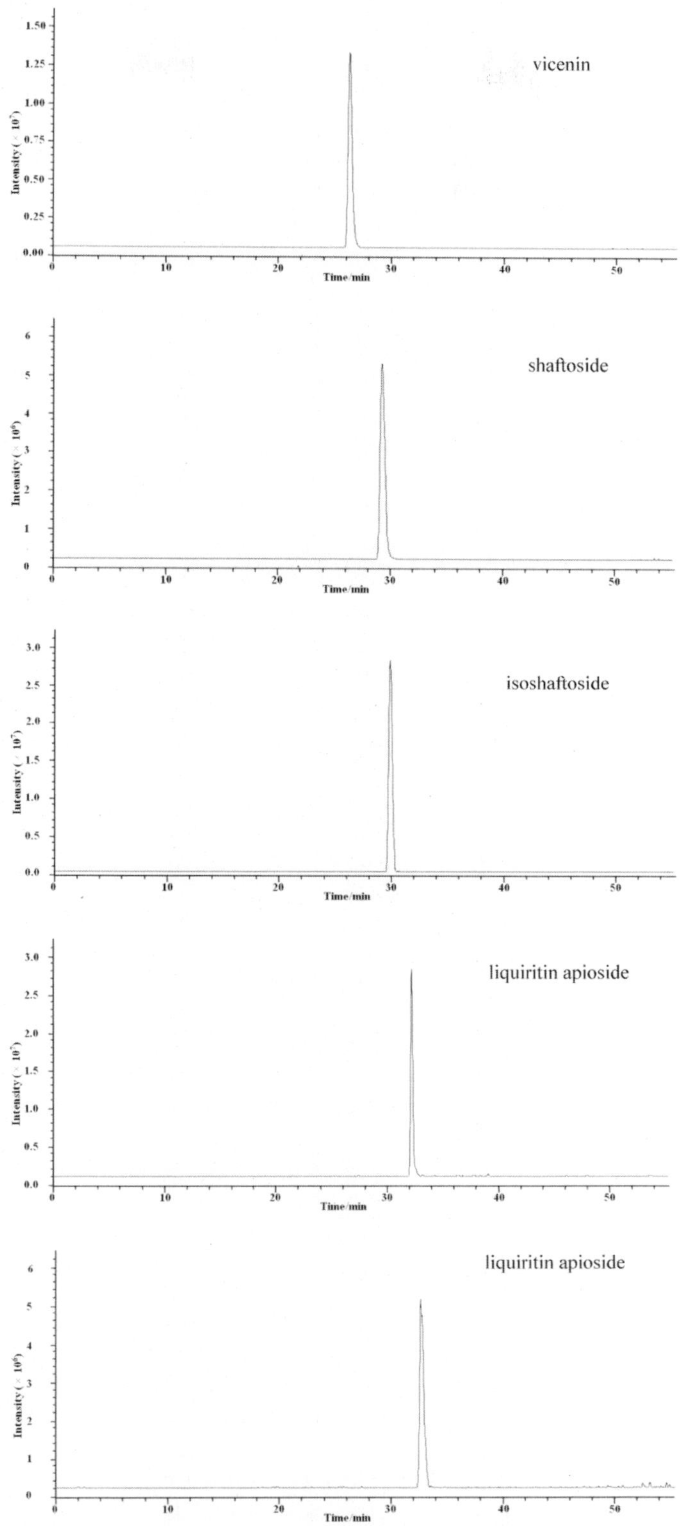

Fig. 7 Total ion current chromatograms of the reference standards of vicenin, shaftoside, isoshaftoside, liquiritin apioside and isoliquiritin apioside

immobilized receptor has the specificity to capture its ligands from complex matrices. The five peaks were identified by MS/MS analysis and the comparison with mass spectrometric behaviors of reference standards (Fig. 7). The peaks at 26.4 min showed an $[M-H]^-$ ion with *m/z* 593.0, which produced daughter ions at *m/z* 503.1, 473.2 and 353.8. This peak was identified as vicenin due to their identical mass patterns. The peaks at 29.2 min and 29.8 min gave same father ion of *m/z* 563.0 $[M-H]^-$. This ion generated daughter ions of *m/z* 503.1, 473.2, 443.5, 383.5 and 353.6. Compared with the retention time and mass behavior of reference standards, we attributed this peak to shaftoside and isoshaftoside. The peaks at 32.9 min and 33.4 min generated the same quasi-molecular ion $[M-H]^-$ of *m/z* 549.0, which gave main fragment ions of *m/z* 417.0, 297.0 and 255.0. Inspired by previous report and the mass patterns of reference standards, we identified the two peaks as liquiritin apioside and isoliquiritin apioside [34, 35]. In addition, we observed several puny peaks in Fig. 6b. At present, we failed to identify these peaks ascribed to lack of corresponding reference standards and their low intensity which was far away from the requirement of MS/MS analysis.

The interaction between the five compounds and β_2-AR was investigated using molecular docking. As displayed in Fig. 8, serine (Ser) ^{169}, Ser^{170} and phenylalanine (Phe)^{256} were found to be the main binding sites of vicenin, shaftoside, isoshaftoside, liquiritin apioside and isoliquiritin apioside to β_2-AR. The driving force of this interaction was the formation of hydrogen bonds between the receptor and the drug.

Discussion

This was aimed to develop a rapid methodology that enables us to screen the ligands of GPCRs. Development of such methodologies is challenging due to the instability of the receptors when they were removed from their native environment. As illustrated in the scheme of Fig. 9, His-tagged β_2-AR was first immobilized onto Fe_3O_4@NH_2 FPs to achieve an affinity selection supporter. Owning to the large surface area and high biocompatibility of the particles, this immobilization improved the stability of β_2-AR. The Fe_3O_4@β_2-AR FPs were used to select bioactive compounds binding to the receptor in a complex prescription. The bound compounds were released from the receptor by competitive displacement using a specific agonist. Finally, HPLC–MS/MS was used to identify the compounds that were released from the Fe_3O_4@β_2-AR FPs. Such procedure is attractive since the recognition and isolation of the target compounds are achieved at the same time.

Morphological characterization of the immobilized β_2-AR demonstrated that both the types of particles displayed a relatively uniform size distribution. Compared with Fe_3O_4@NH_2 FPs, the Fe_3O_4@β_2-AR FPs produced a size growth of 41.6 nm. We attributed this growth to the immobilization of β_2-AR based on the size of the receptor [36]. The hydroxyl content of the Fe_3O_4 FPs was determined to be 384 ± 6.94 μmol/g by acid–base titration. After amino group modification, the hydroxyl content decreased to 43.18 ± 3.21 μmol/g due to reversible Schiff base formation, confirming the covalent modification of Fe_3O_4 FPs by APTES. This change became more significant when APTES-modified FPs were treated with β_2-AR, providing a proof of chemical immobilization of the receptor on the particle surface. The molecular weight of the purified protein was determined to be 66.5 kDa by SDS-PAGE. According to this result, we identified the purified protein to be β_2-AR. The quantity of immobilized β_2-AR was determined by the bicinchoninic acid assay. A calibration curve with a regression equation of $y = (0.825 \pm 0.025)x - (0.0127 \pm 0.002)$ and a correlation coefficient of 0.996 was plotted using bovine serum albumin as the reference standard. Using this curve, the amount of β_2-AR immobilized on the particle surface was determined to be 8.439 ± 0.784 nmol/g. Compared with the immobilization using silica gel as a supporter [37], we declared that the current method was beneficial to achieve a uniform, high density and stable immobilization of the receptor.

Affinity magnetic materials are primarily limited by false positive and false negative results. False positives are caused by nonspecific ligand adsorption, while false negatives are caused by excessive washing steps or manipulation. Considering the mentioned competitive displacement results, we concluded that flushing ligand-Fe_3O_4@β_2-AR FPs two times with ammonium acetate was optimal during the washing step. This buffer was compatible with the receptor, and was effective to remove nonspecifically bound moieties and remain high speed without false positive and false negative results.

As a common prescription, SAD is mainly utilized for relieving cough and asthma symptoms in practice [38]. Pharmacological investigation showed that the treatment of asthma with SAD mainly involves the vasodilatations of bronchial vascular smooth muscle, where β_2-AR is the main drug target [39, 40]. These studies indicated that the five compounds were the main bioactive compounds for asthma treatment through mediating β_2-AR signal pathway. Molecular docking results aligned with a previous report states that three sites contribute to the binding of an agonist to β_2-AR. The sites included an aspartate residue on the third domain, two serine residues on the fifth domain and two phenylalanine residues [41]. The agreement of our results with the report confirms the

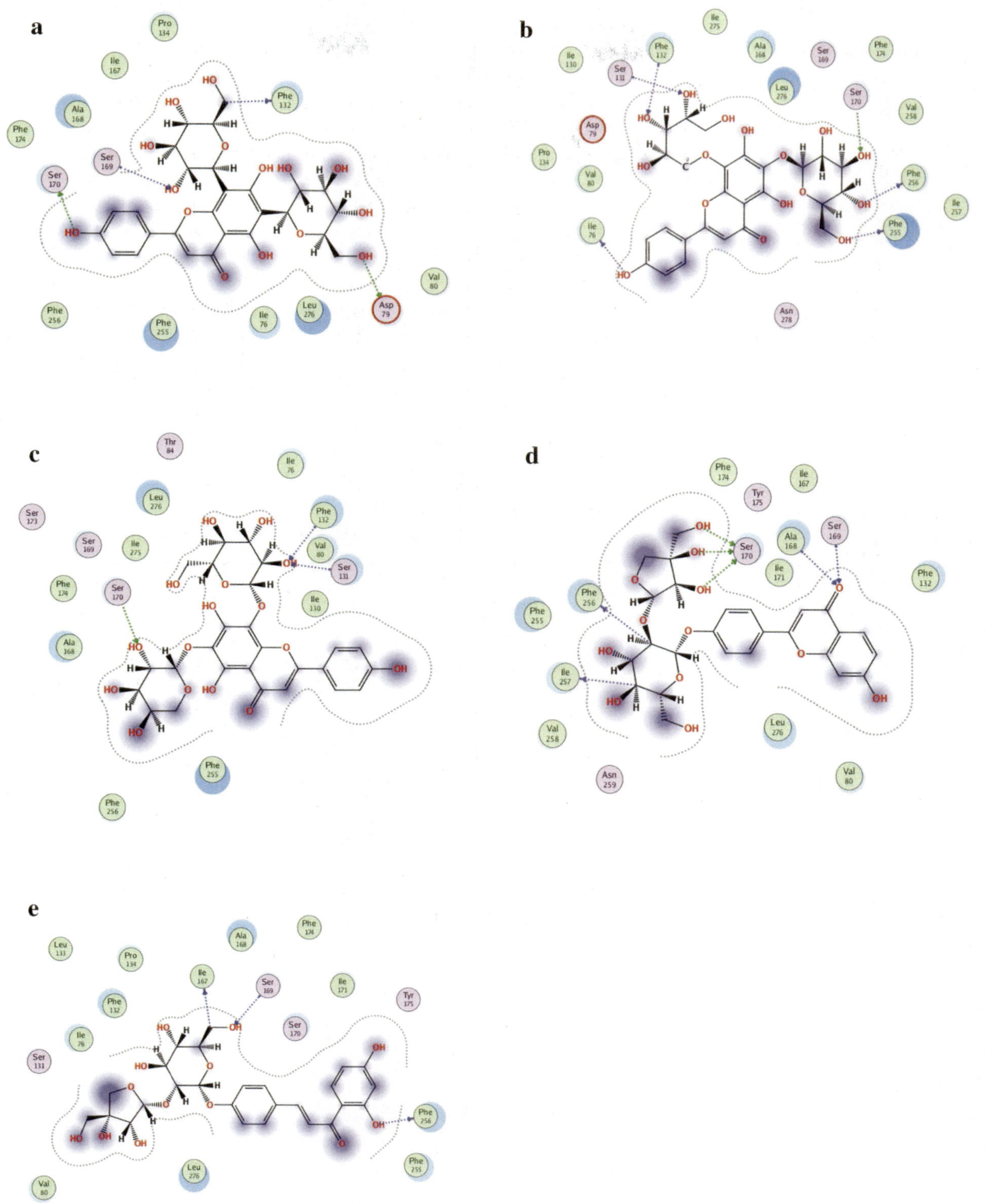

Fig. 8 Two-dimensional overview of docking complexations of ligand/β_2-AR. **a** Vicenin, **b** shaftoside, **c** isoshaftoside, **d** liquiritin apioside, **e** isoliquiritin apioside

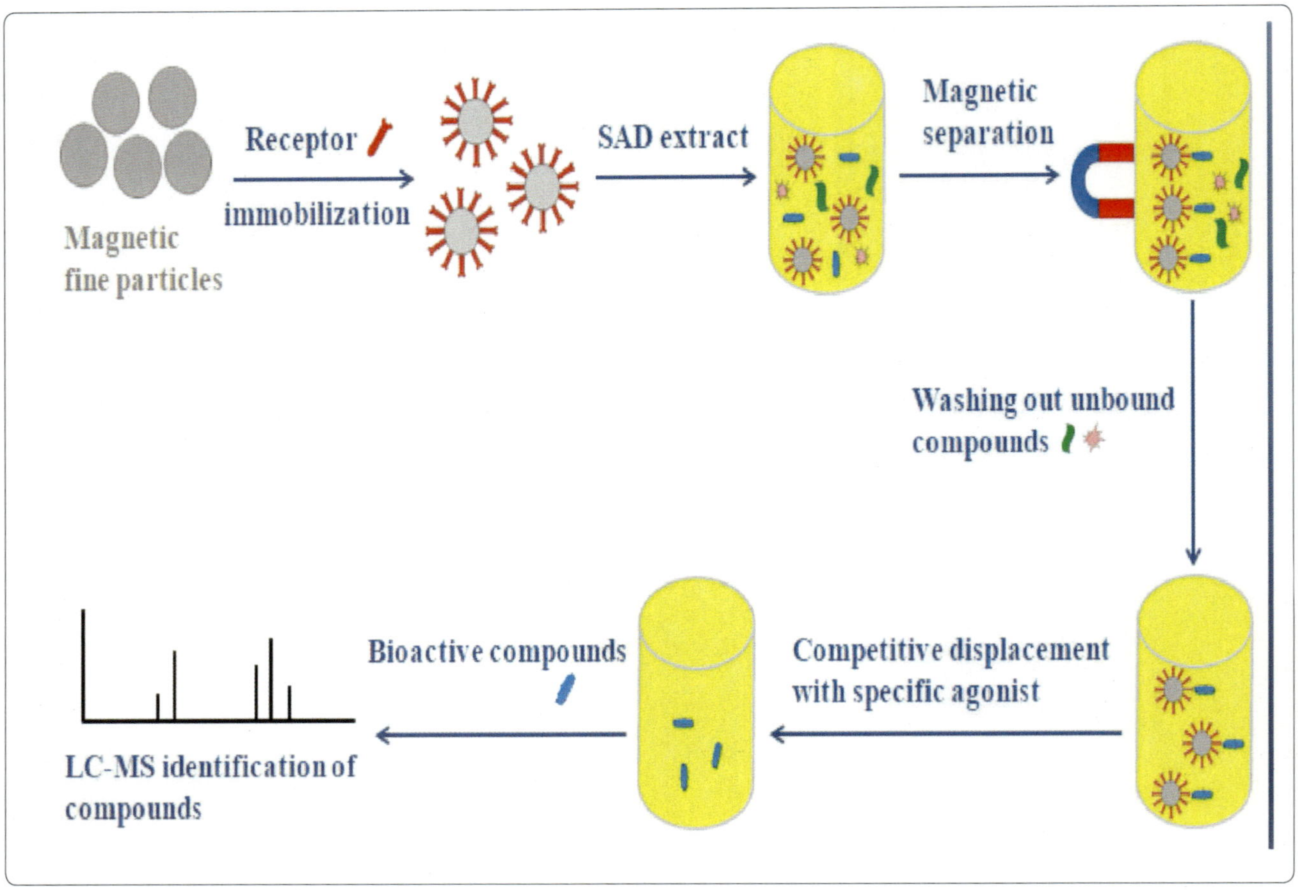

Fig. 9 Schematic overview of $Fe_3O_4@\beta_2$-AR FPs-based ligand screening method. The $Fe_3O_4@\beta_2$-AR FPs were synthesized by immobilizing the receptor onto $Fe_3O_4@NH_2$ using N,N′-carbonyldiimidazole as a linking reagent. The bioactive compounds bound to β_2-AR were achieved by incubating the particles with desired samples and were isolated by a magnet. The bound compounds were released into solution by competitive displacement after the particles were totally rinsed. The compounds released from the particles were analyzed by LC–MS/MS to pursue their structures

feasibility of $Fe_3O_4@\beta_2$-AR FPs in screening bioactive compounds of the receptor from complex matrices including traditional Chinese medicine.

Conclusions

In this work, we synthesized $Fe_3O_4@\beta_2$-AR FPs to fish out bioactive compounds of the receptor from SAD. Bioactive compounds in SAD that targeted β_2-AR were identified as vicenin, shaftoside, isoshaftoside, liquiritin apioside and isoliquiritin apioside by LC–MS/MS. The compound–receptor interactions occurred at Ser^{169}, Ser^{170}, and Phe^{256}. These results indicated that the affinity magnetic particles have the ability to recognize and separate the target compounds plus the probe of their exact binding site on the receptor. This is probably constitute an effective and rapid method for separating and identifying ligands of GPCRs from complex system such as traditional Chinese medicine.

Abbreviations

APTES: aminopropyltriethoxysilane; β_2-AR: beta 2-adrenoceptor; DLS: dynamic light scattering; $Fe_3O_4@NH_2$ FPs: Fe_3O_4 fine particles coupled with NH_2; $Fe_3O_4@\beta_2$-AR FPs: Fe_3O_4 fine particles coupled with the beta 2-adrenoceptor; GPCRs: G protein-coupled receptors; MFPs: magnetic fine particles; OD: optical density; SAD: San-ao decoction; FT-IR: Fourier transform infrared.

Authors' contributions

FF and HS carried out the screening experiments and wrote the manuscript, XC and JL analyzed the data, JW performed the molecular docking, QL thoroughly revised the manuscript, YZ conceived of the study, contributed to the design and interpretation of the research. All authors read and approved the final manuscript.

Acknowledgements

Not applicable.

Competing interests

The authors declare that they have no competing interests.

Consent for publication

Not applicable.

Funding

We thank for the financial support from the National Natural Sciences Foundation of China (Nos. 21775119, 21705126 and 81702832), the Postdoctoral Science Foundation of China (No. 2017M620467).

References

1. Lam W, Bussom S, Guan FL, Jiang ZL, Zhang W, Gullen EA, et al. The four-herb Chinese medicine PHY906 reduces chemotherapy-induced gastrointestinal toxicity. Sci Transl Med. 2010;2(45):45–59.
2. Itokawa H, Morris-Natschke SL, Akiyama T, Lee KH. Plant-derived natural product research aimed at new drug discovery. J Nat Med. 2008;62(3):263–80.
3. Tu Y. The discovery of artemisinin (qinghaosu) and gifts from Chinese medicine. Nat Med. 2011;17(10):1217–20.
4. Berube G. An overview of molecular hybrids in drug discovery. Expert Opin Drug Discov. 2016;11(3):281–305.
5. Zhao XF, Zheng XH, Fan TP, Li ZJ, Zhang YY, Zheng JB. A novel drug discovery strategy inspired by traditional medicine philosophies. Science. 2015;347(6219):S38–9.
6. Newman DJ, Cragg GM. Natural products as sources of new drugs over the 30 years from 1981 to 2010. J Nat Prod. 2012;75(3):311–35.
7. Li LJ, Zhou XW, Li N, Miao S, Lv JX, Xu ZC. Herbal drugs against cardiovascular disease: traditional medicine and modern development. Drug Discov Today. 2015;20(9):1074–86.
8. Jiang WY. Therapeutic wisdom in traditional Chinese medicine: a perspective from modern science. Discov Med. 2005;5(29):455.
9. Yuan R, Lin Y. Traditional Chinese medicine: an approach to scientific proof and clinical validation. Pharmacol Ther. 2000;86(2):191–8.
10. Bagdas D, Muldoon PP, Alsharari S, Carroll FI, Negus SS, Damaj MI. Expression and pharmacological modulation of visceral pain-induced conditioned place aversion in mice. Neuropharmacology. 2016;102:236–43.
11. Zhao XF, Li Q, Bian LJ, Zheng XH, Zheng JB, Zhang YY, et al. Using immobilized G-protein coupled receptors to screen bioactive traditional Chinese medicine compounds with multiple targets. J Pharm Biomed Anal. 2012;70(11):549–52.
12. Wang J, Li F, Zeng KZ, Li Q, Zhao XF, Zheng XH. Bioactive compounds of Shuang–Huang–Lian prescription and an insight into its binding mechanism by β_2-adrenoceptor chromatography coupled with site-directed molecular docking. J Sep Sci. 2017;40(22):4357–65.
13. Ciesla L, Moaddel R. Comparison of analytical techniques for the identification of bioactive compounds from natural products. Nat Prod Rep. 2016;33(10):1131–45.
14. Zhuo RJ, Liu H, Liu NN, Wang Y. Ligand fishing: a remarkable strategy for discovering bioactive compounds from complex mixture of natural products. Molecules. 2016;21(11):1516.
15. Chen CYC. TCM Database@Taiwan: the world's largest traditional Chinese medicine database for drug screening in silico. PLoS ONE. 2011;6(1):e15939.
16. Li ZH, Gao HY, Li JY, Zhang YJ. Identification of bioactive compounds in Shaoyao-Gancao decoction using β_2-adrenoceptor affinity chromatography. J Sep Sci. 2017;40(12):2558–64.
17. Wubshet SG, Brighente IMC, Moaddel R, Staerk D. Magnetic ligand fishing as a targeting tool for HPLC-HRMS-SPE-NMR: alpha-glucosidase inhibitory ligands and alkylresorcinol glycosides from *Eugenia catharinae*. J Nat Prod. 2015;78(11):2657–65.
18. Wang Z, Li XQ, Chen MH, Liu F, Han C, Kong L, et al. A strategy for screening of α-glucosidase inhibitors from Morus alba root bark based on the ligand fishing combined with high-performance liquid chromatography mass spectrometer and molecular docking. Talanta. 2018;180:337–45.
19. Moaddel R, Marszall MP, Bighi F, Yang Q, Duan X, Wainer IW. Automated ligand fishing using human serum albumin-coated magnetic beads. Anal Chem. 2007;79(14):5414–7.
20. Yang ZZ, Zhang YF, Sun LJ, Wang Y, Gao XM, Cheng YY. An ultrafiltration and high performance liquid chromatography coupled with diode array detector and mass spectrometry approach for screening and characterizing thrombin inhibitors from Rhizoma Chuanxiong. J Chromatogr B. 2017;1061–1062:421–9.
21. Qing LS, Xue Y, Zheng Y, Xiong J, Liao X, Ding LS, et al. Ligand fishing from *Dioscorea nipponica* extract using human serum albumin functionalized magnetic nanoparticles. J Chromatogr B. 2010;1217(28):4663–8.
22. Jönsson PE. Superparamagnetism and spin glass dynamics of interacting magnetic nanoparticle systems. Adv Chem Phys. 2003;128(128):191–248.
23. Zhou Q, Li ZQ, Shuang CD, Li AM, Zhang MC, Wang MQ. Efficient removal of tetracycline by reusable magnetic microspheres with a high surface area. Chem Eng J. 2012;210(6):350–6.
24. Yang Y, Zhang W, Yang F, Zhou B, Zeng DH, Zhang N, et al. Ru nanoparticles dispersed on magnetic yolk-shell nanoarchitectures with Fe_3O_4 core and sulfoacid-containing periodic mesoporous organosilica shell as bifunctional catalysts for direct conversion of cellulose to isosorbide. Nanoscale. 2018;10(5):2199–206.
25. Song HP, Chen J, Hong JY, Hao HP, Qi LW, Lu J, et al. A strategy for screening of high-quality enzyme inhibitors from herbal medicines based on ultrafiltration LC–MS and in silico molecular docking. Chem Commun. 2015;51(8):1494–7.
26. Johnson M. Beta2-adrenoceptors: mechanisms of action of beta2-agonists. Paediatr Respir Rev. 2001;2(1):57–62.
27. Liu GX, Wang P, Li Q, Wang J, Sun ZY, Zhao XF, et al. Confirming therapeutic target of protopine using immobilized β_2-adrenoceptor coupled with site-directed molecular docking and the target-drug interaction by frontal analysis and injection amount-dependent method. J Mol Recognit. 2017;30(7):e2613.
28. Ma CH, Qian YF, Fan XS, Shang EX, Yao X, Ma SP. Using UPLC–Q-TOF–MS to analyze the chemical changes between traditional and dispensing granule decoctions of San-Ao-Tang. J Chromatogr Sci. 2014;52(4):277–92.
29. Yang D, Hu JH, Fu SK. Controlled synthesis of magnetite-silica nanocomposites via a seeded sol-gel approach. J Phys Chem C. 2009;113(18):7646–51.
30. Can K, Ozmen M, Ersoz M. Immobilization of albumin on aminosilane modified superparamagnetic magnetite nanoparticles and its characterization. Colloids Surf B Biointerfaces. 2009;71(1):154–9.
31. Zhao XF, Li Q, Xiao CN, Zhang YJ, Bian LJ, Zhao XF, et al. Oriented immobilisation of histidine-tagged protein and its application in exploring interactions between ligands and proteins. Anal Bioanal Chem. 2014;406(12):2975–85.
32. Marszall MP, Bucinski A. A protein-coated magnetic beads as a tool for the rapid drug-protein binding study. J Pharm Biomed Anal. 2010;52(3):420–4.
33. Sun ZY, Wang J, Li Q, Zhao MM, Zhang YY, Xiong XY, et al. A fast affinity extraction methodology for rapid screening of bioactive compounds specifically binding to beta2-adrenergic receptor from Xie-Bai-San. Med Chem Res. 2017;26(10):1–10.
34. Li ZH, Liu T, Liao J, Ai N, Fan XH, Cheng YY. Deciphering chemical interactions between Glycyrrhizae Radix and Coptidis Rhizoma by liquid chromatography with transformed multiple reaction monitoring mass spectrometry. J Sep Sci. 2017;40(6):1254–65.
35. Ren LL, Xue XY, Zhang FF, Xu Q, Liang XM. High performance liquid chromatography–mass spectrometry analysis of protoberberine alkaloids in medicine herbs. J Sep Sci. 2007;30(6):833–42.
36. Zeng KZ, Li Q, Wang J, Yin GW, Zhang YJ, Xiao CN, et al. One-step methodology for the direct covalent capture of GPCRs from complex matrices onto solid surfaces based on the bioorthogonal reaction between haloalkane dehalogenase and chloroalkanes. Chem Sci. 2018;9(2):446–56.
37. Li Q, Bian LJ, Zhao XF, Gao XK, Zheng JB, Li ZJ, et al. Immobilised histidine tagged β_2-adrenoceptor oriented by a diazonium salt reaction and its application in exploring drug–protein interaction using ephedrine and pseudoephedrine as probes. PLoS ONE. 2014;9(4):e94955.
38. Ma CH, Ma ZQ, Fu Q, Ma SP. Pharmacokinetic properties of ephedrine, amygdalin and glycyrrhizic acid after oral gavage of San-Ao-decoction in beagle dogs using a UPLC-MS method. Anal Methods. 2013;5(8):2119–25.

39. Fang R, Cui Q, Sun J, Duan X, Ma X, Wang W, et al. PDK1/Akt/PDE4D axis identified as a target for asthma remedy synergistic with beta(2)-AR agonists by a natural agent arctigeni. Allergy. 2015;70(12):1622–32.
40. Walker JKL, Defea KA. Role for β-arrestin in mediating paradoxical beta(2)-AR and PAR(2) signaling in asthma. Curr Opin Pharmacol. 2014;16:142–7.
41. Sorianoursua MA, Trujilloferrara JG, Correabasurto J, Vilar S. Recent structural advances of β_1 and β_2 adrenoceptors yield keys for ligand recognition and drug design. J Med Chem. 2013;56(21):8207–23.

13

Internationalization of traditional Chinese medicine: current international market, internationalization challenges and prospective suggestions

Annie Xianghong Lin[1], Ging Chan[2], Yuanjia Hu[2], Defang Ouyang[2], Carolina Oi Lam Ung[2], Luwen Shi[1] and Hao Hu[1,2*]

Abstract

Through reviewing the current international market for traditional Chinese medicine (TCM), this paper identified the internationalization challenges for TCM, including unclear therapeutic material basis and mechanism, difficulty of quality control, low preparation level, registration/policy barriers, and shortage of intellectual property. To deal with these challenges, suggestions were given including: (1) product innovation of TCM (study the TCM by using the methods and means of western medicine; innovate the basic theory of TCM; develop TCM health product); (2) standard innovation of TCM; (3) building big data platform of Chinese medicine (big data platform of TCM preparation; big data platform on the quality of TCM).

Keywords: TCM, Internationalization, International market, Quality control, Standardization

Background

Traditional Chinese medicine has an extensive history and, for 5000 years, has been the fruit of the Chinese people's intelligence in the struggles against diseases. With the advancement in medicine and technology, and the quest to better understand the science of natural medicine, the interests in and acceptance of traditional Chinese medicines (TCM) continues to grow. Featured with the long history of use in treating certain challenging diseases resulting in curative effects, comparatively lower costs and reportedly less side effects, the role of TCM in health is widely recognized around the globe [1].

In 1996, China newly introduced the concept of "internationalization of TCM" which comprised of two major aspects: (1) it is important to expand the volume of import and export of TCM in order to push forward the "going abroad" of TCM, to promote the sustainable development of TCM international trade and to foster the TCM market share across the countries; (2) the legal status of TCM in overseas countries has to be appropriately established to ensure reasonable market entry and to enable sustainable development of TCM under the protection of the local laws and regulations [2].

After more than 2 decades of commitment to the internationalization of TCM nationwide, the progress appears to be stagnated. In order to formulate strategies to achieve a break through, the obstacles inhibiting the internationalization of TCM need to be reviewed systematically. However, limited studies on the challenges facing the internationalization of TCM, this paper aims to study the current international market for TCM, to analyze internationalization challenges, and to propose solutions that can help facilitate the internationalization of TCM in the future.

*Correspondence: haohu@umac.mo
[2] State Key Laboratory of Quality Research in TCM, Institute of Chinese Medical Sciences, University of Macau, Room 2057, Building N22, Avenida da Universidade, Taipa, Macao
Full list of author information is available at the end of the article

Analysis of the current international market for TCM

Internationalization of TCM has seen a decline in the volume and value of export. According to the China Customs statistics, the import and export value of TCM in 2016 experienced a negative growth for the first time in nearly 10 years despite a slight increment in the import and export value of Chinese pharmaceutical products compared to 2015. The total value of TCM import and export in 2016 was 4.6 billion USD, accounting for 4.45% of the total value of the import and export of Chinese pharmaceutical products. While the export value of TCM in 2016 dropped by 9.13% compared to 2015 from 3.77 to 3.426 billion USD, the import value achieved a big reversal, increasing 14.50% from $1.025 billion in 2015 to 1.174 billion USD in 2016.

TCM encompasses a wide range of items: traditional Chinese medicinal materials, decoction pieces, Chinese patented medicines, herbal extracts, and health care products. The export volume and values of most of these items have declined over the years. For instance, the export value of Chinese medicinal materials and decoction pieces in 2016 was 1.025 billion USD, a 3.13% decrease in growth rate year-on-year. For the health care products, the export value in 2016 was 249 million USD which was a 13.22% reduction from the same period of the previous year. The export value of the Chinese patent medicines was 225 million USD in 2016 which is equivalent to a decrease by 13.94% as compared with the previous year with the export volume declined greatly. The most significant impact on the declined volume and value of export came from the Chinese herbal extracts. In the past, these extracts were on high demand as the market for new products of essential oil bloomed both nationally and overseas. The Chinese herbal extracts were the largest and fasting growing item among all Chinese pharmaceutical products in 2015, accounted for the largest share of the total export of CM. While the export value of Chinese herbal extracts accounted for 56.2% in 2016, it failed to maintain a growing trend. The export value was only 1.972 billion USD in 2016 which was a decrease of 10.93% compared to that of last year, and the export volume also decreased by 14.3% [3, 4]. The significant downfall in the export value of herbal extracts greatly contributed to the overall negative growth of TCM export.

TCM were exported to 185 countries and regions and its main markets still remained in Asia with the dominant target markets located in Hong Kong, Japan, Malaysia, South Korea and Indonesia. Next to Asia was the United States. In 2016, China exported 526 million USD worth of TCM to the United States, accounting for 15.34% of TCM exports for China. It is anticipated that the United States would soon overtake Hong Kong and Japan and became the largest market of TCM exported from China [5]. Although TCM has a large, promising world market, it also has many obstacles. TCM's entry into the American market requires the approval of the Food and Drug Administration (FDA), which implies large capital (over 100 million USD) and lengthy process (lasting at least 8 years). However, the more stinging problem in the entry process is that the risks of American financing support for TCM enterprises implementing internationalization strategy are still neither clear nor strong enough [6]. With the implementation of "Regulations for Botanical Drug Approval" and "Guidance for Industry: Botanical Drug Development", the United States began to consider botanical drug compounds as a therapeutic drugs. Take "Xuezhikang (XZK)" for an example, with the special fund support for innovation and preparation of major new drugs designated in the 12th 5-year of China, it entered the FDA clinical trial. This is the first time for domestic clinical organizations to participate in registration and clinical study of lipid regulating TCM in FDA. For "Xuezhikang (XZK)" to enter clinical phase successfully, a good clinical trial protocol should be well prepared and the proper indications with supplementary functions to be tested in the clinical trials should be well selected [7].

The drop of the two major markets in Hong Kong and Japan is another major reason for the decline in the overall TCM export value and export volume. Japan was once the largest importer of Chinese medicinal materials and mainly involved Chinese medicinal materials and decoction pieces [8]. But after 1990, Japan began to vigorously develop the herbal medicine base and establish the herbal plantations in order to become self-sufficient of medicinal herbs and to reduce import from China, which led to Japan's falling import of volume and value of Chinese medicinal materials. In 2016, the market began to pick up, embodied in the growth of export volume and value. Today, Japan has become the second largest market for TCM exports next to the United States, with an export value of 505 million USD in 2016, a 6.62% increase over the past year. There are more than 200 Japanese Kampo medicine manufacturers in Japan. These domestic enterprises possess advanced equipment and technology to process Chinese medicinal materials and to manufacture quality-stable TCM under strict standards. The locally manufactured TCM has occupied a considerable share of the markets of Chinese patent medicines and health care products. In South Korea, the drop in the sales of TCM manufactured in China was multifactorial: the issues with the packaging design and promotion strategy of TCM discouraging the use and masking the true value of TCM in health; and concerns over the content of heavy metals and pesticide residues exceeding the national standards, which are a lot more stringent compared to standards alike in many developed countries [9]. In addition, many developed countries have set up high green trade barriers and technical trade barriers for TCM entering their countries, hindering the process of internationalization of TCM.

Another factor discouraging the internationalization of TCM is the high policy thresholds. In certain countries such as Russia, Vietnam and Australia, TCM is sold as a pharmaceutical drug. In many other countries and regions, however, TCM are approved for sales as health care product, active pharmaceutical ingredient (API), or dietary supplement. On 1st May 2011, the European Union's 2004/24/EC EU Directive on traditional herbal medicine (namely the EU botanical drug approval and continuity clause) came into force. This directive of the European Union provides a simplified registration procedure for traditional herbal medicines, and gives a 7-year transition period of the traditional herbal medicine sold in the EU market before 2004. However, after 7 years, all unregistered traditional herbal medicines will be removed from the EU market [10]. At present, Diaoxinxuekang capsule, which is developed and manufactured by Chengdu Diao Pharmaceutical Group Company, is the only one China-manufactured traditional herbal medicine marketed and sold in the EU market. It is approved as the secondary-types of TCM new drugs and carries Chinese independent intellectual property rights. This exceptional product helped demonstrate how a high policy threshold is translated into great obstacles to the entry of TCM into the international market, greatly reducing the export volume of TCM in the EU market especially the British market.

Internationalization challenges for TCM

The therapeutic material basis and mechanism of TCM are key to the quality, effectiveness and safety of TCM, and are the fundamental prerequisite for the internationalization of TCM. The effective substance basis of TCM is the general name of chemical components that bring about the clinical efficacy of the medicine. Due to the diversity and complexity of compound structures, a TCM is a natural "combinatorial chemical sample library." There are more than 200,000 known compounds in TCM, but currently only a few compounds such as artemisinin and arsenious acid have been studied thoroughly and clearly for their pharmacological action and biological mechanism. The targets and biological mechanisms of most compounds still remain unknown.

On the other hand, each TCM consisting of multiple compounds is a complex chemical system. Its characteristics of synergistic reaction of multi-components, multichannels and multi-targets are difficult to be elucidated by the study model of "single component and single target" in modern medicine. The uncertainties in the effective substance basis and the mechanism of TCM further make it difficult to formulate a scientific and effective system for evaluating the efficacy and safety of TCM. International communities always find it hard to recognize and adopt the quality standards and the standards of production management of TCM. As a result, Chinese patent medicines lose their competitiveness the international market [11].

The quality control of TCM is directly related to the safety and effectiveness of TCM and is critical to the internationalization of TCM. China has set up a quality inspection technology system focusing on chemical marker detection. This method has gradually developed into quality analysis mode of quantitative analysis, chromatographic fingerprint, and discriminant analysis from the initial sensory experience. However, the research pattern of the quality control of TCM is still relying on the analysis method research. This requires careful determination of focusing on the quality inspection of Chinese traditional medicine and ignoring the quality control during the production process; paying attention to the chemical markers detection and ignoring the biomarkers; and emphasizing the drug quality analysis and evaluation and ignoring the study on the medicines regulation system. The scientific and reliable quality assurance system complying with the characteristics of TCM are yet to be fully constructed [12]. Meanwhile, assurance of TCM safety is also a difficult task added to the quality control of TCM. Many countries have added test items of microbes, preservatives, pesticide residues, heavy metals and aflatoxin for traditional medicines and herbal health foods, and formulated their national standards presenting significant cross-country variations. Although China has strengthened the quality control in microorganisms, pesticide residues, heavy metals and arsenic salts, there is still a large gap between Chinese and international standards.

The low level of dosage form is one of the important factors that restrict TCM internationalization. The modernization level of the TCM formulation is relatively backward. Tablets, capsules and granules accounted for more than half of current TCM dosage form. The advanced dosage form for TCM such as sustained-release, controlled-release and targeted preparations are still in the research stage. The majority of small and medium-sized TCM enterprises still use the traditional excipients, which makes it difficult for the TCM formulation to meet the international standard requirements. The basic research on TCM formulation is backward, especially the researches on pharmacokinetics, stability, dose–response relationships, etc. are relatively scarce.

The internationalization of TCM is also faced with a number of registration/policy barriers. Along with the gradual expansion of the international market of natural medicines, some developed countries have implemented trade protectionism in order to protect the interests of the domestic pharmaceutical companies and related medical services, set up a multitude of technical barriers to trade and continue to strengthen the management measures of the import Chinese patent medicines, which seriously hampered the process of the internationalization of TCM. These technical barriers to trade are various, such as technical standard barriers, technical regulation barriers, patent technology barriers, green barriers, etc., which makes Chinese products fail to enter or forced to withdraw from the target market due to shortcomings in technology, environmental protection, and other areas mandated by the policy and regulations.

The intellectual property of TCM is also the weak link of the internationalization of TCM. There are multiple issues related to the patents of TCM: low international patent application, low effective patents, numerous invalid patents, low patent quality and fast growth of application volume not transformed into a rapid growth of market share and so on [13]. At the same time, there are also many problems in the technology transfer of TCM, including lacking of original innovation, lacking of basic research, serious shortage of R&D investment, dislocation of R&D subjects, imperfect market transformation and industrialization mechanism, and weak service links.

Suggestions for further internationalization of TCM

The cross integration of multidisciplinary and innovative drug research and development have brought new opportunities for the development of TCM [14].

Product innovation of TCM

Study TCM by using the methods and means of western medicine

With the continuous development and progress of modern science and technology, the technology of quality identification, extraction and separation, analysis and detection of TCM is becoming more and more mature, and its action of mechanism and active components are becoming increasingly clear. In addition, the modern chemistry, biology, physics, information science and other disciplines have continuously permeated the field of research and development of TCM, which provides a new model for the research and development of TCM [15]. Academician Zhang once suggested that "the development of new varieties of TCM should focus on the research and development of TCM with high technology content such as component medicine and drug monomers, etc.; special attention should be paid to the research of new formulations of Chinese herbal preparation; attempts should be made to achieve breakthrough on traditional dosage forms such as bolus, powder, plaster, and pellet, and develop new formulations with high bioavailability, convenient administration and high level of quality control" [16]. In addition to the innovative research and development of monomeric drugs and dosage forms, the methods and means of western medicines can also be adopted in the research of TCM prescription as deemed appropriate. Prescription of TCM is not just a combination of TCM ingredients. There are new ingredients generated in the formation of prescriptions, which warrants thorough analysis of the active components and the extractions. This is considered conducive to the rapid development of TCM research and development [15].

Innovate the basic theory of TCM

TCM has its own connotations and it is not simply equivalent to botanical drug. If the TCM pursues westernization and abandons the theory of TCM, the research road of the TCM will be narrower and narrower [17]. Different from the western medicine which starts from the molecular biology, TCM is researched and developed based on systematic biology. After a long time of use, the toxicity and efficacy of TCM becomes clearer [18]. Rather than exploring from the very beginning and exploring pharmacological action from pharmacological experiments, the most important thing in TCM research and development is to explore and utilize ancient medicine literatures and thousands of years of clinical experience.

The improvement of clinical research of TCM can also drive the innovation and development of TCM. This provides a ground where the concepts and methods of evidence-based medicine, the principles of international clinical research, and the characteristics of TCM clinical research can all be combined. In recent years, sufficient experiences in the exploration of the clinical research of TCM has been accumulated for the design of measures that promote the improvement of the overall levels leading to many landmark achievements. For example, apricot Shi Gan Tang with Yinqiao powder for the treatment of H1N1, etc. [19].

In order to demonstrate the scientific, technological and economical values of the TCM industry for its sustainable development, academician Zhang introduced the concept of the secondary development of TCM. This concept refers to the re-development of the TCM products which have good clinical efficacy and significant market share in order to promote the redesign of the TCM product, accelerate the cultivation of famous Chinese medicine varieties and develop China's own "blockbuster" drug [20]. With the help of modern science and technology, the development of a safe, effective, stable and controllable compound Chinese medicine is promising [21].

Development of TCM health product

Globally, one of the sunrise industries pivot towards health care products, which are referred to as "health-care food", "functional food" and "food supplement" in different countries. With the 1000 years of usage history, the TCM healthcare products have huge international market potential and room for expansion [22]. Healthcare products of TCM provide a great potential route for TCM to enter the international market. Chen Shilin pointed out that "TCM has the homology tradition of medicine and food". Among them, many Chinese herbal medicine and decoction pieces can enter the market as health products. However, the TCM are facing many challenges including export volume decreasing, uneven distribution of export areas, and less proportion of developed regions such as in the US and EU as well as lacking of brands winning the trust of the customers" [23]. The industry of TCM health products should strive to establish a sound quality management system, seek protection of the processing technology, establish quality identification and intellectual property rights, and select appropriate promotion and sales strategy [24].

Standard innovation of TCM

In order to enter the international market, the key step of promoting TCM is to optimize our own standard to make it acceptable to the international market [25]. The important method is to include the standard of TCM in the national pharmacopoeias such as the US Pharmacopoeia or the European Pharmacopoeia. More than 140 countries in the world have adopted the US pharmacopoeia, while the European Pharmacopoeia standard is widely used among all the European Union country members. Being included in these two Pharmacopoeia indicates a global acceptance of the TCM standards which will greatly benefit the internationalization of these products. In recent years, 27 standards of "9 varieties" such as salvia miltiorrhiza, pseudo-ginseng and ganoderma have been included in the US Pharmacopoeia, and a number of standards have entered the US Pharmacopoeia audit procedure [19]. More than 10 TCM standards including uncaria and platycodon entered the European pharmacopoeia or forum. These achievements have proved to the world that TCM can also be evaluated according to international standards, which brings new prospects for the entry of TCM into the international market.

Building big data platform of TCM

Big data platform of TCM preparation

A systematic and transparent preparation of large data information platform of TCM preparation is key to comprehensive mining of the vast amounts of information on TCM and its preparation field, professional processing of data—drawing of scientific knowledge map, tracing patent data, digging and analyzing of clinical trial data and marketed drug data, drawing the navigational chart of TCM and its preparation in the era of big data. The establishment of the platform will effectively integrate all aspects of TCM research and development, serve the needs of multiple demand groups including enterprises, government regulators, academic research institutions, and so on, and greatly shorten the development time of new varieties of Chinese medicine and its preparation.

Big data platform on the quality of TCM

The quality data platform of TCM includes the quality standards of Chinese medicinal materials, decoction pieces, and Chinese patent medicine, so as to enhance the research on the technical standards and specifications of varieties, quality, planting, collecting, processing, preparing of decoction pieces and extraction of TCM. For example, the DNA barcode species identification system that was jointly established by the National Key Laboratory of TCM quality in Macao University and Beijing Union Medical College won the second place of the 2016 National Science and Technology Progress Award. This barcode species identification system has established a "genetic identity card" for TCM. The achievement also established the world's largest TCM DNA barcode identification database, which contains more than 1.70 million DNA sequences, and may achieve rapid identification to almost all herbal species included in CP, USP, JP, EP, South Korea Pharmacopoeia and India Pharmacopoeia, etc., and promote TCM identification study to enter into the standardized gene identification era.

Concluding remarks

To promote the internationalization of TCM, the government, academic institutions and industry must cooperate closely, and establish an international platform for the development and communication of TCM rather than just the domestic efforts limited in China. The establishment of the international cooperation platform is not only conducive to the internationalization of TCM but also provides opportunities for other countries and regions to develop traditional medicines, so as to better promote the traditional medicines to serve the global health.

Abbreviations

TCM: traditional Chinese medicine; FDA: Food and Drug Administration; API: active pharmaceutical ingredient.

Authors' contributions
LS and HH conceived and designed the review. ALX, GC, YH, DO and COLU wrote the manuscript. All authors read and approved the final manuscript.

Author details
[1] International Research Center for Medicinal Administration, Peking University, Beijing, China. [2] State Key Laboratory of Quality Research in TCM, Institute of Chinese Medical Sciences, University of Macau, Room 2057, Building N22, Avenida da Universidade, Taipa, Macao.

Acknowledgements
Not applicable.

Competing interests
The authors declare that they have no competing interests.

Consent for publication
All of authors consent to publication of this work in *Chinese Medicine*.

Funding
Not applicable.

References

1. Zhang H, Wang N, Zheng L. The influence of acceding to WTO on progress of modernization of Chinese materia medica in the 21st century. China Pharm. 2000;11(2):51–3.
2. Wu G. International opportunities and challenges of Chinese medicine. Co-op Econ Sci. 2015;11:83–4.
3. Medical network. The export of Chinese medicine decreased by 10% in 2016 [EB/OL]. 2016. http://news.pharmnet.com.cn/news/2017/02/15/463976.html. Accessed 15 Feb 2017.
4. The ancient prescription of traditional Chinese medicine network. Import and export trade mixed in 2015 [EB/OL]. 2015. http://www.cn939.com/zysc/zymy/2016/03/31/109721.html. Accessed 31 Mar 2016.
5. Sohu health. The United States became the largest market for Chinese medicine exports in 2016 [EB/OL]. 2016. http://mt.sohu.com/health/d20170228/127506057_377310.shtml. Accessed 28 Feb 2017.
6. Zhang L. Discuss on the export barriers and Countermeasures of traditional Chinese medicine. Chin Bus Trade. 2011;7:204–5.
7. Li Y. The way Chinese medicine goes out is a long and tortuous way. China's Foreign Trade. 2013;7:92–3.
8. Yin L, Zhao Y, Zhang L, Xu X. Analysis on export competitiveness and strategy of Chinese herbal medicines. J Anhui Agric Sci. 2010;38(25):14091–3.
9. Wu S. When will the traditional Chinese medicine dominate the international market. China Inspection Quarantine. 2013;3:49–50.
10. Li C. Research on the current situation and Countermeasures of Chinese medicine in the international market. J Qiqihar Univ Med. 2013;34(4):567–8.
11. Wang X. Methodology for systematic analysis of in vivo efficacy material base of traditional Chinese medicine—Chinmedomics. China J Chin Materia Med. 2015;40:13–7.
12. Shen J, Wang K, Hu Q, Su J, Zhang W. Establishment quality control method of traditional Chinese medicine based on efficacy and safety. Modernization Trad Chin Med Materia Med. 2014;3:502–5.
13. Wang L. On the protection of intellectual property rights of Chinese medicine. Legal Econ. 2014;7:110–2.
14. Chen K. Innovative drug research and development into an era of revolutionary change. China's Strategic Emerg Ind. 2016;23:96.
15. Zhang M, Chang Y. On the research and development mode of the combination of Chinese and Western pharmacy. Lishizhen Med Materia Med Res. 2007;18(3):737–8.
16. Zhang B, Zhang J. Twenty years' review and prospect of modernization research on traditional Chinese medicine. China J Chin Materia Med. 2015;40(17):3331–4.
17. Liu C. Reflections on TCM modernization and TCM international development. China Pharm. 2016;27(11):1441–4.
18. Zhang B. A proposal of the establishment of technology system of review and registration in conformity with the characteristics traditional Chinese medicine. Modernization Trad Chin Med Materia Med. 2016;18(12):2031–3.
19. Zhang B. For the future: the world needs traditional Chinese medicine. J Fourth Mil Med Univ. 2016;37(1):1–4.
20. Zhang B, Fan X, Liu Y, Qu H, Zhang J, Cheng Y. Strategy and core technologies for the secondary development of Chinese patent medicine. China J Chin Materia Med. 2013;38(22):3797–800.
21. Zhang B, Zhang J. The relevation of that Chief Researcher of Tu Youyou won 2015 Nobel Prize in physiology and medicine. Sci Sin Vitae. 2015;45(11):1153–5.
22. Zhong F. The current development status and prospect on Chinese medicine health foods. China Health Ind. 2014;11(10):187–8.
23. Hua M. Factors affecting the export of Chinese medicine health care products and Countermeasures. J Nant Text Vocat Technol Coll. 2011;11(4):41–3.
24. He Y. The status and countermeasures health and health care tourism of traditional Chinese medicine in Yunnan province. Tour Res. 2017;9(2):16–21.
25. Zhao Z, Chen H, Xiao P, Guo P, Hong X, Huang L, Liang Z, Bai X, Liu J. Inheritance and innovation of traditional Chinese medicinal authentication. China J Chin Materia Med. 2015;40(17):3385–90.

14

Cupping therapy versus acupuncture for pain-related conditions: a systematic review of randomized controlled trials and trial sequential analysis

Ya-Jing Zhang[1†], Hui-Juan Cao[1†], Xin-Lin Li[1], Xiao-Ying Yang[1], Bao-Yong Lai[1], Guo-Yang Yang[3] and Jian-Ping Liu[1,2*]

Abstract

Background: Both cupping therapy and acupuncture have been used in China for a long time, and their target indications are pain-related conditions. There is no systematic review comparing the effectiveness of these two therapies.

Objectives: To compare the beneficial effectiveness and safety between cupping therapy and acupuncture for pain-related conditions to provide evidence for clinical practice.

Methods: Protocol of this review was registered in PROSPERO (CRD42016050986). We conducted literature search from six electronic databases until 31st March 2017. We included randomized trials comparing cupping therapy with acupuncture on pain-related conditions. Methodological quality of the included studies was evaluated by risk of bias tool. Mean difference, risk ratio, risk difference and their 95% confidence interval were used to report the estimate effect of the pooled results through meta-analysis or the results from each individual study. Trial sequential analysis (TSA) was applied to adjust random errors and calculate the sample size.

Results: Twenty-three randomized trials with 2845 participants were included covering 12 pain-related conditions. All included studies were of poor methodological quality. Three meta-analyses were conducted, which showed similar clinical beneficial effects of cupping therapy and acupuncture for the rate of symptom improvement in cervical spondylosis (RR 1.13, 95% CI 1.01 to 1.26; n = 646), lateral femoral cutaneous neuritis (RR 1.10, 95% CI 1.00 to 1.22; n = 102) and scapulohumeral periarthritis (RR 1.31, 95% CI 1.15 to 1.51; n = 208). Results from other outcomes (such as visual analogue and numerical rating scale) in each study also showed no statistical significant difference between these two therapies for all included pain-related conditions. The results of TSA for cervical spondylosis demonstrated that the current available data have not reached a powerful conclusion. No serious adverse events related to cupping therapy or acupuncture was found in included studies.

Conclusion: Cupping therapy and acupuncture are potentially safe, and they have similar effectiveness in relieving pain. However, further rigorous studies investigating relevant pain-related conditions are warranted to establish comparative effectiveness analysis between these two therapies. Cost-effectiveness studies should be considered in the future studies to establish evidence for decision-making in clinical practice.

Keywords: Acupuncture, Cupping therapy, Randomized controlled trial, Systematic review, Trial sequential analysis

*Correspondence: Liujp@bucm.edu.cn; Jianping_l@hotmail.com
†Ya-Jing Zhang and Hui-Juan Cao contributed equally to this work
[1] Centre for Evidence-Based Chinese Medicine, Beijing University of Chinese Medicine, 11 Bei San Huan Dong Lu, Beijing 100029, China
Full list of author information is available at the end of the article

Background

Traditional Chinese non-pharmaceutical therapies, such as acupuncture, are applied under the guidance of the Traditional Chinese Medicine (TCM) theory of syndrome differentiation. As an important part of TCM, these therapies mainly use manual or technique stimulations at specific body parts (especially acupoints) to dredge the meridian system. Generally, non-pharmaceutical therapies, including acupuncture, cupping therapy, moxibustion, massage (*tuina*), and *guasha*, are more likely to be accepted by patients since they have been used in treating numerous diseases or conditions and may have fewer side effects than drugs [1]. Acupuncture, as one of the most popular non-pharmaceutical therapy, has been widely used to treat diseases by regulating the functions of *qi* (vital energy) and blood of the organs through puncturing certain acupoints of meridians in the body with needles, to strengthen the resistance of the body against diseases [2]. A current clinical guideline issued by the American College of Physicians (ACP) recommends non-pharmacologic treatments (such as acupuncture, massage and superficial heat) as the priority treatments to patients with acute, subacute or chronic low back pain [3]. In addition, systematic reviews have reported that acupuncture was indicated for the treatment of chronic pain, mainly headaches, migraines, cervical pain, back pain, and pain from osteoarthritis [4–9].

Cupping therapy also belongs to TCM non-pharmaceutical therapy, which has been used for long time [10]. Cupping practitioners utilize the flaming heating power to achieve suction (minus pressure) inside the glass cups to make them apply on the desired part of the body, and this suction on selected acupoints produces hyperemia or hemostasis, which may result in a therapeutic effect [11]. There are different types of cupping including retained cupping, flash cupping, moving cupping, wet cupping, medicinal cupping, and needling cupping [12]. Since a report about the Olympic swimmer Michael Phelps using cupping therapy to relieve his muscular discomfort, this treatment has become more and more popular outside China. However, although beneficial effects of cupping therapy have been reported in treating various diseases/conditions, there is lack of high-quality evidence to confirm its efficacy [13]. Our previous systematic reviews on cupping for pain-related conditions also identified no high-quality evidence to prove its effectiveness [14, 15].

Both acupuncture and cupping therapy are commonly used in treating similar conditions, especially pain-related conditions. Though the mechanism of acupuncture and cupping therapy may be different, both, therapies employ the meridian and acupoints to activate blood stasis and regulate the flow of *qi* to relieve pain. Cupping therapy has more advantages than acupuncture, such as a non-invasive therapy with relatively shorter treatment duration and potential less treatment cost. It is worthy to critically review the evidence of the comparison of these two therapies to inform clinical practice. Herein, to the objective of this review is to comprehensively review the evidence from randomized controlled trials (RCTs) comparing cupping therapy with acupuncture for pain-related conditions.

Methods

The protocol of this review was registered in PROSPERO (CRD42016050986) on 15th November 2016 (Achieved at http://www.crd.york.ac.uk/PROSPERO/). Since pain-related conditions were most commonly treated by cupping therapy and acupuncture, we limited the target conditions (such as musculoskeletal pain, tissue pain and neuralgia pain) in this review to reduce the clinical heterogeneity among included studies.

Inclusion criteria

RCTs comparing cupping therapy with acupuncture were included. Pain-related conditions were classified by the type of tissue according to international statistical classification of disease and health related problems by World Health Organization [16], including musculoskeletal system pain (such as spondylopathies, lumbar spondylosis, knee osteoarthritis, acute tissue pain), and neurologic pain (such as lateral femoral cutaneous nerve and herpes zoster pain). Acupuncture is defined as the insertion of fine needles, sometimes in conjunction with electrical stimulus, to influence physiological functioning of the body. In this review, we included both manual acupuncture (including auricular therapy, scalp needle, and abdominal acupuncture) and electro-acupuncture. Cupping is defined that practitioners utilize the flaming heating power to achieve suction (minus pressure) inside the glass cups to make them apply on the desired part of the body. In this review, all types of cupping (i.e. wet cupping, herbal cupping, moving cupping, flash cupping or retained cupping) were included. Primary outcome measures included severity of pain, functional capacity, quality of life (QoL). Secondary outcomes included depression, rate of symptom improvement and adverse effects. There was no limitation on language and publication type.

Identification and selection of studies

We searched China Network Knowledge Infrastructure (CNKI), Chinese Scientific Journal Database (VIP), Wan Fang Database, PubMed, EMBASE, and the Cochrane Library, all the searches ended at March 2017. The search terms included acupuncture-related terms (i.e. "acupuncture", "acupoint", "needle", "electroacupuncture", "manual acupuncture", "auricular needling", "scalp needle", or "abdominal acupuncture"), combined with cupping-related terms (i.e. "cupping therapy", "bleeding cupping", "wet cupping", "dry cupping", "flash cupping", "herbal cupping", "moving cupping" or "retained cupping") and pain-related terms (i.e. "ache", "pain", "painful", or "analgesic"). Two authors (XY Yang and BY Lai) selected studies for eligibility and checked against the inclusion criteria independently.

Data extraction and risk of bias assessment

Two authors (YJ Zhang and XL Li) extracted the data from the included studies independently. The methodological quality of RCTs was assessed according to the criteria from the Cochrane Handbook for Systematic Reviews of Interventions [17]. The quality of studies was categorized into low, unclear, or high risk of bias according to the risk for each important outcome within included studies, including adequacy of generation of the allocation sequence, allocation concealment, blinding, whether there were incomplete outcome data and selected reporting the results. Studies which met all criteria were categorized to low risk of bias, studies which meet none of the criteria were categorized to high risk of bias, and those were categorized to unclear risk of bias if insufficient information acquired to make the judgment.

Data analysis

Data were extracted and calculated for frequency using Microsoft Excel 2007 (American: The Microsoft Corporation, 2007). Binary outcomes were summarized using risk ratio (RR) with 95% confidence intervals (CI) for relative effect and risk difference (RD) with 95% CI for absolute effect. The continuous outcomes were summarized using mean difference (MD) with 95% CI. Revman 5.3 (Copenhagen: The Nordic Cochrane Centre, The Cochrane Collaboration, 2016) was used for data analyses. Meta-analysis was used if the studies had similar clinical characteristics (such as study design, participants, interventions, control, and outcome measures) and acceptable statistical heterogeneity. Random-effect model was used for meta-analysis. Statistical heterogeneity was detected by I^2 test, an $I^2 > 50\%$ indicates the possibility of statistical heterogeneity among the studies. If I^2 was larger than 75%, which means there was obviously statistical heterogeneity among studies, only results from each single study were present respectively rather than pooling analysis. Funnel plot analysis was planned to be generated to detect publication bias.

Trial sequential analysis (TSA)

TSA can be performed if there are more than 5 included studies in the meta-analysis. We applied TSA version 0.9.5.5 (Copenhagen: The Copenhagen Trial Unit, Center for Clinical Intervention Research, 2016) to calculate the required sample size in a meta-analysis and to detect the robustness of the result. We used the diversity-adjusted required information size estimated from a control event proportion of the included studies and a priori intervention effect of 5%, and the diversity which was estimated in the included studies.

Results

Basic information of included studies

After primary searches from the 6 databases, 3102 studies were identified. After screening title and abstract, the majority of studies were not included due to obvious ineligibility, and full texts of 3079 studies were retrieved. Finally, 23 RCTs [18–40] were included in this review, 21 of which were published in Chinese and the remaining 2 [21, 40] were published in English. All of the 23 studies were conducted in China (see Fig. 1).

Description of interventions

All the included studies compared cupping therapy with acupuncture. In the cupping group, 20 (86.96%) studies used wet cupping, and 3 [33, 36, 40] (13.04%) studies used at least two types of cupping methods. Treatment frequency in 3 [33, 36, 37] (13.04%) studies was once daily, in 8 [19, 25, 27, 29, 31, 32, 38, 39] (34.78%) studies was once every 2 days, in 1 [21] (4%) study was twice weekly, in 6 [18, 20, 22–24, 40] (26.08%) studies was 3 times weekly and in other 2 [34, 35] studies (8.6%) was once weekly. The remaining 3 [26, 28, 30] (13.04%) studies not reported the frequency of the treatment. The treatment duration per session in 22 (95.7%) studies was 3–10 min, and in the remaining 1 [27] study was 30 min. In the acupuncture group, 22 (95.6%) studies used manual acupuncture, and 1 (4.3%) study used electroacupuncture. Treatment frequency in 13 [18–20, 22–24, 29, 31, 32, 34–36, 38] (56.52%) studies was once a day, in 4 [27, 28, 30, 39] (17.39%) studies was once 2 days, in 1 [21] (4.3%) study was once weekly, in another 1 [40] (4.3%) study was 3 times weekly. The remaining 4 (17.39%) studies not reported the treatment frequency. The treatment duration per session was 20–30 min (Table 1).

Description of acupoints

In the cupping group, 22 (95.7%) studies used wet cupping on tender points (Ashi), and 1 [38] (4.3%) studies chose the acupoints on the meridians passing the pain area. In the acupuncture group, 4 [31, 37, 39, 40] (17.3%) studies only used tender points (Ashi) the remaining 19 (82.6%) studies chose the acupoints on the meridian of pain and acupoints according to syndrome differentiation.

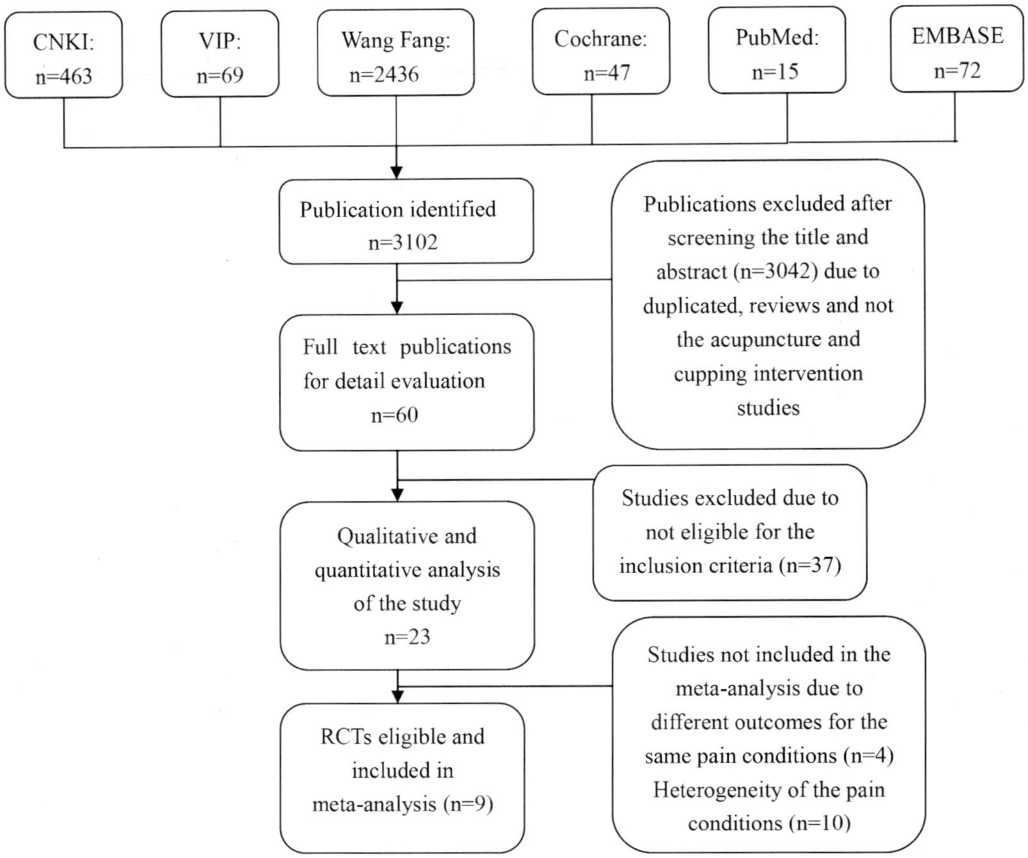

Fig. 1 Flow chart of the study

In general, the number of acupoints in acupuncture group is more than that in cupping therapy. According to the included studies of this review, it's interesting to find that acupuncturists often selected acupoints according to syndrome differentiation, as well as the tender points (Ashi), while cupping therapy practitioners were more likely to choose the tender points (Ashi) for retaining cupping.

Distribution of diseases/conditions

Twelve diseases or conditions were treated in the included RCTs (Table 1). The top 6 diseases/conditions are cervical spondylosis [18–24], knee osteoarthritis [20, 21], lateral femoral cutaneous neuritis [27, 28], lumber disk herniation [29, 30], postherpetic neuralgia [31, 32] and scapulohumeral periarthritis [34, 35].

The pain-related conditions included locomotor pain (cervical spondylosis, lumber disk herniation, scapulohumeral periarthritis and knee osteoarthritis); tissue injury (soft tissue contusion, acute ankle joint); muscle pain (muscles fibrositis and fibromyalgia), neuralgia pain (lateral femoral cutaneous neuritis and postherpetic neuralgia) and acute pain (toothache). Relieving pain was the main goal of the treatments for the included trials, and the study purposes of them were to compare the effectiveness on pain reduction between acupuncture and cupping therapy.

Outcome assessment

Twenty studies (86.95%) used the rate of symptom improvement as the primary outcome, which was defined as the rate of the sum of the cured, markedly effective and effective improvement. Symptom improvement was categorized into four grades (i.e. cured, markedly effective, effective, and ineffective) according to the changes or improvement of the symptoms. 'The cured' was the disappearance of the pain symptoms, 'markedly effective' was the almost disappearance of the symptoms, 'effective' was symptoms alleviation, and 'ineffective' was no changes in symptoms. Besides, 8 [18, 19, 21, 26, 29, 30, 32, 40] studies (34.78%) used numerical scales to evaluate the severity of the symptoms, including the Visual Analogue Scale (VAS) for pain, the neck disability index (NDI), the Clinical Assessment Scale (CAS), the Western Ontario and McMaster Universities osteoarthritis index (WOMAC), the Joint Operational Area (JOA) Scores for

Table 1 Characteristics of 23 included trials comparing cupping therapy and acupuncture for pain-related conditions

Study ID	Diseases	Sample size (Rx/C)	Age Year (Rx/C)	Gender M/F	Cupping group	Acupuncture group	Treatment duration (days)	Outcomes
Dong [18]	Cervical spondylosis of vertebral artery type	60/60	40.62 ± 14.57 41.15 ± 13.34	33/27 34/26	Wet cupping on Haoyi acupoint. If not effect, wet cupping on Zhengumai acupoint after 3 days and evaluate the effect on the seventh day	Acupuncture on bilateral cervical (C3–7), Jiaji (EX-B2) points, Dazhui (DU14), Fengchi (GB20), Neiguan (PC6), Hegu (LI4) with stimulation. 1×/day	15	Symptom score, total effective rate
Zhou [19]	Cervical spondylosis	100/100	20–60	Not reported	With Zhuang medicine lotus needle pricking and cupping therapy. 1×/2 days	Acupuncture on bilateral cervical (C3–7), Jiaji (EX-B2) points, Dazhui (DU14), Fengchi (GB20), Neiguan (PC6), Hegu (LI4) with stimulation. 1×/day	20	VAS, symptom improvement rate
Hu [20]	Cervical spondylosis of vertebral artery type	20/20	40.9 ± 3.5 42.8 ± 1.6	12/8 10/10	Wet cupping on Haoyi acupoint. If not effect, wet cupping on Zhengumai acupoint after 3 days and evaluate the effect on the seventh day	Acupuncture on bilateral cervical (C3–7), Jiaji (EX-B2) points, Dazhui (DU14), Fengchi (GB20), Neiguan (PC6), Hegu (LI4) with stimulation 30 min. 1×/day	15	Symptom improvement rate
Mou [21]	Cervical spondylotic radiculopathy	68/56	46.4 ± 11.6 47.8 ± 11.9	34/34 24/32	Wet cupping on Dazhui (GV14) and Jianjing (GB21) acupoint 2×/week	Acupuncture on bilateral cervical (C3–7), Jiaji (EX-B2) points and Jianjing (GB 21) on the affected side, 30 min, 2×/week	60	VAS, NDI, CAS
A [22]	Cervical spondylosis	43/43	45.3 ± 9.4 44.2 ± 9.2	23/20 22/21	Wet cupping on Haoyi acupoint. If not effect, wet cupping on Zhengumai acupoint after 9 days	Acupuncture on bilateral cervical (C3–7), Jiaji (EX-B2) points, Dazhui (DU14), Fengchi (GB20), Neiguan (PC6), Hegu (LI4) with stimulation, 1×/day, 25 min	14	Symptom improvement rate
Wang [23]	Cervical spondylosis	72/72	45.9 ± 8.7 45.1 ± 7.9	79/65	Wet cupping on Haoyi acupoint for 10 min. If not effect, wet cupping on Zhengumai acupoint after 3 days	Acupuncture on Fengchi (GB20), Wangu (GB12), Sishencong (EX-HN1), Baihui (GV20), Tianzhu (BL10), Yunting, Jiaji (EX-B2), 1×/day, 25 min	14	Symptom improvement rate
Na [24]	Cervical spondylosis	28/28	45.1 ± 8.5 44.3 ± 8.9	15/13 17/11	Wet cupping on Haoyi acupoint. If not effect, wet cupping on Zhengumai acupoint after 9 days and evaluate the effect on the 12 day	Acupuncture on bilateral cervical (C3–7), Jiaji (EX-B2) points, Dazhui (DU14), Fengchi (GB20), Neiguan (PC6), Hegu (LI4) with stimulation, 1×/day, 25 min	14	Symptom improvement rate

Table 1 continued

Study ID	Diseases	Sample size (Rx/C)	Age Year (Rx/C)	Gender M/F	Cupping group	Acupuncture group	Treatment duration (days)	Outcomes
Wang [25]	Knee osteoarthritis	40/40	42–68	62/58	Wet cupping on tender point (Ashi), Xiyan (EX-LE5), Heding (EX-LE2), Yanglingwquan (GB34), Liangqiu (ST34), 1×/2 days	Acupuncture: abdominal acupuncture on Zhongwan (N12), Guanyuan (N4), Shuifen (RN9), Qipang, Waling, Xiafengshidian, Xiafenshineidian with stimulation, 30 min	23	Symptom improvement rate
Wang [26]	Knee osteoarthritis	89/82	59 ± 9 61 ± 8	18/71 21/61	Wet cupping on Xiyan (EX-LE2), tender acupoints (Ashi) for 5–10 times	Acupuncture on Xiyan (EX-LE2), tender acupoints (Ashi), 20 min for 5–10 times	28	VAS, WOMAC
Shu [27]	Lateral femoral cutaneous neuritis	25/25	50.32 ± 10.44 50.88 ± 9.27	14/11 12/13	Wet cupping on tender point and Yanglingquan (GB34), 30 min, 1×/2 days	Local multiple superficial needling, 30 min, 1×/2 days	21	Symptom improvement rate
Zhang [28]	Lateral femoral cutaneous neuritis	26/26	46.9 47.6	20/6 21/5	Wet cupping on tender point	Local Multiple superficial needling, 30 min, 1×/2 days	21	Symptom improvement rate
Wang [29]	Lumber disk herniation	32/30	20–60	48/45	Wet cupping in tender point (Ashi) and surface reflect lesion site and retained for 5–1 min, 1×/2 days	Acupuncture on traditional site, 30 min, 1×/day.	28	JOA score, symptom improvement rate
Zhou [30]	The third lumber vertebral transverse process syndrome	60/60	35.1 35.9	38/22 34/26	Wet cupping on tender point (Ashi) and retained cupping for 5 min	Acupuncture on Ashi, Jiaji (EX-B2), Huantiao (GB30), Weizhong (BL40), 20 min, 1×/2 days	28	VAS, Symptom improvement rate
Zhang [31]	Postherpetic neuralgia	20/20	61 ± 7 60 ± 7	12/8 13/7	Wet cupping on Ashi for 3–10 min, 1×/2 days	Acuponcture around the pain site for 20–30 mins, 1×/day	10	Symptom improvement rate
Huang [32]	Postherpetic neuralgia	49/47	65.35 64.28	28/21 25/22	Wet cupping with Zhuang lotus needle on Longji, Jiaji (EX-B2), Jianjing (GB21), Ashi and retained cupping for 5–10 min, 1×/2 days	Acupuncture on Quchi (LI11), Hegu (LI4), Taichong (LR3), Sanyinjiao (SP6), Xuehai (SP10), Zusanli (ST36) and tender points (Ashi), 25 min. 1×/day	30	Symptom improvement rate, VAS
Wu [33]	Toothache	204/203	Not reported	Not reported	Wet cupping on Dazhui (DU14), Jiaji (EX-B2) and flash cupping around Dazhui for 10–15 min, 1×/day	Acupuncture on traditional site	Not Reported	Symptom improvement rate

Table 1 continued

Study ID	Diseases	Sample size (Rx/C)	Age Year (Rx/C)	Gender M/F	Cupping group	Acupuncture group	Treatment duration (days)	Outcomes
Bao [34]	Scapulohumeral periarthritis	52/52	57.1 ± 7.9 56.2 ± 8.6	28/24 26/26	Wet cupping on Jian, Jianqian, Jianhou and Ashi, 1×/week	Acupuncture on Jinayu (LI15), Jianzhen (SI9), Jianliao (SJ14), Jinaqian, Quchi (LI11), Waiguan (SJ5), Yanglingquan (GB34), 30 min, 1×/day	15	Symptom improvement rate
Sha [35]	Scapulohumeral periarthritis	52/52	51.1 ± 5.8 51.3 ± 6.5	28/24 29/23	Wet cupping on Jian, Jianqian, Jianhou and Ashi, 1×/week	Acupuncture on Jinayu (LI15), Jianzhen (SI9), Jianliao (SJ14), Jinaqian, Quchi (LI11), Waiguan (SJ5), Yanglingquan (GB34), 30 min, 1×/day	15	Symptom improvement rate
Liu [36]	Muscles fibrositis	38/38	30–60	19/19 23/15	Flash cupping on tender points and retained for 10–15 min, 1×/day	Electricacupuncture on traditional acupoints. 1×/day	16	Symptom improvement rate
Huang [37]	Soft tissue contusion	132/132	4–69	107/157	Wet cupping on Ashi. 1×/day	Resistance acupuncture on the contusion site	7	Symptom improvement rate
Zhou [38]	Acute lumbar sprain	26/26	41.27 ± 8.76 39.38 ± 8.12	9/17 12/14	Wet cupping on waist area of the bladder meridian for 5 mins, 1×/2 days	Acupuncture on bladder meridian for 30 min, 1×/day	10	Symptom improvement rate, temperature difference of body surface
Wang [39]	Acute ankle joint	47/73	9–60	36/37 25/22	Wet cupping on Ashi, 10 min 1×/2 days	Acupuncture on Ashi or surrounding acupoint, 1×/2 days	20	Symptom improvement rate
Cao [40]	Fibromyalgia	29/27	Not reported	Not reported	Cupping for tender points, 3×/week	Acupuncture for tender points, 3×/week	35	VAS, SF36, HAMD

VAS Visual Analogue Scale, *NDI* neck disability index (physical therapy), *CAS* the Clinical Assessment Scale, *WOMAC* the Western Ontario and McMaster Universities osteoarthritis index, *JOA* the Joint Operational Area, *SF-36* the MOS item short from health survey, *HAMD* the Hamilton Depression Scale joint mobility, the MOS item short from health survey (SF-36), and the Hamilton Depression Scale (HAMD) for social activity.

Risk of bias assessment

According to our pre-defined methodological quality criteria, no study was evaluated as low risk of bias, 8 [19–21, 26, 29, 31, 32, 40] studies unclear risk of bias, and the remaining 15 studies high risk of bias. The sample size in each study varied from 40 to 407 participants with an average of 56 patients per group. None of the studies specified the sample size calculation. Eleven studies described the details of randomization procedure. Among them, 6 studies [19–21, 26, 29, 32] used a random number table to generate the random allocation. One study [27] was declared as 'randomized controlled trial', however, it used a quasi-randomization method by dividing participants into two groups based on the sequence of the registration order. Only 1 [26] of the above 11 studies reported using sealed envelope to implement allocation concealment. Three studies [31, 39, 40] mentioned they used blinding method, in which 2 studies [31, 40] reported that they blinded outcome assessors, while the other one did not specify who were blinded. Two studies [21, 26] reported the number of dropouts, but none of them used intention-to-treat analysis or other appropriate methods to deal with the missing data (Fig. 2).

There were 19 (82.6%) studies reported the comparability of baseline, but only 1 [40] study reported the baseline data of both the outcomes and the demographic characteristics of participants. Nine [19, 21, 26, 29, 31, 32, 34, 39, 40] (39.13%) studies reported the inclusion criteria, and 9 [18, 19, 21, 26, 29, 31, 32, 38, 40] (39.13%) studies reported the exclusion criteria. Seventeen (73.91%) studies reported the diagnostic criteria (as we mentioned before). Only one protocol of a study [40] was available which was registered in Clinicaltrials.gov, thus we acquired the protocol to supporting the judgment of reporting bias of this study and it was of low risk.

Effect estimates

Results from individual trials

Due to the variations in study quality, participants' characteristics and outcome measures of the included RCTs, data from 14 studies could not be synthesized by meta-analysis. Among them, 11 [21, 25, 29–33, 36–38, 40] studies (78.5%) reported that there was no statistical significant difference between cupping and acupuncture on the rate of symptom improvement for specific conditions, including cervical spondylotic radiculopathy, lumber disk herniation, knee

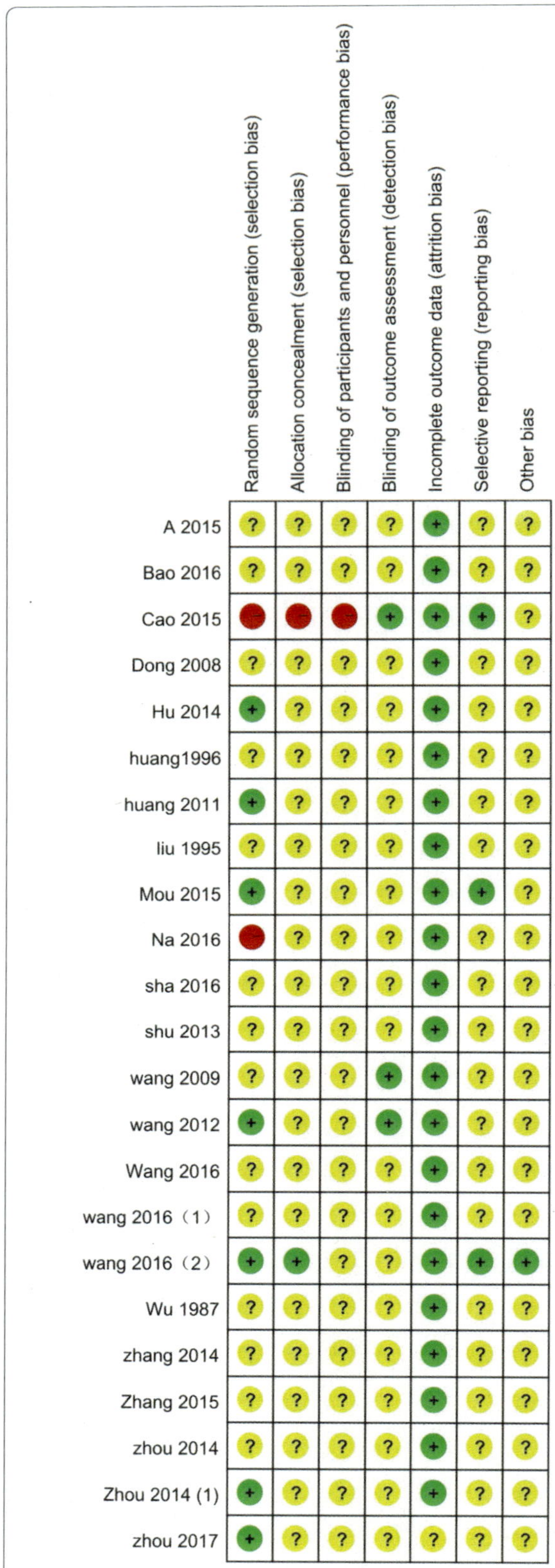

Fig. 2 Risk of bias summary

osteoarthritis, toothache, muscles fibrositis, soft tissue contusion, acute lumber sprain, postherpetic neuralgia and fibromyalgia. Three [19, 26, 39] studies reported cupping might have better effects than acupuncture on increasing the total effective rate in acute ankle joint knee osteoarthritis, acute lumbar sprain and the third lumber vertebral transverse process syndrome according to the VAS scores. Table 2 shows the detailed results of the 14 studies.

Results from pooling analyses

Seven studies [18–24] compared acupuncture and cupping therapy for cervical spondylosis, 2 [19, 21] of them reported VAS scores and found cupping therapy was superior to acupuncture on pain relief, however, data could not be pooled due to the statistical heterogeneity ($I^2 = 93\%$). One [18] of these two studies reported that cupping had better effect on reducing VAS scores (MD

Table 2 Estimate effect of cupping therapy and acupuncture for pain-related conditions

Study ID	Sample size	Disease	Estimate effect	P	Outcomes
Zhou [19]	200	Cervical spondylosis	MD −1.70, 95% CI −1.94 to −1.46	P < 0.00,001	VAS for pain
Mou [21]	124	Cervical spondylotic radiculopathy	MD 0.11, 95% CI −0.78 to 1.00 MD 4.33, 95% CI −3.14 to 11.80 MD 1.59, 95% CI −1.17 to 4.35	P = 0.81 P = 0.26 P = 0.26	VAS Neck disability index (physical therapy) CAS
Wang [25]	80	Knee osteoarthritis	RR 1.29, 95% CI 0.32 to 5.19 RD 0.03, 95% CI −0.11 to 0.16	P = 0.72 P = 0.72	Symptom improvement rate
Wang [26]	171	Knee osteoarthritis	MD −0.97, 95% CI −1.56 to −0.38 MD −1.35, 95% CI −1.91 to −0.79 MD −1.01, 95% CI −1.87 to −0.15 MD −0.17, 95% CI −0.52 to 0.18 MD −2.92, 95% CI −6.18 to 0,34 MD −4.14, 95% CI −8.49 to 0.21 MD −1.66, 95% CI −2.48 to −0.84 MD −0.35, 95% CI −0.68 to −0.02 MD −4.93, 95% CI −7.97 to −1.89 MD −6.93, 95% CI −11.0 to −12.85	P = 0.001 P < 0.00001 P = 0.02 P = 0.34 P = 0.08 P = 0.06 P < 0.0001 P = 0.04 P = 0.001 P = 0.0009	VAS VAS (follow at 4 weeks) WOMAC—pain scores WOMAC—stiff scores WOMAC—difficult of life scores WOMAC —total scores WOMAC—pain scores (follow at 4 weeks) WOMAC—stiff scores (follow at 4 weeks) WOMAC—difficult of life scores (follow at 4 weeks) WOMAC total scores (follow at 4 weeks)
Wang [29]	62	Lumber disk herniation	MD 1.88, 95% CI −0.24 to 4.00 RR 0.89, 95% CI 0.63 to 1.27 RD −0.07, 95% CI −0.31 to 0.16	P = 0.08 P = 0.53 P = 0.53	JOA scores Symptom improvement rate
Zhou [30]	120	The third lumber vertebral transverse process syndrome	RR 1.05, 95% CI 0.96 to 1.15 RD 0.05, 95% CI −0.03 to 0.13 MD −1.58,95% CI −2.04 to −1.12	P = 0.25 P = 0.24 P < 0.00001	Symptom improvement rate VAS scores
Zhang [31]	40	Postherpetic neuralgia	RR 0.95, 95% CI 0.83 to 1.09 RD −0.05, 95% CI −0.18 to 0.08 MD 0.10, 95% CI −0.51 to 0.70	P = 0.47 P = 0.44 P = 0.75	Symptom improvement rate VAS
Huang [32]	96	Postherpetic neuralgia	RR 1.16, 95% CI 1.00 to 1.33 RD 0.13, 95% CI 0.01 to 0.25 MD −1.17, 95% CI −1.67 to −0.67	P = 0.05 P = 0.04 P < 0.00001	Symptom improvement rate VAS
Wu [33]	407	Toothache	RR 1.04, 95% CI 1.00 to 1.08 RD 0.03, 95% CI 0.00 to 0.07	P = 0.03 P = 0.03	Symptom improvement rate
Liu [36]	76	Muscles fibrositis	RR 1.05, 95% CI 0.96 to 1.15 RD 0.05, 95% CI −0.03 to 0.14	P = 0.24 P = 0.22	Symptom improvement rate
Huang [37]	264	Soft tissue contusion	RR 0.99, 95% CI 0.93 to 1.05 RD −0.01, 95% CI −0.06 to 0.05	P = 0.79 P = 0.79	Symptom improvement rate
Zhou [38]	46	Acute lumbar sprain	RR 1.09, 95% CI 0.90 to 1.33 RD 0.08, 95% CI −0.10 to 0.25	P = 0.39 P = 0.38	Symptom improvement rate
Wang [39]	120	Acute ankle joint	RR 1.18, 95% CI 1.04 to 1.33 RD 0.15, 95% CI 0.04 to 0.25	P = 0.009 P = 0.005	Symptom improvement rate
Cao [40]	56	Fibromyalgia	MD −4.06, 95% CI −5.4 to 13.72 MD −5.93, 95% CI −7.89 to 19.75 MD −0.42, 95% CI −4.09 to 4.93		VAS Quality of life HAMD

VAS Visual Analogue Scale, *MD* mean difference, *CAS* the Clinical Assessment Scale, *WOMAC* the Western Ontario and McMaster Universities osteoarthritis index, *JOA* the Joint Operational Area, *SF-36* the MOS item short from health survey, *HAMD* the Hamilton Depression Scale

1.70 cm, 95% CI 1.46 to 1.94, n = 200) and the other one [20] reported that cupping and acupuncture had similar effects on decreasing VAS scores (MD −0.11 cm, 95% CI −1.0 to 0.78, n = 64). A meta-analysis was conducted with the data from 6 [18–20, 22–24] studies which reported the symptom improvement rate. The result showed that cupping had better effects on increasing symptom improvement rate (RR 1.13, 95% CI 1.01 to 1.26, P = 0.04, I^2 = 67%; n = 646, 6 trials) than that of acupuncture (Fig. 3). Symptom improvement rate of cupping therapy was 10% higher than acupuncture (RD 0.1, 95% CI 0.01 to 0.19, P = 0.03, I^2 = 67%; n = 646, 6 trials) (Fig. 3). The remaining 1 study [21] found no significant difference between the two therapies on changing of the VAS (MD −0.11 cm, 95% CI −0.92 to 2.62; n = 124), NDI (MD 4.33, 95% CI −3.14 to 11.80; n = 124), and CAS scores (MD 1.59, 95% CI −1.17 to 4.35; n = 124).

Two studies [27, 28] assessed cupping therapy compared with acupuncture for lateral femoral cutaneous neuritis. The meta-analysis showed similar effects between cupping and acupuncture on increasing symptom improvement rate (RR 1.10, 95% CI 1.00 to 1.22, P = 0.71, n = 100, 2 trials; RD 0.10, 95% CI 0.10 to 0.19, P = 0.71, n = 100, 2 trials).

Two studies [34, 35] assessed cupping therapy compared with acupuncture for scapulohumeral periarthritis. The meta-analysis showed similar effects between cupping and acupuncture on symptom improvement rate (RR 1.31, 95% CI 1.51 to 1.51, P = 0.84; n = 208, 2 trials). Cupping therapy was 22% higher than that of acupuncture (RD 0.22, 95% CI 0.12 to 0.32, P < 0.0001; n = 208, 2 trials) in symptom improvement.

Funnel plot analysis could not be conducted due to the insufficient number of included trials in each meta-analysis.

Trial sequential analysis

TSA was conducted with the data from 6 [18–20, 22–24] studies which reported the symptom improvement rate for cervical spondylosis. TSA illustrated that the cumulative Z-curve (blue curve) only across the traditional boundary of 5% significance (horizontal red line) but did not cross the monitoring boundaries (red inward sloping curves), which is needed to obtain firm evidence controlling for the risk of random error. This resulted in a required information size of 2847 participants. TSA of all included trials suggests that about 18 high quality RCTs (2201 participants) were required to confirm possible intervention effect (Fig. 4).

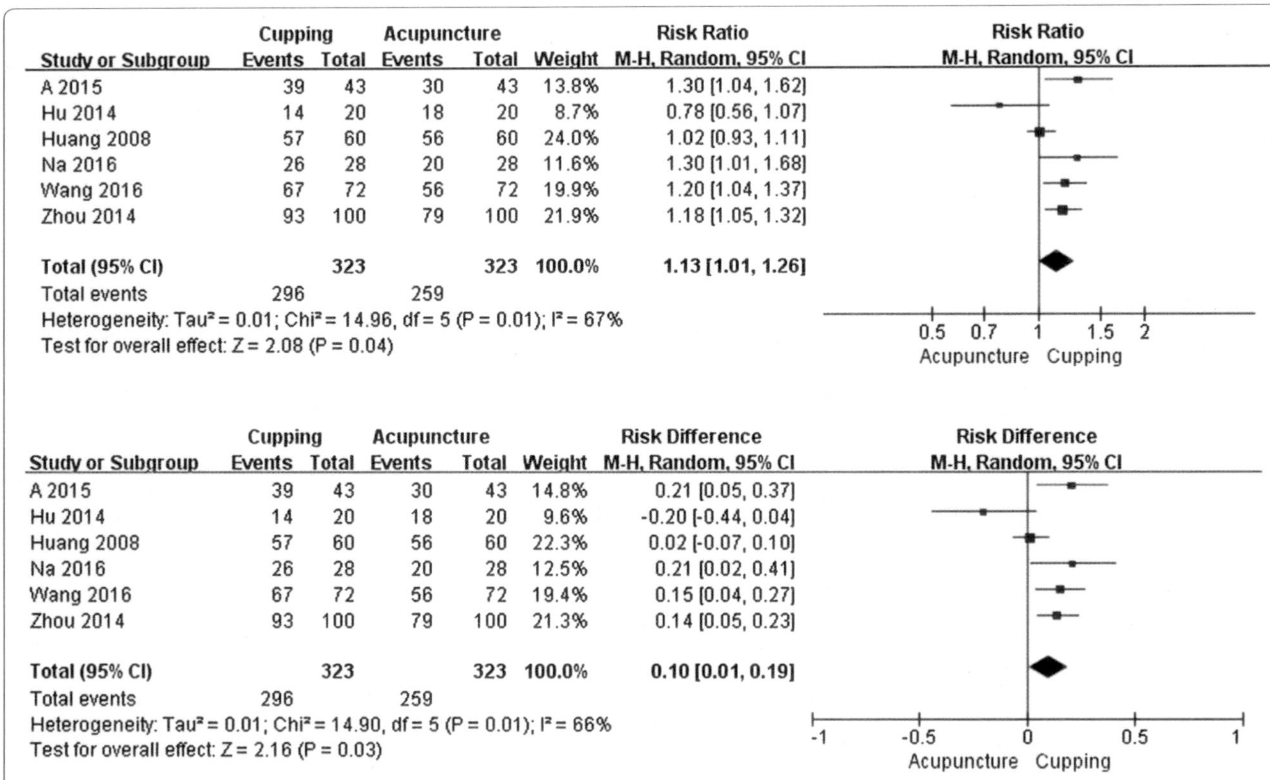

Fig. 3 Forest plot. Cupping therapy versus acupuncture for symptom improvement in patients with cervical spondylosis

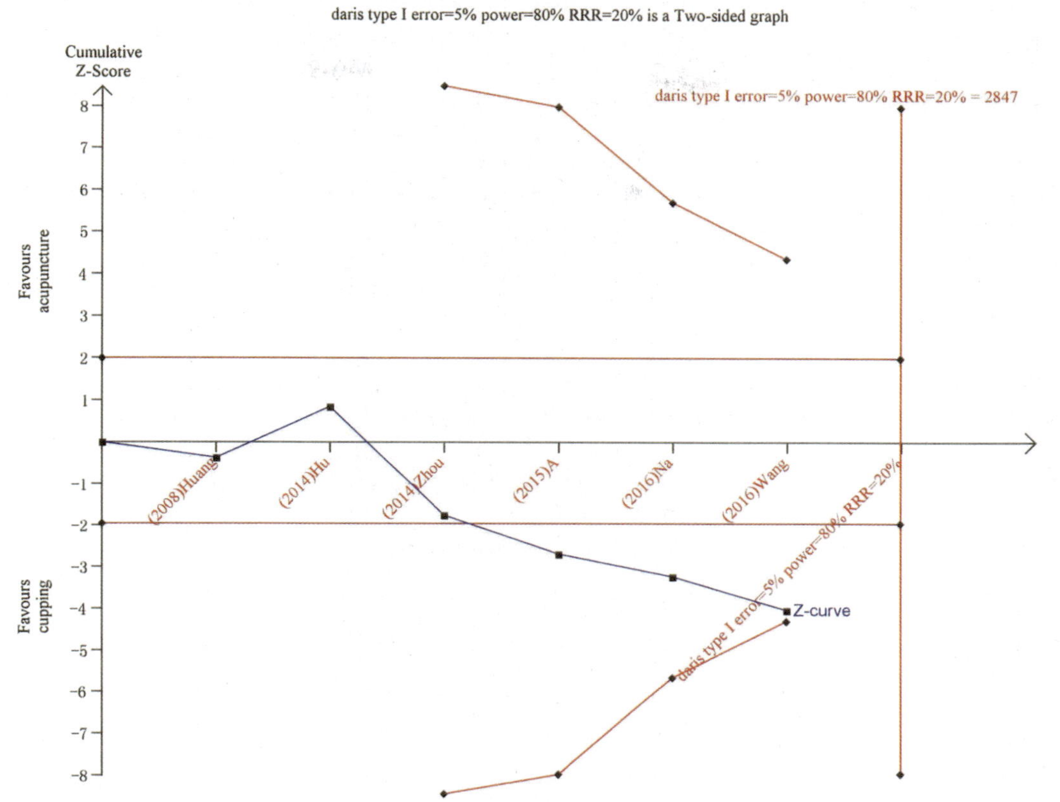

Fig. 4 Trial sequential analysis on cupping therapy versus acupuncture for symptom improvement rate in patients with cervical spondylosis

Adverse events

Seventeen (73.92%) out of the 23 studies did not report the outcome on adverse event, and other 6 [24–27, 31, 32] (26.08%) studies reported that there was no adverse event in both groups during the treatment.

Discussion

Summary of main findings

Twenty-three RCTs with 12 pain-related conditions were included in this review. The majority of the included studies had poor methodological quality according to cochrane risk of bias assessment. Manual or electro-acupuncture were compared with cupping therapy (including wet cupping, moving cupping, flash cupping and retaining cupping) in these studies. Due to the obvious clinical or statistical heterogeneity, only data from ten studies could be pooled in three meta-analyses for cervical spondylosis, lateral femoral cutaneous neuritis and scapulohumeral periarthritis. It should be point out that though some of the included trials reported statistical significant differences between the two therapies according to the symptom improvement rate or pain relieve assessed by scales (such as VAS), according to clinical experience these differences have not achieved clinically meaningful difference between cupping therapy and acupuncture since the differences were too small (RR less than 2 or MD of the VAS less than 3 cm) [41] and the result of TSA for cervical spondylosis also indicated the character available data has not reached a powerful conclusion. All of included studies showed similar effects of these two therapies on increasing symptom improvement rate and other pain reduction for the covered diseases/conditions. No serious adverse events were reported from both groups.

Strengths and weakness

To the best of our knowledge, this review is the first systematic review comparing cupping therapy with acupuncture for pain-related conditions. The findings of our review might provide evidence-based information of the therapeutic effects of the two therapies to support clinical treatment decisions on pain-related conditions.

There are some limitations of this review. Only 23 RCTs covering 12 conditions were included, thus for most of the conditions we got only 1 or 2 small studies for each to compare the effect of cupping therapy and acupuncture. Furthermore, the sample size of the included participants was too small to provide a powerful evidence. In addition, only three meta-analyses could be conducted with 2–6 studies in each. Though funnel plot analysis could not be conducted, most of the included studies were conducted and published in China, and outcomes of the original studies all got 'positive' conclusions, though some of which did not show any clinically meaningful difference between the two therapies. Therefore, the 'uncertainty principle' might be destroyed due to the 'preference' of the researchers and lead to publication bias.

Implication for clinical practice

Regardless the potential bias and limitations of this review, all of the included studies showed that cupping therapy had similar therapeutic effects with acupuncture in treating pain-related conditions (such as cervical pain, back pain, osteoarthritis, and acute soft tissue injury).

For pain-related conditions, cupping therapy and acupuncture have different choice of acupoints. Based on our review, acupuncture often use two basic acupoints which are tenderness point (Ashi) and the meridians passing through the pain area; while for cupping therapy, wet cupping uses special acupoints (such as Haoyi for cervical spondylopathy) for local pain, and flash cupping combined with moving cupping often use the meridians passing through the pain area for widespread pain.

Considering the similar therapeutic effects of these two therapies, clinical practitioners may consider to choose any of them, based on their own clinical experience and the preference of patients.

Implications for future research

The methodological quality of included studies was general poor, therefore more well designed, conducted and reported RCTs are warranted in the future. According to the Consolidated Standards of Reporting Trials (CONSORT) [42], randomization methods need to be clearly described and fully reported. Although blinding of patients and practitioners might be very difficult for cupping therapy and acupuncture, we strongly suggest the blinding of outcome assessors should be attempted to minimize assessment bias. We also suggest future researchers to select outcome measures based on international consensus for relevant pain conditions. The study protocol is strongly suggested to be registered in authoritative registration plat form [43], such as WHO international Clinical Trial Registration Platform (WHO ICTRP) or Clinicaltrial.com. The reporting of sample size calculation, and using intention-to-treat analysis to deal missing data might be considered.

In addition, due to different treatment durations and variations of the cupping therapy and acupuncture, it is worthy developing cost-effectiveness analyses to further comparing these two TCM non-pharmaceutical therapies, in order to find more economic clinical procedure. Clinical equivalence trials with large sample size will be needed to confirm the non-significant difference of effectiveness between acupuncture and cupping therapy. In addition, compliance, satisfaction and preference of participants to treatment would be considered to employ as outcome measurements in future study.

Conclusion

Currently, there are limited evidence shows that cupping therapy and acupuncture has similar effect on relieving pain and improving other symptoms of pain-related conditions. Larger and rigorously designed RCTs are needed to confirm this conclusion. Economic studied might be considered in the future to further compare the cost-effectiveness of cupping therapy and acupuncture.

Abbreviations

CI: confidence intervals; CAS: the Clinical Assessment Scale; HAMD: the Hamilton Depression Scale; JOA: the Joint Operational Area; MD: mean difference; NDI: neck disability index (physical therapy); RCT: randomized controlled trial; RD: risk difference; RR: risk ratio; REM: random-effect model; SF-36: the MOS item short from health survey; TCM: Traditional Chinese Medicine; TSA: trial sequential analysis; VAS: Visual Analogue Scale; WOMAC: the Western Ontario and McMaster Universities osteoarthritis index.

Authors' contributions

HJC participated in the design of the study and drafted the manuscript. YJZ participated in extracted data, assessed study quality, analyzed data, performed the statistical analysis and drafted the manuscript. XYY, BYL participated in searched literature, identified clinical studies for inclusion and extracted data. XLL participated in extracted data and assessed study quality. GYY participated in the modification of the manuscript. JPL conceived of the study, and co-developed the full text of the review and is the corresponding author. All authors read and approved the final manuscript.

Author details

[1] Centre for Evidence-Based Chinese Medicine, Beijing University of Chinese Medicine, 11 Bei San Huan Dong Lu, Beijing 100029, China. [2] The National Research Center in Complementary and Alternative Medicine (NAFKAM) Department of Community Medicine, Faculty of Health Science, UiT, The Arctic University of Norway, 9037 Tromsø, Norway. [3] National Institute of Complementary Medicine, Western Sydney University, Sydney, NSW 2751, Australia.

Acknowledgements

We greatly thank Sun Jin for professional assistance in writing the manuscript and Yun Xia for expert assistance during the process of Trial sequential analysis.

Competing interests

The authors declare that they have no competing interests.

Consent for publication

Not applicable.

Funding

HJ Cao is supported by Beijing Municipal Organization Department talents project (2015000020124G083). This work is partially supported by the Project for Capacity Building of TCM Clinical Researchers (No. 201207007).

References

1. Xu XQ, Xu QL, Xie SP, et al. Practice and consideration of non-drug therapy in AIDS prevention and treatment. Chin J Tradit Chin Med Pharm. 2016;31:4912–5.
2. Shi XM. Acupuncture and moxibustion therapy. Beijing: People's Medical Publishing House; 2001. p. 3.
3. Qaseem A, Wilt TJ, Mclean RM, et al. Noninvasive treatments for acute, subacute, and chronic low back pain: a clinical practice guideline from the American College of Physicians. Ann Intern Med. 2017. doi:10.7326/M16-2367.
4. MacPherson H, Vickers A, Bland M, et al. Acupuncture for chronic pain and depression in primary care: a programme of research. Southampton (UK): NIHR Journals Library; 2017. doi: 10.3310/pgfar05030.
5. Rubinstein SM, van Middelkoop M, Kuijpers T, et al. A systematic review on the effectiveness of complementary and alternative medicine for chronic non-specific low-back pain. Eur Spine J. 2010;19:1213–28.
6. Munoz-ortego J, Solans-Domenech M, Carrion C. Medical indications for acupuncture: systematic review. Med Clin. 2016;147:250–6.
7. Qin ZS, Wu JN, Tian JH, et al. Network meta-analysis of the efficacy of acupuncture, alpha-blockers and antibiotics on chronic prostatitis/chronic pelvic pain syndrome. Sci Rep. 2016;6:35737.
8. Deare JC, Zheng Z, Xue CCL, et al. Acupuncture for treating fibromyalgia. Cochrane Database Syst Rev. 2013;5:CD007070. doi:10.1002/14651858.
9. Linde K, Allais G, Brinkhaus B, et al. Acupuncture for migraine prophylaxis. Cochrane Database Syst Rev. 2009;21:CD001218. doi:10.1002/14651858.
10. Gao LW. Practical cupping therapy (2004). Beijing: Academy Press; 2004. p. 5.
11. Chirali IZ. The cupping procedure. Traditional Chinese Medicine Cupping Therapy. London: Churchill Livingstone. 1999. p. 73–86.
12. Cao HJ, Han M, Li X, et al. Clinical research evidence of cupping therapy in China: a systematic literature review. BMC Complement Altern Med. 2010;10:70–80.
13. Cao H, Han M, Zhu X, Liu J. An overview of systematic reviews of clinical evidence for cupping therapy. J Tradit Chin Med Sci. 2015;2:3–10.
14. Cao H, Li X, Liu J. An updated review of the efficacy of cupping therapy. PLoS ONE. 2012;7:e31793.
15. Cao HJ, Zhu CJ, Liu JP. Wet cupping therapy for treatment of herpes zoster: a systematic review of randomized controlled trials. Altern Ther Health Med. 2010;16:48–54.
16. World Health Organization. International statistical classification of diseases and health related problems. Geneva: World Health Organization; 2008.
17. Higgins JPT, Green S, et al. Cochrane handbook for systematic reviews of interventions, version 5.0.1 [updated September 2008]. The Cochrane Collaboration. 2008. http://www.cochrane-handbook.org. Accessed 27 Mar 2010.
18. Dong YL, Ari GT. Clinical study of bloodletting therapy in the treatment of cervical spondylosis of vertebral artery type. Inn Mong Med J. 2008;04:409–11.
19. Zhou H, Huang GH, Li XM, et al. Lotus needling cupping of Zhuang medicine by clinical observation of 100 cases of blood stasis in treatment of cervical spondylosis. Sichuan J Tradit Chin Med. 2014;12:142–3.
20. Huge JLT, Hexi GBT. Mongolian medicine therapy treatment of vertebral artery type cervical spondylosis, theory study and clinical analysis. Latest Med Inf Abstr. 2014;04:208–9.
21. Mou MY, Pu SA, Meng XW, et al. Thorn complex therapy curative effect observation of treatment of cervical spondylosis of nerve root type. J Acupunct Tuina Sci. 2015;04:236–41.
22. Amu GL. Clinical observation of 43 cases of bleeding and cupping therapy in the treatment of cervical spondylosis. Chin J Natl Med. 2015;11:8–9.
23. Wangsu RKLT. Mongolian medicine cupping bloodletting therapy to treat 72 cases of cervical spondylosis clinical observation. Chin J Med. 2016;9:27–8.
24. Nayin HY. Clinical observation of 28 cases of bleeding and cupping therapy in the treatment of cervical spondylosis. Chin Folk Med. 2016;2:6.
25. Wang PL. Observation of abdominal acupuncture combined with plum blossom needle therapy and cupping therapy in the treatment of knee osteoarthritis curative effect. Clin J Chin Med. 2016;8:100–2.
26. Wang B, Liu XR, Hu ZH, et al. The "Yang" pricking and cupping therapy for knee osteoarthritis: a multicenter randomized controlled study. Zhong Guo Zhen Jiu. 2016;36:113–8.
27. Shu Q, Jiao Y. Plum blossom needle combined with cupping bloodletting in treating 25 cases of lateral femoral cutaneous neuritis. Hunan J Tradit Chin Med. 2013;6:71–2.
28. Zhang W, Wang XQ. Plum blossom needle and 26 cases of lateral femoral cutaneous neuritis treated with flash cupping. Hunan J Tradit Chin Med. 2014;04:96–7.
29. Wang H, Wang L, Zhang XL, et al. Clinical observation of acupuncture and cupping in the treatment of lumbar disc herniation. Shandong J Tradit Chin Med. 2012;12:875–6.
30. Zhou SD, Li J, Liang Z. 60 cases of bloodletting therapy in the treatment of the third lumbar transverse process syndrome. Guiding J Tradit Chin Med. 2014;16:93–4.
31. Zhang YX. Comparison of different methods of acupuncture treatment of residual neuralgia of herpes zoster. Shanghai J Acu-mox. 2015;34:620–2.
32. Huang JM, Han HT, Li J, et al. To observe the curative effect of the treatment of postherpetic neuralgia of lotus needle cupping. Guangxi Tradit Chin Med. 2011;01:31–2.
33. Wu JS. To explore the treatment and mechanism of acupuncture and cupping toothache. China, Beijing: the establishment of the world federation of acupuncture and moxibustion and the first international symposium on acupuncture and moxibustion. 1987.
34. Bao S, Wuyun QQG. Clinical research on Mongolian medicine bloodletting therapy in treating 52 cases of scapulohumeral periarthritis. Chin J Natl Med. 2016;11:8–9.
35. Sharen YT. The bleeding and cupping therapy in the treatment of periarthritis of shoulder: clinical observation of 52 cases. Chin J Natl Med. 2016;02:7–8.
36. Liu LJ. 40 cases of cellulitis electroacupuncture plus cupping treatment of muscle fiber. Zhong Guo Zhen Jiu. 1995;02:20.
37. Huang W. To observe the resistance of acupuncture and pricking blood purification blood in the treatment of soft tissue contusion curative effect. Chin J Sports Med. 1996;01:74–5.
38. Zhou X, Ao H, Mao X, et al. Seven Star needle buckle thorn cupping clinical observation on the treatment of acute lumbar sprain. J Emerg Tradit Chin Med. 2017;26:103–5.
39. Wang WZ. Cupping treatment of acute ankle sprain in 73 cases. Shanghai J Acupunct Moxibustion. 2009;05:282.
40. Cao HJ, Liu J, Li T, Hu H. Cupping therapy for fibromyalgia: interim results from a partially randomized patient preference study. Integr Med Res. 2009;4(1):14.
41. Guyatt GH, Oxman AD, Sultan S, Glasziou P, AKl EA, Alonso-Coello P, Atkins D, Kunz R, Brozek J, Montori V, Jaeschke R. GRADE guidelined: 9. Rating up the quality of evidence. J Clin Epidemiol. 2011;64(12):1311–6.
42. CONSORT Statement 2001-Checklist: Items to include when reporting a randomized trial. (http://www.consort-statement.org).
43. Laine C, Horton R, DeAngelis CD, Drazen J, Frizelle F, Godlee F, et al. Clinical trial registration looking back and moving ahead. N Engl J Med. 2007;356:2734–6.

15

Isorhynchophylline alleviates learning and memory impairments induced by aluminum chloride in mice

Hui-Qin Li[1], Siu-Po Ip[1,2], Guo-Qing Zheng[3], Yan-Fang Xian[1,2*] and Zhi-Xiu Lin[1,2,4*]

Abstract

Background: To evaluate the effect of Isorhynchophylline (IRN) on the learning and memory impairments induced by aluminum chloride ($AlCl_3$) in mice.

Methods: Fifty male Balb-c mice (4-month-old) were randomly divided into five groups: control, $AlCl_3$ plus vehicle, $AlCl_3$ plus IRN (20 mg/kg), $AlCl_3$ plus IRN (40 mg/kg) and $AlCl_3$ plus donepezil (5 mg/kg). Learning and memory impairments were induced in mice by subcutaneously injecting with $AlCl_3$ (50 mg/kg) once a day for 8 consecutive weeks. At the same time, mice were intragastrically given vehicle or IRN (20 and 40 mg/kg) or donepezil (5 mg/kg) 30 min before each $AlCl_3$ injection. The spatial learning and memory function was assessed using radial arm maze. After sacrificed, the parameters of oxidative stress and cholinergic system in the brain tissues were examined with ELISA kits. Moreover, the expression of nuclear factor kappa B (NF-κB) signaling pathway was analyzed with western blotting.

Results: The results showed that treatment with IRN could significantly ameliorate the cognitive deficits induced by $AlCl_3$ in mice. In addition, treatment with IRN was found to reduce the level of malondialdehyde, enhance the activities of superoxide dismutases and catalase, increase the level of glutathione, and markedly inhibit the activity of acetylcholinesterase (AChE) in the brain tissues of the $AlCl_3$-treated mice. Moreover, IRN significantly suppressed the phosphorylation of NF-κB p65 and IκBα in the brain tissues of $AlCl_3$-treated mice. However, IRN did not show significant effect on the activity of butyrylcholinesterase.

Conclusion: Our findings demonstrated for the first time that IRN could alleviate learning and memory impairments induced by $AlCl_3$ in mice. The neuroprotective effect of IRN against $AlCl_3$-induced AD is probably mediated, at least in part, through inhibiting the AChE activity and reducing the oxidative damage of brain tissue via suppress the NF-κB signaling pathway. These results contributed to a better understanding of the in vivo anti-AD mechanism of IRN. It was concluded that IRN could protect the learning and memory function.

Keywords: Isorhynchophylline, Aluminum chloride, Learning and memory impairments, Oxidative stress, Cholinergic system, Nuclear factor kappa B pathway

Background

Alzheimer's disease (AD) is a neurodegenerative disease characterized by progressive memory dysfunction and cognitive deficiency [1]. As the world's population ages, we face a looming global epidemic of AD; and by 2050 the number of AD patients is estimated to be 106.4 million globally [2]. Although beta-amyloid (Aβ) accumulation and tau protein malformation are generally accepted to be the causal factors of AD, the cellular and molecular pathology and etiology of AD have not been fully understood, largely due to the fact that AD is a multifactorial disease involving genetic, epigenetic, and environmental factors [3]. Furthermore, present treatments available for AD are usually limited to symptomatic management, and no satisfactory therapeutic agents are available for AD patients [4–6]. Thus, novel therapies with better efficacy

*Correspondence: lisaxian@cuhk.edu.hk; linzx@cuhk.edu.hk
[1] School of Chinese Medicine, Faculty of Medicine, The Chinese University of Hong Kong, Hong Kong, SAR, People's Republic of China
Full list of author information is available at the end of the article

and safety profiles are urgently needed to modify the natural history of AD.

Aluminum, which can cross the blood brain barrier (BBB) [7], is a well-known neurotoxin that has close association with AD pathogenesis [8]. Based on the studies on the hippocampal neurons of AD patients, aluminum was found to be involved in the formation of neurofibrillary tangles in neurons, and therefore considered as a causative factor for AD [9]. Moreover, studies have also shown that exposure to aluminum can cause memory impairment in animal models [10, 11]. The underlying mechanisms for aluminum to induce AD-like behaviors are believed to involve oxidative damage [11], formation of hyperphosphorylated tau [12], aggregation of amyloid beta protein [13], increase in AChE activity [14] and neuronal apoptosis [13]. In addition to neuronal dysfunction, aluminum could also lead to brain dysfunction via glial alterations [15]. Given that aluminum exposure could eventually result in neuropathological and neurobehavioral changes, and impaired learning and memory, $AlCl_3$-induced model is therefore used as an established AD animal model and often used for testing the efficacy of therapeutic agents for AD.

Uncaria rhynchophylla is a component herb of many popular herbal formulae commonly prescribed for the treatment of AD [16, 17]. Recently, many studies have showed that ethanol extract of *U. rhynchophylla* has neuroprotective effect on different in vivo and in vitro AD models [18, 19]. Isorhynchophylline (IRN, the chemical structure is shown in Fig. 1), a c-22 oxindole alkaloid richly presented in the ethanol extract of *U. rhynchophylla*, is the main active chemical ingredient for its biological activities [20]. Our previous studies revealed that IRN could ameliorate the neurotoxicity induced by $A\beta_{25-35}$ on PC12 cells via PI3K/Akt/GSK-3β signaling pathway [21], improve the memory deficits induced by $A\beta_{25-35}$ in rats via inhibition of neuronal apoptosis and tau protein hyperphosphorylation [22], and reduce the memory deficits induced by D-galactose in mice through enhancing the antioxidant status and anti-inflammatory effect in brain tissues via nuclear factor kappa B (NF-κB) signaling pathway [23]. Moreover, it was found that the LD_{50} values of IRN in mice are about 510, 217 and 80 mg/kg, respectively, with oral, intraperitoneal and intravenous administration, indicating that IRN is at least 10 times less toxic than other known anti-AD drugs, and is a safer chemical compound for AD treatment [24]. All these studies implied that IRN is a promising neuroprotective agent for AD treatment warranting further investigation. However, whether IRN has therapeutic effect on $AlCl_3$-treated mice and the underlying mechanisms have not been studied yet. The present study aimed to investigate the neuroprotective effects of IRN on cognitive function in the $AlCl_3$-treated mice and to elucidate the underlying mechanisms of action.

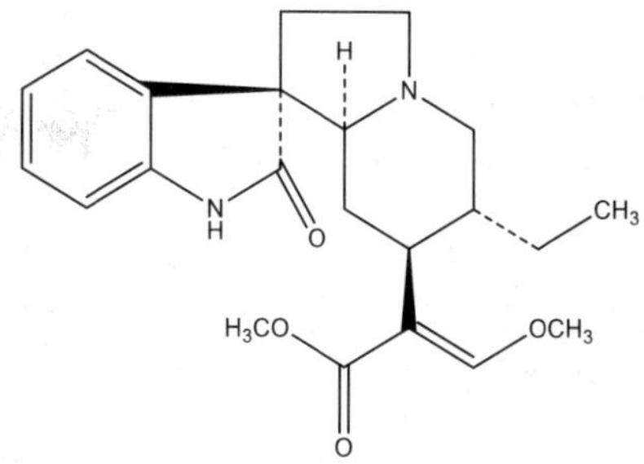

Fig. 1 Chemical structure of isorhynchophylline (IRN)

Methods

The minimum standards of reporting checklist (Additional file 1) contains details of the experimental design, statistics, and resources used in this study.

Drugs and reagents

Isorhynchophylline (IRN, purity ≥ 98%) was purchased from Chengdu Mansite Pharmaceutical Co. Ltd. (Chengdu, Sichuan, China). Aluminum chloride hexahydrate ($AlCl_3$) and donepezil hydrochloride (referred to simply as donepezil thereafter) were purchased from Sigma-Aldrich (St. Louis, MO, USA). All other reagents and chemicals used in the study were of analytical grade.

Animals

Fifty male Balb-c mice (4-month-old, weighing 25–30 g) were obtained from the Laboratory Animal Services Center, The Chinese University of Hong Kong. The animals were maintained on a 12 h light/dark cycle under controlled temperature (22 ± 2 °C) and humidity (50 ± 10%), and given standard diet and water ad libitum.

Animal groupings and drug treatment

The mice were randomly assigned into five groups of 10 animals each: (a) control; (b) $AlCl_3$ plus vehicle; (c) and (d) $AlCl_3$ plus IRN (20 and 40 mg/kg); and (e) $AlCl_3$ plus donepezil (5 mg/kg), which was used as the positive control [22]. The dosages of IRN were selected based on our previous studies [22, 23]. $AlCl_3$ was dissolved in sterile physiological saline at the concentration of 5 mg/mL, and subcutaneously injected into the mice at a dosage of 50 mg/kg once a day for 8 consecutive weeks before the behavioral assessments were started. The duration and dosage of aluminum was selected based on the previous published studies with minor modification [25]. In the control group, mice were subjected to the same injection schedule except using physiological saline instead of $AlCl_3$. At the same time, IRN and donepezil were suspended in 0.5% sodium carboxymethyl cellulose (CMC-Na), then given to the mice intragastrically daily 30 min before each $AlCl_3$ injection, while the control group and $AlCl_3$ plus vehicle control group were given the same volume of 0.5% CMC-Na. Behavioral assessments were carried out after the $AlCl_3$ injection was finished. During the behavioral assessment, the treatment was ongoing until the working and reference memory tasks test, which was undertaken at day 64. Detailed experimental schedules were depicted in Fig. 2.

Radial arm maze (RAM) test

Spatial learning and memory changes in mice were determined by the RAM test. A modular radial arm maze with SuperMaze V2.0 video tracking software (Shanghai Xinruan Information Technology Co. Ltd, Shanghai, China) was used for this experiment. The maze consisted of eight arms, numbered from 1 to 8 (35 cm long, 5 cm wide and 10 cm high), extending radially from a central platform (22 cm in diameter). The radial arm maze test was conducted as described previously with minor modifications [26, 27]. In the room, several visual extra-maze cues were provided close (10–30 cm) to the maze in a fixed configuration. A circular food well (1 cm in diameter, 0.5 cm deep) was positioned at the end of each arm. During behavioral training and testing, to stimulate hunger, the animals were kept on restricted diet with only water being available ad libitum and the body weight was maintained at about 85–90% of their free-feeding level. Initially, animals received two 10 min habituation trials, 24 h apart, with free access to all arms on the first 2 days. At the beginning of each habituation trial, three or four mice were simultaneously placed in the central platform and all arms were baited with several approximately 10 mg food pellets. Then, mice were trained for 5 consecutive days, one trial per day, to run to the end of the arms and consume the bait. At the beginning of each training trial, only one mouse was placed in the central platform and only four constant arms were randomly selected and baited with one approximately 10 mg food pellet, which was placed in a food cup that prevented visual detection. A trial was ended when all the four baits had been consumed or after a maximum of 10 min had elapsed. An arm entry was counted when all four limbs of the mice were within an arm. At the eighth day, the mice were subjected to working and reference memory tasks, in which the same four arms were baited as each daily training trial, and the following behavioural measurements were recorded: (1) number of reference memory errors (RMEs), i.e. entries into a non-baited arm, (2) number of working memory errors (WMEs), i.e. reentries into an already visited baited arm, (3) number of total entries to complete the test.

Preparation of brain samples

Twenty-four hours after the RAM test, mice were decapitated under anesthesia and the brain tissues were removed quickly. After washed with normal saline over the ice, brains were immediately stored at −80 °C until assay.

Measurement of oxidative stress

To evaluate the effect of IRN on oxidative stress status, the levels of malondialdehyde (MDA) and glutathione (GSH) and the activities of superoxide dismutases (SOD) and catalase (CAT) were measured. For these biochemical analyses, 10% (w/v) brain homogenate was prepared in 0.9% sterile normal saline using a potter homogenizer at a speed of 1200 rpm. The homogenate was centrifuged at 3000×*g* for 10 min at 4 °C and then the supernatant

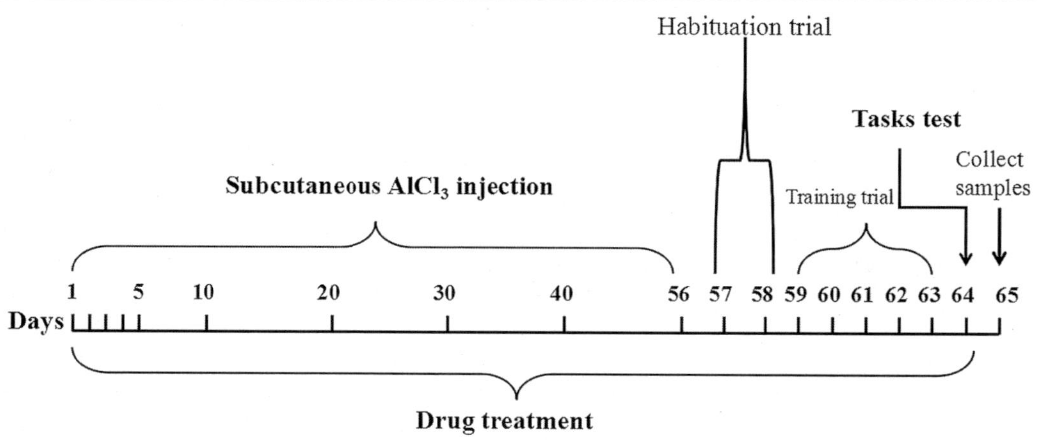

Fig. 2 Experimental design and treatment schedule

was collected. The supernatant was separated and tested with SOD assay kit, GSH assay kit, CAT assay kit and MDA assay kit (Cat. A001-3, A006-1, A007-1 and A003-1, respectively, Nanjing Jiancheng Institute, Jiangsu, China) following the manufacturer's protocols. CAT activity was determined by the rate of decomposition of 1 μM H_2O_2 and expressed as U/mgprot. SOD activity was determined by the amount of enzyme required to produce 50% inhibition and expressed as U/mgprot. Reduced GSH was determined based on the formation of a yellow colored complex with 5,5′-dithiobis-(2-nitrobenzoic acid) (DTNB) and the level of GSH in tissue was expressed as mgGSH/gprot. Reduced MDA was determined based on the formation of a red colored complex with thiobarbituric acid (TBA) and the level of MDA in tissue was expressed as nmol/mgprot. All samples were measured in duplicate.

Measurement of the activities of acetylcholinesterase (AChE) and butyrylcholinesterase (BuChE)

The activities of AChE and BuChE in the brain tissues were examined. At first, 10% (w/v) brain homogenate was prepared in 0.9% sterile normal saline using a potter homogenizer at a speed of 1200 rpm. The homogenate was centrifuged at 3000×*g* for 10 min at 4 °C and then the supernatant was collected. The supernatant was separated and tested with the AChE assay kit and BuChE assay kit (Cat. A024 and A025, respectively, Nanjing Jiancheng Institute, Jiangsu, China) following the manufacturer's instructions. The activities of AChE and BuChE were determined based on the formation of Sym-Trinitrobenzene (TNB), which is a yellow colored complex, and the results were both expressed as U/mg protein. All samples were measured in duplicate.

Western blotting analysis

For preparation of whole cell protein lysate, the brain tissues were homogenized in RIPA lysis buffer (50 mM Tris–HCl (pH 8.0), 150 mMNaCl, 1% NP-40, 0.1% SDS, 0.5% sodium deoxycholate and 1% Protease/Phosphatase Inhibitor Cocktail) (Cell Signaling Technology, USA) for 30 min on ice, then centrifuged at 12,000 rpm at 4 °C, and then the supernatant was collected. Protein concentrations were determined using Bradford method with protein assay dye reagent (Bio-Rad, USA). Equal amounts of protein of different samples were separated by sodium dodecyl sulfate polyacrylamide gel electrophoresis (SDS-PAGE), and then transferred to PVD membranes. After blocked with 5% (w/v) non-fat milk in TBS-T (50 mM Tris, 150 mM NaCl and 0.1% Tween-20, pH 7.4) at room temperature for 2 h, the PVD membranes were incubated overnight at 4 °C in NF-κB p65 (p65), phospho-NF-κB p65 (p-p65), phospho-IκBα (p-IκBα), IκBα or β-actin primary antibody (1:1000, Cell Signaling Technology, #6956S, 3033S, 2859S, 9242S or 3700S, respectively). Rinsed with TBS-T for 5 min × 3 times, the PVD membranes were then incubated with secondary antibody for 2 h at room temperature, and then rinsed again with TBS-T for 5 min × 3 times. The protein bands were visualized by the ECL western blotting detection reagents (Amersham Biosciences, Buckinghamshire, UK). The intensity of each band was analyzed using Image J software (NIH Image, MD, USA).

Statistical analysis

All data were presented as the mean ± standard error of the mean (SEM). Multiple group comparisons were performed using one-way analysis of variance (ANOVA) followed by Post-hoc Dunnett's test to detect inter-group differences. GraphPad Prism software (Version 5, GraphPad Software, Inc., CA, USA) was used to perform the statistical analysis. A difference was considered statistically significant when the $p < 0.05$.

Results

IRN ameliorated the cognitive deficits induced by $AlCl_3$ in mice

After 7 days of training, the mice were subjected to working and reference memory tasks. Figure 3a shows the effect of IRN on the number of total entries to complete the maze. The results showed that $AlCl_3$ + vehicle group markedly increased the number of total entries when compared with the control group ($F (4, 33) = 4.694$, $p < 0.01$), while treatment with IRN (40 mg/kg) significantly decreased the number of total entries when compared with the $AlCl_3$ + vehicle group ($p < 0.01$). Donepezil (5 mg/kg) treatment also decreased the number of total entries ($p < 0.05$) when compared with the $AlCl_3$ + vehicle group.

The effects of IRN on reference memory errors (RMEs) and the working memory errors (WMEs) were shown in Fig. 3b, c, respectively. The results showed that $AlCl_3$ plus vehicle group elevated the RMEs ($F (4, 33) = 3.895$, $p < 0.05$) and WMEs ($F (4, 33) = 4.416$, $p < 0.01$) to complete the task when compared with the control group, while treatment with IRN (40 mg/kg) significantly reduced the RMEs ($p < 0.05$) and WMEs ($p < 0.01$) when compared with the $AlCl_3$ + vehicle group. Donepezil (5 mg/kg) treatment also significantly reduced the RMEs ($p < 0.05$) and WMEs ($p < 0.05$) when compared with the $AlCl_3$ + vehicle group. On the other hand, IRN treatment at dosage of 20 mg/kg/day showed no significant difference in the number of the total entries ($p > 0.05$), RMEs ($p > 0.05$) or WMEs ($p > 0.05$) when compared with the $AlCl_3$ + vehicle group.

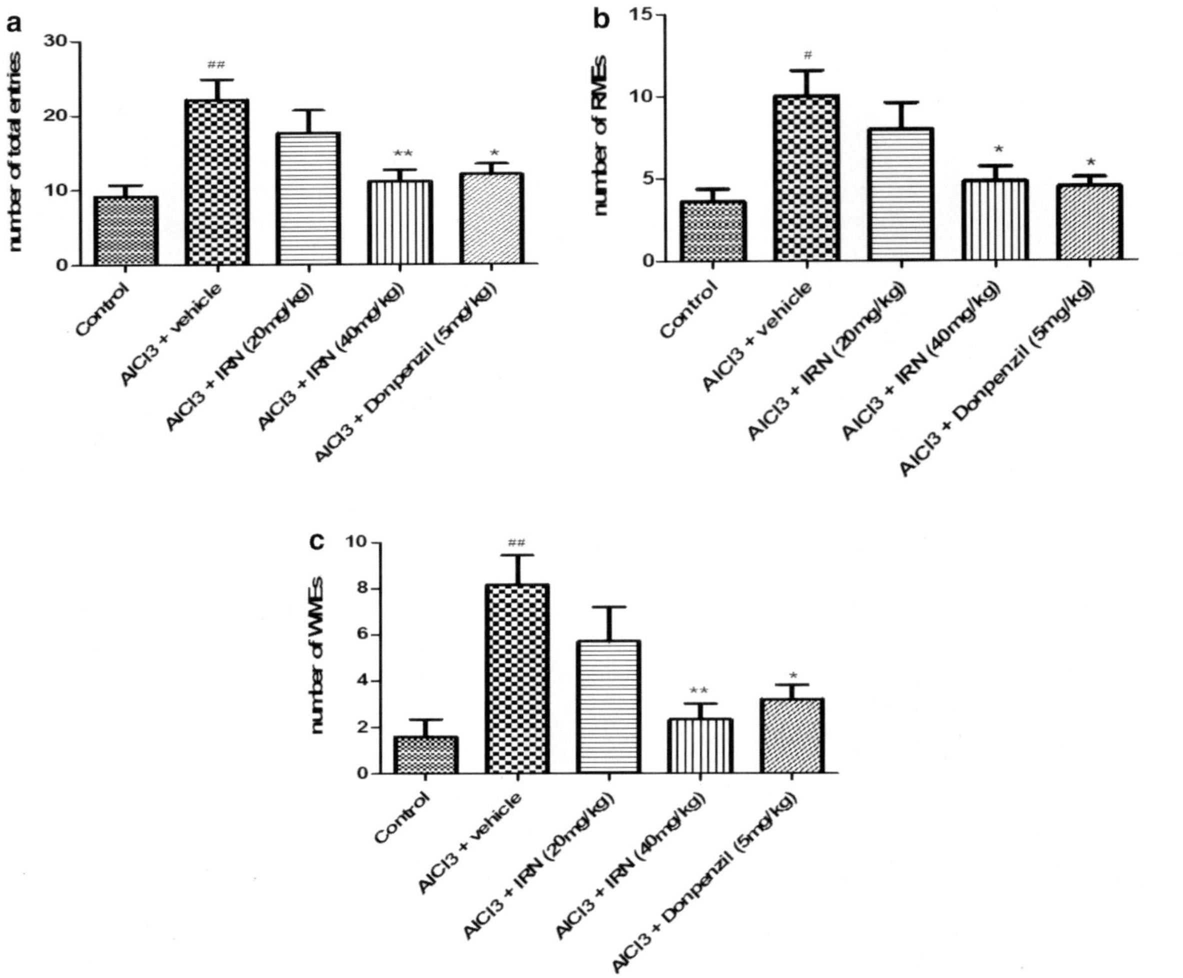

Fig. 3 Effects of IRN on spatial learning and memory of mice as evaluated by the RAM test after 7 days of training. The total entrances to complete the task (**a**), the reference memory errors (RMEs) (**b**), and the working memory errors (WMEs) (**c**). Data were expressed as mean ± SEMs (n = 6–10). $^{\#}p < 0.05$ and $^{\#\#}p < 0.01$ compared with the control group; $^{*}p < 0.05$ and $^{**}p < 0.01$ compared with the $AlCl_3$ + vehicle group

IRN reduced the oxidative damage induced by $AlCl_3$ in mice

The oxidative stress of brain tissue was assessed by measuring the level of MDA, a lipid peroxidation product (Fig. 4a), and antioxidants including GSH (Fig. 4b), SOD (Fig. 4c) and CAT (Fig. 4d).

Figure 4a showed that the MDA level was significantly higher in $AlCl_3$ + vehicle group than the control group (F (4, 34) = 6.585, $p < 0.05$], while treatment with IRN (40 mg/kg) significantly decreased the MDA level when compared with the $AlCl_3$ + vehicle group ($p < 0.05$). Donepezil (5 mg/kg) treatment also inhibited the MDA level when compared with $AlCl_3$ + vehicle group ($p < 0.01$).

As shown in Fig. 4b, the GSH level was significantly lower in the $AlCl_3$ + vehicle group than the control group (F (4, 34) = 4.06, $p < 0.01$), while treatment with IRN (40 mg/kg) significantly increased the GSH level when compared with the $AlCl_3$ + vehicle group ($p < 0.05$). Donepezil (5 mg/kg) treatment also increased the GSH level when compared with the $AlCl_3$ + vehicle group ($p < 0.01$).

Figure 4c showed that the SOD activity was significantly suppressed in the $AlCl_3$ + vehicle group when compared with the control group (F (4, 34) = 5.571, $p < 0.001$), while treatment with IRN (40 mg/kg) significantly increased the SOD activity when compared with the $AlCl_3$ + vehicle group ($p < 0.05$). Donepezil (5 mg/kg) treatment also increased the SOD activity when compared with the $AlCl_3$ + vehicle group ($p < 0.05$).

Moreover, Fig. 4d showed that the CAT activity was significantly decreased in the $AlCl_3$ + vehicle group when compared with the control group (F (4,

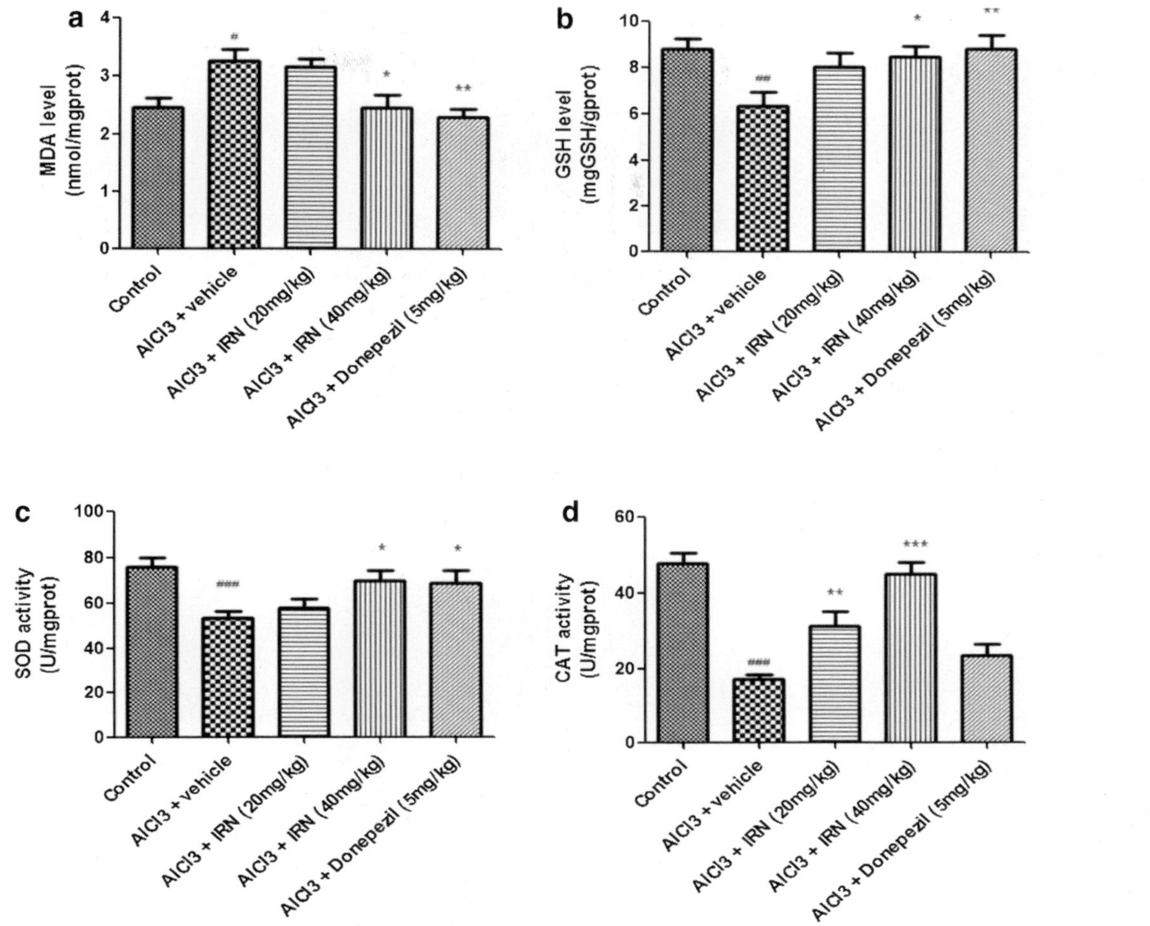

Fig. 4 Effect of IRN treatment on the levels of MDA (**a**) and GSH (**b**) and the activities of SOD (**c**) and CAT (**d**) in the brains of $AlCl_3$-treated mice. Data were expressed as mean ± SEMs (n = 6–9). $^{\#}p < 0.05$, $^{\#\#}p < 0.01$ and $^{\#\#\#}p < 0.001$ compared with the control group; $^{*}p < 0.05$, $^{**}p < 0.01$ and $^{***}p < 0.001$ compared with the $AlCl_3$ + vehicle group

34) = 18.29, $p < 0.001$), while the treatment with IRN (20 and 40 mg/kg) significantly increased the CAT activity when compared with the $AlCl_3$ + vehicle group, ($p < 0.01$ and $p < 0.001$, respectively). However, donepezil (5 mg/kg) treatment did not show significant effect ($p > 0.05$) on the activity of CAT.

IRN inhibited the cholinesterase activity in the brain of $AlCl_3$-treated mice

The effect of IRN on cholinesterase activity was assessed by measuring the activities of AChE (Fig. 5a) and BuChE (Fig. 5b). Figure 5a showed that the AChE activity was significantly increased in the $AlCl_3$ + vehicle group when compared with the control group (F (4, 34) = 4.144, $p < 0.05$], while treatment with IRN (40 mg/kg) significantly decreased the AChE activity when compared with the $AlCl_3$ + vehicle group ($p < 0.05$). Donepezil (5 mg/kg) treatment also decreased the AChE activity when compared with the $AlCl_3$ + vehicle group ($p < 0.01$). On the other hand, Fig. 5b showed that the BuChE activity was significantly increased in the $AlCl_3$ + vehicle group when compared with the control group, but treatment with IRN (20 and 40 mg/kg) did not show significant effect on BuChE activity when compared with the $AlCl_3$ + vehicle group ($p > 0.05$ for both). Donepezil (5 mg/kg) treatment markedly decreased the BuChE activity when compared with the $AlCl_3$ + vehicle group ($p < 0.05$).

IRN inhibited the activation of NF-κB signaling pathway in the brain of $AlCl_3$-treated mice

Effect of IRN treatment on the NF-κB signaling pathway in the brain tissues of $AlCl_3$-treated mice were determined by Western blotting (Figs. 6a and 7a). Relative density of p-p65/p65 and p-IκBα/IκBα were shown in Figs. 6b and 7b, respectively. Figure 6b showed that the relative density of p-p65/p65 was significantly increased in the $AlCl_3$ + vehicle group when compared with the control group (F (4, 34) = 9.896, $p < 0.001$],

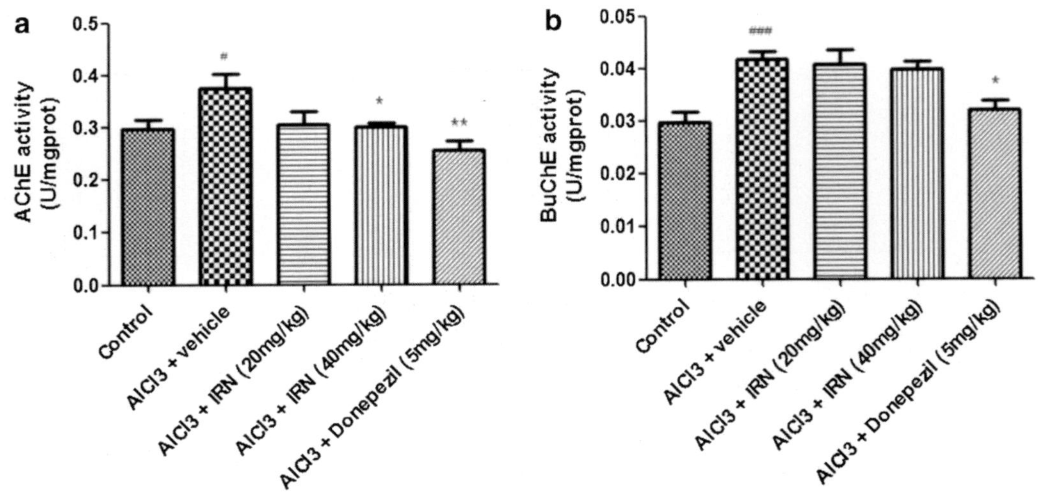

Fig. 5 Effect of IRN treatment on the activities of AChE (**a**) and BuChE (**b**) in the brain of the $AlCl_3$-treated mice. Data were expressed as mean ± SEMs (n = 6–9). #$p < 0.05$ and ###$p < 0.001$ compared with the control group; *$p < 0.05$ and **$p < 0.01$ compared with the $AlCl_3$ + vehicle group

while treatment with IRN (20 and 40 mg/kg) significantly decreased the relative density of p-p65/p65 when compared with the $AlCl_3$ + vehicle group ($p < 0.01$ and $p < 0.01$, respectively). Donepezil (5 mg/kg) treatment also decreased the relative density of p-p65/p65 when compared with $AlCl_3$ + vehicle group ($p < 0.01$). On the other hand, Fig. 7b showed that the relative density of p-IκBα/IκBα was significantly increased in the $AlCl_3$ + vehicle group when compared with the control group (F (4, 23) = 7.125, $p < 0.001$), while the treatment with IRN (20 and 40 mg/kg) significantly decreased the relative density of p-p65/p65 when compared with the $AlCl_3$ + vehicle group ($p < 0.01$ and $p < 0.01$, respectively). Donepezil (5 mg/kg) treatment also decreased the relative density of p-p65/p65 when compared with the $AlCl_3$ + vehicle group ($p < 0.01$).

Discussion

The present study investigated the neuroprotective effects of IRN on the $AlCl_3$-induced cognitive impairment in mice. In our experiment, radial arm maze test was conducted to assess the spatial learning and memory functions of the mice. The results showed that $AlCl_3$ treatment impaired the spatial learning and memory functions of the mice, enhanced the oxidative stress,

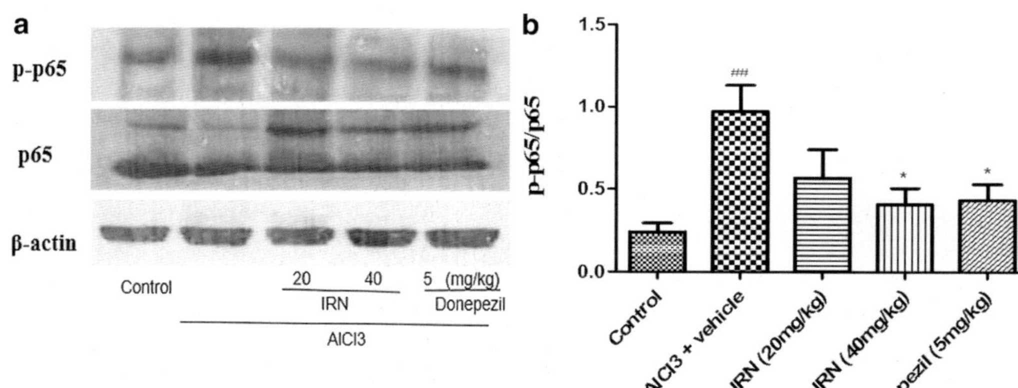

Fig. 6 Effect of IRN treatment on NF-κB p65 (p65) and phospho-NF-κB p65 (p-p65) expressions in the brain of the $AlCl_3$-treated mice were determined by Western blotting (**a**). The relative density of p-p65/p65 (**b**) were analyzed by Image J. software. Data were expressed as mean ± SEMs (n = 4–6). ###$p < 0.01$ compared with the control group; **$p < 0.05$ compared with the $AlCl_3$ + vehicle group

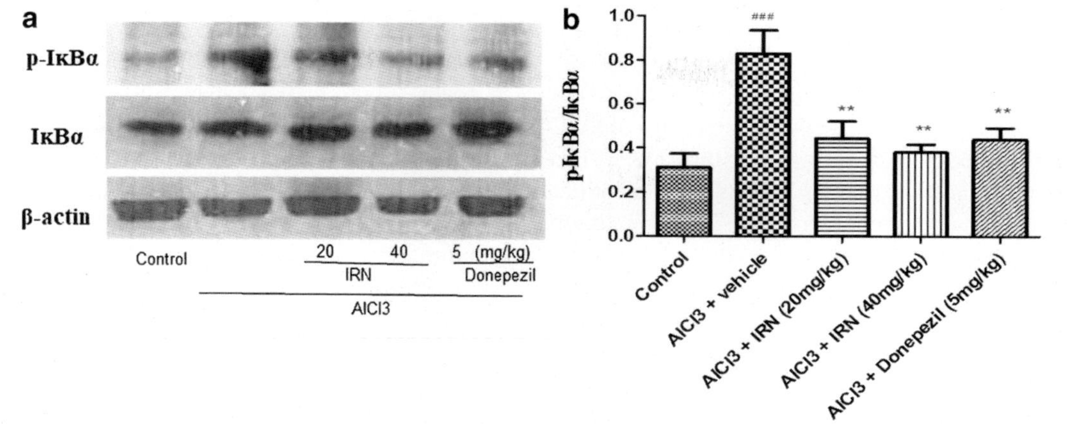

Fig. 7 Effect of IRN treatment on IκBα and phospho-IκBα (p-IκBα) expressions in the brain of the $AlCl_3$-treated mice were determined by Western blotting (**a**). The relative density of p-IκBα/IκBα (**b**) were analyzed by Image J. software. Data were expressed as mean ± SEMs (n = 4–6). $^{###}p < 0.001$ compared with the control group; $^{**}p < 0.01$ compared with the $AlCl_3$ + vehicle group

damaged the cholinergic system, and activated the NF-κB signaling pathway in the brain. On the other hand, treatment with IRN significantly reversed these changes induced by $AlCl_3$ in mice, suggesting that IRN is a potential anti-AD agent for the treatment of AD.

So far, several cognitive domains found disrupted in AD have been modeled, and the two most extensively modeled and assessed domains are working memory and reference memory [28]. The RAM test was firstly introduced by Olton in 1976 [29]. It is one of the most commonly used animal behavioral tasks to assess working memory and reference memory, just as the Morris water maze [28]. In the RAM test, the number of total entries to complete the maze is considered as an overall measure of learning and memory [30]. As previously reported, a reference memory error was noted if an animal enters an arm that never contained a food reward, and a working memory error was noted if an animal enters a baited arm previously visited during the same trial [31, 32]. The higher numbers of RMEs and WMEs are recorded, the worse the reference memory and working memory are indicated. In the present study, $AlCl_3$ + vehicle group showed significant increases in RMEs and WMEs to complete the task when compared with the control group, indicating that $AlCl_3$ induced significant impairments on reference memory and working memory in mice. IRN treatment reduced both of RMEs and WMEs when compared with the $AlCl_3$ + vehicle group, indicating that IRN could improve the reference memory and working memory.

It has been reported that chronic exposure to aluminum at a dose of 1.6 mg/kg/day, equivalent to the high end of the human dietary aluminum range, could lead to oxidative damage in the brain and cause AD-like behaviors in rats [12]. However, short exposure to aluminum could only lead to transient memory impairment in Morris water maze [33], and low doses of aluminum may fail to observe impairment of performance in RAM test [34]. Therefore, to ensure well-established biochemical and behavioral deficits, suitable duration and dose of $AlCl_3$ should be selected. In our preliminary study, we found that about 70% mice died after treatment with $AlCl_3$ at a dose of 100 mg/kg/day for 8 consecutive weeks (data not shown), suggesting that the dose of $AlCl_3$ (100 mg/kg/day) is too high. Therefore, in this present study, the dosage of 50 mg/kg/day of $AlCl_3$ was used to induce the AD-like behaviors and the duration of exposure was set for 8 weeks.

Oxidative stress is an imbalance state between the generation and detoxification of reactive oxygen species (ROS) products [35]. It could be assessed by measuring peroxidation products of ROS, such as lipid peroxidation, and antioxidant levels [35]. Oxidative stress in human increases with age [36]. Oxidative stress is known to play an important role in the initiation of AD [37]. High lipid peroxidation and decreased antioxidant defenses are found to be presented in mild cognitive impairment (MCI) patients, implying that oxidative stress represents a sign of AD pathology and could be an early event in the progression of MCI to AD [38]. In addition, oxidative damage is found not only in the vulnerable neurons of brain affected in this disease [39], but also throughout the body in AD patients [40]. Moreover, many line of evidence showed that oxidative stress could cause marked accumulation of Aβ and phosphorylated tau protein in vitro and in vivo [41–43], which are considered to be the two main causal factors for AD. Given its close correlation, oxidative stress is even considered as a primary progenitor of AD, not merely an epiphenomenon. Thus, novel drug with anti-oxidative effects could be a preventative cure for the disease [44]. The present study showed that in the brains of the $AlCl_3$+vehicle mice, the MDA level was significantly higher, while the activities of SOD and CAT and the GSH level were significantly lower than control group, suggesting that $AlCl_3$ was able to induce high oxidative stress in mice. However, IRN treatment decreased this oxidative damage induced by $AlCl_3$, indicating it is a potential antioxidant for AD. In the present study, donepezil did not show effect on CAT activity. Donepezil is known as cholinesterase inhibitor for AD treatment. Although there is evidence that donepezil also affected the levels of GSH and MDA [45], but no evidence showed donepezil had effect on the activity of CAT, which is an antioxidant. Donepezil may suppress oxidative stress by affecting the levels of GSH and MDA, as well as the activity of SOD, but not CAT activity.

As is known, the cholinergic pathway in basal forebrain plays an important role in mnemonic processes, memory, conscious awareness and attention [46]. Evidence showed acetylcholine involved in spatial information processing [47]. Degeneration and loss of cholinergic neurons in the basal forebrain nuclei cause deficit of acetylcholine, then cause disturbances in presynaptic cholinergic terminals in the hippocampus and neocortex, leading to memory disturbances and other cognitive symptoms associated with AD [48]. Thus, acetylcholine is considered as an important neurotransmitter for memory in brains, and preventing the decrease of the level of acetylcholine may be an effective treatment strategy for AD. AChE is the primary cholinesterase that breaks down acetylcholine in the body, and activation of AChE will aggravate the deficit of acetylcholine. Cholinesterase inhibitors, such as donepezil, delay the breakdown of acetylcholine via suppressing the activity of AChE, more or less restore the cortical concentration of acetylcholine, and thus temporarily ameliorate the cognitive symptoms of AD [49]. Aluminum exposure was reported to be associated with impairment in the cholinergic system as a strong activator of AChE [50]. Our results showed that activity of AChE in the brain of $AlCl_3$+vehicle group was significantly higher than control group. On the other hand, IRN treatment significantly inhibited the AChE activity, but not BuChE. Although both of AChE and BuChE are cholinesterase, they differ in location, substrate specificity and kinetics [51]. IRN showed effect on AChE activity but not BuChE activity, indicating it is a potential selective AChE inhibitor for treatment of AD.

NF-κB, a collective name for inducible dimeric transcription factors, is involved in activation of many genes in response to infections, inflammation and other stressful situations requiring rapid reprogramming of gene expression [52]. Evidence showed that NF-κB is involved in brain function, particularly following injury and in neurodegenerative conditions such as AD, and is activated in neurons in certain regions of the brain during neurogenesis [53]. Furthermore, studies suggested that NF-κB plays a critical role in initiating and regulating the inflammation or oxidative stress in AD [54]. Increase of NF-κB p65 level could be found both in the temporal and frontal cortices of human AD brains [55]. It is now known that NF-κB preexists in the cytoplasm of cells in an inactive form bound to the inhibitor, IκB, as NF-κB:IκB complex [56]. Under certain circumstances, stimulation of cells by diverse inducers causes phosphorylation of cytosolic NF-κB:IκB complex, then NF-κB is activated by phosphorylation of IκBα and released to the nucleus [57, 58]. In the nucleus, NF-κB dimers bind to target DNA elements and activate transcription of genes encoding proteins involved with innate immune or inflammation responses [59]. Thus, inhibition of the phosphorylation of IκBα and NF-κB p65 may be a valuable drug target to reduce stressful damage for AD patients. The most abundant form of the NF-κB family is the heterodimeric p65–p50 complex [57] and the best-characterized IκB proteins is IκBα [56]. Our result revealed that the levels of phosphorylation of NF-κB p65 and IκBα were significantly accentuated in the brain of $AlCl_3$+vehicle mice. IRN treatment decreased the phosphorylation of NF-κB p65 and IκBα, suggesting that IRN inhibited the activation of NF-κB signaling pathway induced by $AlCl_3$ in mice.

Conclusions

Our experimental results for the first time demonstrated that IRN alleviated learning and memory impairments induced by $AlCl_3$ in mice. The protective effect of IRN against $AlCl_3$-induced cognitive deficits is probably mediated, at least in part, through inhibiting the AChE activity and reducing the oxidative damage of brain tissue via inhibiting the activation of NF-κB signaling pathway. These results further confirmed the in vivo anti-AD effect of IRN and suggested that IRN exhibits multi-target therapeutic potential for the treatment of AD. It was concluded that IRN could protect the learning and memory function. Further investigations are needed to reveal the anti-AD effect mechanisms of IRN.

Abbreviations

AChE: acetylcholinesterase; AD: Alzheimer's disease; $AlCl_3$: aluminum chloride; BuChE: butyrylcholinesterase; CAT: catalase; DTNB: 5,5′-dithiobis

(2-nitrobenzoic acid); CMC-Na: sodium carboxymethyl cellulose; GSH: glutathione; IRN: isorhynchophylline; MDA: malondialdehyde; MCI: mild cognitive impairment; NF-Kb: nuclear factor kappa B; p-IκBα: phospho-IκBα; p-p65: phospho-NF-κB p65; RAM: radial arm maze; ROS: reactive oxygen species; RMEs: reference memory errors; SDS-PAGE: sodium dodecyl sulfate polyacrylamide gel electrophoresis; SEM: standard error of the mean; SOD: superoxide dismutases; TBA: thiobarbituric acid; TNB: Sym-Trinitrobenzene; WMEs: working memory errors.

Authors' contributions

LZX and XYF conceived and designed the study. LHQ performed the in vivo studies and collected the data. LHQ and XYF analyzed the data. LHQ wrote the manuscript. LZX, XYF, ZGQ and ISP revised the manuscript. All authors read and approved the final manuscript.

Author details

[1] School of Chinese Medicine, Faculty of Medicine, The Chinese University of Hong Kong, Hong Kong, SAR, People's Republic of China. [2] Brain Research Centre, School of Chinese Medicine, Faculty of Medicine, The Chinese University of Hong Kong, Hong Kong, SAR, People's Republic of China. [3] Department of Neurology, The Second Affiliated Hospital and Yuying Children's Hospital of Wenzhou Medical University, Wenzhou, Zhejiang Province, People's Republic of China. [4] Institute of Integrative Medicine, Faculty of Medicine, The Chinese University of Hong Kong, Hong Kong, SAR, People's Republic of China.

Acknowledgements

Not applicable.

Competing interests

The authors declare that they have no competing interests.

Consent for publication

Not applicable.

Fundings

This work was supported by the General Research Fund from Research Grants Council of Hong Kong (Project No. 14110814) and the CUHK Direct Grant (Project No. 2015.1.081).

References

1. Lecanu L, Papadopoulos V. Modeling Alzheimer's disease with non-transgenic rat models. Alzheimers Res Ther. 2013;5:17.
2. Brookmeyer R, Johnson E, Ziegler-Graham K, Arrighi HM. Forecasting the global burden of Alzheimer's disease. Alzheimers Dement. 2007;3:186–91.
3. Apter JT, Shastri K, Pizano K. Update on disease-modifying/preventive therapies in Alzheimer's disease. CurrGeriatr Rep. 2015;4:312–7.
4. Rygiel K. Novel strategies for Alzheimer's disease treatment: An overview of anti-amyloid beta monoclonal antibodies. Indian J Pharmacol. 2016;48:629.
5. Kumar A, Singh A, Ekavali. A review on Alzheimer's disease pathophysiology and its management: an update. Pharmacol Rep. 2015;2:195–203.
6. Honig LS, Vellas B, Woodward M, Boada M, Bullock R, Borrie M, Hager K, Andreasen N, Scarpini E, Liu-Seifert H, et al. Trial of Solanezumab for Mild Dementia Due to Alzheimer's Disease. N Engl J Med. 2018;4:321–30.
7. Priest N. The biological behaviour and bioavailability of aluminium in man, with special reference to studies employing aluminium-26 as a tracer: review and study update. J Environ Monit. 2004;6:375–403.
8. Kawahara M, Kato-Negishi M. Link between aluminum and the pathogenesis of Alzheimer's disease: the integration of the aluminum and amyloid cascade hypotheses. Int J Alzheimers Dis. 2011;2011:276393.
9. Walton J. Aluminum in hippocampal neurons from humans with Alzheimer's disease. Neurotoxicology. 2006;27:385–94.
10. Walton J. Functional impairment in aged rats chronically exposed to human range dietary aluminum equivalents. Neurotoxicology. 2009;30:182–93.
11. Yu L, Jiang R, Su Q, Yu H, Yang J. Hippocampal neuronal metal ion imbalance related oxidative stress in a rat model of chronic aluminum exposure and neuroprotection of meloxicam. Behav Brain Funct. 2014;10:6.
12. Walton J. An aluminum-based rat model for Alzheimer's disease exhibits oxidative damage, inhibition of PP2A activity, hyperphosphorylated tau, and granulovacuolar degeneration. J InorgBiochem. 2007;101:1275–84.
13. Prakash D, Sudhandiran G. Dietary flavonoid fisetin regulates aluminium chloride-induced neuronal apoptosis in cortex and hippocampus of mice brain. J NutrBiochem. 2015;26:1527–39.
14. Prakash A, Kumar A. Effect of N-Acetyl Cysteine against Aluminium-induced Cognitive Dysfunction and Oxidative Damage in Rats. Basic ClinPharmacolToxicol. 2009;105:98–104.
15. Erazi H, Sansar W, Ahboucha S, Gamrani H. Aluminum affects glial system and behavior of rats. C R Biol. 2010;333:23–7.
16. Iwasaki K, Satoh-Nakagawa T, Maruyama M, Monma Y, Nemoto M, Tomita N, Tanji H, Fujiwara H, Seki T, Fujii M. A Randomized, observer-blind, controlled trial of the traditional Chinese medicine Yi-Gan San for improvement of behavioral and psychological symptoms and activities of daily living in dementia. J Clin Psychiatry. 2005;66:248–52.
17. Watanabe H, Zhao Q, Matsumoto K, Tohda M, Murakami Y, Zhang SH, Kang TH, Mahakunakorn P, Maruyama Y, Sakakibara I. Pharmacological evidence for antidementia effect of Choto-san (Gouteng-san), a traditional Kampo medicine. PharmacolBiochemBehav. 2003;75:635–43.
18. Xian YF, Lin ZX, Mao QQ, Hu Z, Zhao M, Che CT, Ip SP. Bioassay-guided isolation of neuroprotective compounds from Uncaria rhynchophylla against beta-amyloid-induced neurotoxicity. Evid Based Complement Alternat Med. 2012;2012:802625.
19. Xian YF, Lin ZX, Zhao M, Mao QQ, Ip SP, Che CT. Uncaria rhynchophylla ameliorates cognitive deficits induced by D-galactose in mice. Planta Med. 2011;77:1977–83.
20. Kang TH, Murakami Y, Takayama H, Kitajima M, Aimi N, Watanabe H, Matsumoto K. Protective effect of rhynchophylline and isorhynchophylline on in vitro ischemia-induced neuronal damage in the hippocampus: putative neurotransmitter receptors involved in their action. Life Sci. 2004;76:331–43.
21. Xian YF, Lin ZX, Mao QQ, Chen JN, Su ZR, Lai XP, Ip PS. Isorhynchophylline protects PC12 cells against beta-amyloid-induced apoptosis via PI3K/Akt signaling pathway. Evid Based Complement Alternat Med. 2013;2013:163057.
22. Xian YF, Mao QQ, Wu JC, Su ZR, Chen JN, Lai XP, Ip SP, Lin ZX. Isorhynchophylline treatment improves the amyloid-β-induced cognitive impairment in rats via inhibition of neuronal apoptosis and tau protein hyperphosphorylation. J Alzheimers Dis. 2014;39:331–46.
23. Xian YF, Su ZR, Chen JN, Lai XP, Mao QQ, Cheng CH, Ip SP, Lin ZX. Isorhynchophylline improves learning and memory impairments induced by D-galactose in mice. Neurochem Int. 2014;76:42–9.
24. Ozaki Y. Pharmacological studies of indole alkaloids obtained from domestic plants, Uncaria rhynchophylla Miq. and Amsonia elliptica Roem. et Schult. Nihon YakurigakuZasshi. 1989; 94:17–26.
25. Abdel-Aal RA, Assi AA, Kostandy BB. Rivastigmine reverses aluminum-induced behavioral changes in rats. Eur J Pharmacol. 2011;659:169–76.
26. Crusio WE, Schwegler H, Brust I. Covariations Between Hippocampal Mossy Fibres and Working and Reference Memory in Spatial and Non-spatial Radial Maze Tasks in Mice. Eur J Neurosci. 1993;5:1413–20.
27. Foyet HS, Asongalem AE, Oben EK, Cioanca O, Hancianu M, Hritcu L. Effects of the methanolic extract of Vitellaria paradoxa stem bark against scopolamine-induced cognitive dysfunction and oxidative stress in the rat hippocampus. Cell MolNeurobiol. 2016;36:1139–49.
28. Webster SJ, Bachstetter AD, Nelson PT, Schmitt FA, Van Eldik LJ. Using mice to model Alzheimer's dementia: an overview of the clinical disease and the preclinical behavioral changes in 10 mouse models. Front Genet. 2014;5:88.
29. Olton DS, Samuelson RJ. Remembrance of places passed: Spatial memory in rats. J Exp Psychol Anim Behav Process. 1976;2:97.

30. Evola M, Hall A, Wall T, Young A, Grammas P. Oxidative stress impairs learning and memory in apoE knockout mice. PharmacolBiochemBehav. 2010;96:181–6.
31. Hashimoto M, Hossain S, Agdul H, Shido O. Docosahexaenoic acid-induced amelioration on impairment of memory learning in amyloid beta-infused rats relates to the decreases of amyloid beta and cholesterol levels in detergent-insoluble membrane fractions. Biochim Biophys Acta. 2005;1-3:91–8.
32. Mhatre M, Nguyen A, Kashani S, Pham T, Adesina A, Grammas P. Thrombin, a mediator of neurotoxicity and memory impairment. Neurobiol Aging. 2004;6:783–93.
33. Jamil A, Mahboob A, Ahmed T. Ibuprofen targets neuronal pentraxins expresion and improves cognitive function in mouse model of AlCl3-induced neurotoxicity. ExpTher Med. 2016;11:601–6.
34. Connor DJ, Jope RS, Harrell LE. Chronic, oral aluminum administration to rats: cognition and cholinergic parameters. PharmacolBiochemBehav. 1988;31:467–74.
35. Wang X, Wang W, Li L, Perry G, Lee HG, Zhu X. Oxidative stress and mitochondrial dysfunction in Alzheimer's disease. BiochimBiophys Acta. 2014;1842:1240–7.
36. Li Z, Chen X, Lu W, Zhang S, Guan X, Li Z, Wang D. Anti-Oxidative Stress Activity Is Essential for Amanita caesarea Mediated Neuroprotection on Glutamate-Induced Apoptotic HT22 Cells and an Alzheimer's Disease Mouse Model. Int J Mol Sci. 2017;18:1623.
37. Nunomura A, Perry G, Aliev G, Hirai K, Takeda A, Balraj EK, Jones PK, Ghanbari H, Wataya T, Shimohama S, et al. Oxidative damage is the earliest event in Alzheimer disease. J NeuropatholExp Neurol. 2001;60:759–67.
38. López N, Tormo C, De Blas I, Llinares I, Alom J. Oxidative stress in Alzheimer's disease and mild cognitive impairment with high sensitivity and specificity. J Alzheimers Dis. 2013;33:823–9.
39. Casadesus G, Smith MA, Basu S, Hua J, Capobianco DE, Siedlak SL, Zhu X, Perry G. Increased isoprostane and prostaglandin are prominent in neurons in Alzheimer disease. MolNeurodegener. 2007;2:2.
40. Torres LL, Quaglio NB, de Souza GT, Garcia RT, Dati LMM, Moreira WL, de Melo Loureiro AP, Smid J, Porto CS, de Campos Bottino CM. Peripheral oxidative stress biomarkers in mild cognitive impairment and Alzheimer's disease. J Alzheimers Dis. 2011;26:59–68.
41. Bonda DJ, Castellani RJ, Zhu X, Nunomura A, Lee HG, Perry G, Smith MA. A novel perspective on tau in Alzheimer's disease. Curr Alzheimer Res. 2011;8:639–42.
42. LaFerla FM, Green KN, Oddo S. Intracellular amyloid-β in Alzheimer's disease. Nat Rev Neurosci. 2007;8:499–509.
43. Leuner K, Schütt T, Kurz C, Eckert SH, Schiller C, Occhipinti A, Mai S, Jendrach M, Eckert GP, Kruse SE. Mitochondrion-derived reactive oxygen species lead to enhanced amyloid beta formation. Antioxid Redox Signal. 2012;16:1421–33.
44. Bonda DJ, Wang X, Perry G, Nunomura A, Tabaton M, Zhu X, Smith MA. Oxidative stress in Alzheimer disease: A possibility for prevention. Neuropharmacology. 2010;59:290–4.
45. Saxena G, Singh SP, Agrawal R, Nath C. Effect of donepezil and tacrine on oxidative stress in intracerebral streptozotocin-induced model of dementia in mice. Eur J Pharmacol. 2008;3:283–9.
46. Terry AV Jr, Buccafusco JJ. The cholinergic hypothesis of age and Alzheimer's disease-related cognitive deficits: recent challenges and their implications for novel drug development. J Pharmacol Exp Ther. 2003;3:821–7.
47. Deiana S, Platt B, Riedel G. The cholinergic system and spatial learning. Behav Brain Res. 2011;2:389–411.
48. Whitehouse PJ, Price DL, Clark AW, Coyle JT, DeLong MR. Alzheimer disease: evidence for selective loss of cholinergic neurons in the nucleus basalis. Ann Neurol. 1981;10:122–6.
49. Blennow K, de Leon MJ, Zetterberg H. Alzheimer's disease. Lancet. 2006;368:387–403.
50. Bilkei-Gorzo A. Neurotoxic effect of enteral aluminium. Food ChemToxicol. 1993;31:357–61.
51. Greig NH, Utsuki T, Yu Q, Zhu X, Holloway HW, Perry T, Lee B, Ingram DK, Lahiri DK. A new therapeutic target in Alzheimer's disease treatment: attention to butyrylcholinesterase. Curr Med Res Opin. 2001;3:159–65.
52. Karin M, Ben-Neriah Y. Phosphorylation meets ubiquitination: the control of NF-κB activity. Annu Rev Immunol. 2000;18:621–63.
53. O'Neill LA, Kaltschmidt C. NF-kB: a crucial transcription factor for glial and neuronal cell function. Trends Neurosci. 1997;20:252–8.
54. Zou J, Cai PS, Xiong CM, Ruan JL. Neuroprotective effect of peptides extracted from walnut (Juglans Sigilata Dode) proteins on Aβ25-35-induced memory impairment in mice. J HuazhongUniv Sci Technolog Med Sci. 2016;36:21–30.
55. Kitamura Y, Shimohama S, Ota T, Matsuoka Y, Nomura Y, Taniguchi T. Alteration of transcription factors NF-κB and STAT1 in Alzheimer's disease brains. Neurosci Lett. 1997;237:17–20.
56. Ghosh S, May MJ, Kopp EB. NF-κB and Rel proteins: evolutionarily conserved mediators of immune responses. Annu Rev Immunol. 1998;16:225–60.
57. Chen CH, Zhou W, Liu S, Deng Y, Cai F, Tone M, Tone Y, Tong Y, Song W. Increased NF-κB signalling up-regulates BACE1 expression and its therapeutic potential in Alzheimer's disease. Int J Neuropsychopharmacol. 2012;15:77–90.
58. Kaltschmidt B, Uherek M, Volk B, Baeuerle PA, Kaltschmidt C. Transcription factor NF-kappaB is activated in primary neurons by amyloid beta peptides and in neurons surrounding early plaques from patients with Alzheimer disease. Proc Natl Acad Sci U S A. 1997;94:2642–7.
59. Baldwin AS Jr. The NF-κB and IκB proteins: new discoveries and insights. Annu Rev Immunol. 1996;14:649–81.

16

Temporal divergence of changes in pain and pain-free grip strength after manual acupuncture or electroacupuncture: an experimental study in people with lateral epicondylalgia

Jaewon Jeon, Erin Bussin and Alex Scott*

Abstract

Background: The objective of this study was to examine, in individuals with lateral epicondylalgia (LE), the acute time course of acupuncture-induced hypoalgesia and change in pain-free grip strength (PFGS).

Methods: This was an experimental study, conducted at a single research center in Vancouver, BC. Twenty-one participants with unilateral LE lasting more than 6 weeks duration were enrolled. Participants received a single treatment of acupuncture (either electroacupuncture, 10–30 Hz, or manual acupuncture, assigned randomly). The primary outcome measure was pain level (0–10) during tendon loading (while making a fist) immediately after treatment, and over a 72 h follow-up period. Secondary outcome measures included pain-free grip strength (N).

Results: There was a small but statistically significant reduction in participants' perceived pain level immediately after acupuncture (mean improvement of 1.2, 95% CI 0.45–1.9). This change in pain was not accompanied by a change in PFGS. No difference was observed between the two types of acupuncture at any time point.

Conclusions: The use of acupuncture or electroacupuncture, as administered in the current study, is unlikely to acutely enhance the ability of people with LE to engage in pain-free rehabilitation exercise.

Keywords: Acupuncture, Tendinitis, Tendon, Tendinopathy, Musculoskeletal

Background

Lateral epicondylalgia (LE, or tennis elbow) is a condition characterized by lateral elbow pain and pathology in the common wrist extensor tendons. Pathology is visible on ultrasound as swelling, disorientation of collagen fibre bundles, and increased blood flow [1, 2]. Under the microscope, the pathology is heterogeneous, containing areas of angiofibroblastic reaction as well as acellular regions of degenerate morphology [3]. The pain of LE is thought to involve nociception from the pathological tendon and associated tissues [4, 5], along with peripheral and central sensitization leading to widespread mechanical hyperalgesia [2, 6], with or without referred pain [7]. People with LE experience various types of pain, including resting pain (which may disturb sleep), as well as pain which is worsened by gripping activities such as holding a cup or carrying a bag [8]. A contemporary model of LE emphasizes the interactions among three pathophysiological processes: tissue pathology, changes in the pain system, and changes in motor function [9]. It has been proposed that integrated treatment for people with LE

*Correspondence: ascott@interchange.ubc.ca
Centre for Hip Health and Mobility, Vancouver Coastal Health Research Institute and Department of Physical Therapy, University of British Columbia, 2635 Laurel Street, Vancouver, BC V5Z3M9, Canada

should address observed changes in all three of these domains [9].

The majority of patients with chronic LE recover within 1 year, with or without intervention [10], however resistance exercise has been shown to improve the medium-term outcomes for patients with LE [11]. Multimodal physiotherapy including resistance training has also been found to be superior to a wait-and-see approach in the medium term [10], and is associated with fewer recurrences in the long term than corticosteroid injections [12]. However, pain can hinder active participation in rehabilitation [13]. Exercise programs are, for that reason, often combined with hypoalgesic therapies (e.g. bracing/taping, manual therapy) to allow greater loads to be prescribed without exacerbating pain [14]. Some authors [15] have suggested combining acupuncture with an exercise-based rehabilitation program, however there is no study yet which has examined the potential utility of this approach for people with LE.

Acupuncture has been systematically reviewed with regard to its ability to induce analgesia for a variety of conditions, including fibromyalgia [16], cancer pain [17], peripheral joint OA [18], idiopathic bowel syndrome [19], ankle sprain [20], chronic pain in people with spinal cord injury [21], migraine [22], shoulder pain [23], rheumatoid arthritis [24], low back pain [25], labour pain [26], and lateral epicondylalgia [27]. Of these conditions, sufficient evidence on which to base conclusions was reported for fibromyalgia and chronic episodic migraine. For migraine, acupuncture was more successful than sham needling at reducing the frequency of headaches, although the effect was noted to be small [22].

Acupuncture is one of the treatments that has been suggested to provide short-term analgesia for people with LE [28], although the Cochrane collaboration has concluded that the evidence to support this treatment approach is limited by a high risk of bias [27]. The clinical approach for people with LE depends on the practitioner's training and approach to assessment (e.g. TCM vs medical acupuncture) and also varies depending on an individuals' symptoms. Treatment typically involves the insertion of several small gauge needles to a depth of 1 cm or more into points in the vicinity of the painful area, and can also include needling into tender spots of associated musculature, as well as regional points including the neck and bilateral upper and lower extremities [29]. Acupuncture stimulates afferent nerve pathways [30], culminating in the activation of neurons in the brain related to pain processing [31]. Early studies in humans (e.g. [32]) showed a significant role of endogenous opioids in acupuncture-induced analgesia, but this has not been consistently observed by subsequent studies [33, 34]. Electroacupuncture (EA; the stimulation of sensory nerves using electrical current delivered via acupuncture needles) may invoke additional analgesic mechanisms compared to needling alone; animal studies have suggested a relation between the frequency of electrical stimulation (in Hz) and the amount of opioids released in the brain and spinal cord [35]. An additional proposed mechanism of acupuncture, consistent with fMRI studies, includes the inhibition of ascending nociceptive information (discussed in [31]). In spite of the above, there are no studies which have directly examined the impact of EA and manual acupuncture (MA) for LE using clinically relevant outcome measures for pain and motor function, while controlling important sources of bias. A key paper [36] reported an average reduction in pain of 55.8% in 24 LE participants treated with manual acupuncture. Pain relief was maximal immediately after treatment, and displayed an average duration of 20 h. The key finding of this paper (immediate pain relief for LE in 79% of the patients treated with non-segmental acupuncture, GB34, 5 min treatment duration, peaking immediately after treatment) has never been replicated to our knowledge. Furthermore, the impact of acupuncture on elbow function has not been examined.

PFGS is a sensory threshold test for mechanically-induced pain in people with LE, with excellent reliability, validity, and sensitivity to change [37]. PFGS provides the clinician a method to monitor the threshold of pain onset during gripping (in N) during rehabilitation [37]. Despite this, a recent systematic review of the effects of acupuncture on sensory thresholds did not identify any studies which used PFGS as the outcome measure [38]. In particular, no study to our knowledge has examined acute changes in PFGS following acupuncture treatment of LE, as exists for bracing [39], taping [40], or manual therapy [41] (all of which induce clinically meaningful levels of hypoalgesia in people with LE). It would be useful to know whether acupuncture has a similar magnitude and time course of effect as these other modalities, as this knowledge would inform current models of clinical reasoning for rehabilitation of people with LE [15].

The overall objective of this study was to explore the acute time course of improvements in pain and PFGS in people with LE following a treatment of MA or EA. We hypothesized that both MA and EA would induce a small, short-term hypoalgesic effect, and that this effect would be associated with a simultaneous improvement in PFGS.

Methods

Study design

The Minimum Standards of Reporting Checklist (Additional file 1) contains details of the experimental design, and statistics, and resources used in this study.

This was a randomized, double-blinded, parallel-group experiment conducted at the Centre for Hip Health and Mobility in Vancouver, British Columbia, Canada. This study started in May 2015 and ended in December 2015. All outcome measures which were collected are reported here.

Recruitment and eligibility criteria

Participants were recruited from the general community by advertising in community centres, gyms, tennis facilities, medical clinics and coffee shops in Vancouver, British Columbia. Interested participants contacted the study team either by telephone or email and underwent a telephone interview to screen for the minimal eligibility criteria. A consent form was emailed to those who met the eligibility criteria; and individuals who decided to participate were invited to the Centre for Hip Health and Mobility for further screening and treatment.

Inclusion criteria were: (1) unilateral elbow pain at or around the lateral epicondyle of the humerus for more than 6 weeks, (2) elbow pain provoked by palpation of the lateral humeral epicondyle and by gripping, (3) elbow pain triggered by either resisted wrist extension or resisted middle finger extension [15], between 19 and 65 years old, and (4) fluent in English.

Exclusion criteria were: (1) any other concurrent neck, shoulder, elbow, or arm disorders, (2) history of any injections for LE (e.g. corticosteroid, autologous whole blood, PRP, or prolotherapy), (3) received acupuncture for LE, (4) pregnant, (5) pacemakers or other electrical device implanted in the body, (6) history of seizures or epilepsy, (7) untreated hemorrhagic disorders, (8) infected tissues, osteomyelitis, or wounds around the elbow, (9) active deep vein thrombosis or thrombophlebitis, (10) impaired sensation at and around the elbow, (11) not able to give accurate and timely feedback due to cognition or communication impairment, (12) cancerous lesions at or around the elbow, (13) radiation therapy around the elbow within the previous 6 months, (14) impaired circulation around the elbow, (15) surgery or bone fracture at or around the elbow previously, (16) needle phobia, (17) inflammatory rheumatic diseases, and (18) opioid medications.

Sample size

For this pilot study, we actively recruited over an 8-month period. 21 adults with LE participated. All available participants during this period that met all the eligibility criteria were included in this study. To detect a reduction in pain during gripping of 30% (which is a provisional benchmark for a moderately important clinical change [51]) with a SD of 40 and power of 0.80, a sample size of 16 was required. This calculation was based on a within-group change over time.

Procedures and interventions

After obtaining written informed consent from participants, they were screened for their eligibility for the study by a clinician (JJ).

Before their first visit, participants were asked to: (1) refrain from taking NSAIDs or analgesia for 3 days prior to the study until its completion; (2) avoid any therapy for 3 days prior to the study until its completion; (3) avoid excessive caffeine intake (no more than 2 cups of coffee) 24 h before the study and during the 72 h follow-up; and (4) avoid any activities that aggravate elbow pain for 72 h after treatment.

After the baseline measurements, participants received acupuncture on LI 4, TE 5, LU 5, LI 10, LI 12, SP 6, and GB 34 [36, 42–44]. Needling was done only on the affected arm and ipsilateral leg. Only sterile, single-use, disposable stainless steel needles were used (Seirin L-type, 40 mm × 0.25 mm) for both treatment groups. Participants' skin at the needling sites was cleaned with antiseptic prior to needling. After inserting acupuncture needles into the skin to the required depth (1.5–3.5 cm), the clinician manipulated the acupuncture needles until the patients reported deqi ("arrival of qi"). Deqi is a subjective feeling of a patient at the region where an acupuncture needle is inserted into the acupoint and it is characterized by aching, soreness, numbness, tingling, pressure, or heaviness—this is typically ascribed to stimulation of peripheral sensory nerves [45].

Participants who were allocated in the EA group received electro-stimulation between two pairs of acupoints: one pair between LI 10 (−ve lead) and LI 12 (+ve lead) and the other pair between LI 4 (−ve lead) and SJ 5 (+ve lead). Electro-stimulation was applied using an electro-acupuncture unit (ES-160) (ITO physiotherapy and rehabilitation, Japan). The frequency was set as alternating between 10 and 30 Hz (alternating between two frequencies every 3 s). The pulse width was set as 400 μs. The intensity was set and maintained at a point at which participants received a sensory stimulus, such as tingling or numbness sensation, without visible muscle contraction. Electro-stimulation was applied for 30 min [46, 47].

Participants in the MA group received sham EA: the wires with metal clips were connected to acupuncture needles the same way as in EA group. However, the intensity dials that were connected to these two wires were not manipulated. Instead, the other intensity dials, which were not connected with wires, were turned on so that the ES-160 would still make stimulus sounds as if participants were receiving electrical stimulation. Participants were told that they may or may not feel a tingling sensation due to the use of micro-currents in the study. The electro-stimulator was placed in an opaque box so that participants were not able to watch how the clinician controlled the machine. In order to find out whether the blinding method was successful or not, participants were asked in the survey "Which group do you think you were belonged to, the EA or MA group?" at the end of the their participation.

Acupuncture needles were left in place for 30 min in both treatment groups. Acupuncture points located on the leg (GB 34, SP 6) were re-stimulated with a twirling method, in both treatment groups, once during the middle of treatment. Manipulation of the needles during the treatment was to stimulate acupuncture points, which in turn stimulates peripheral sensory nerves to create pain relief. All acupuncture was performed by a clinician (JJ) who was a registered acupuncturist in British Columbia with over 10 years of experience in clinical practice and teaching acupuncture.

A randomization list of 20 equally weighted, unblocked allocations was uploaded to clinical data management software (REDCAP) prior to the start of the study. The randomization sequence was concealed from the clinician and assessor, and the randomization was stratified by sex. To avoid clinician bias, the participants' treatment group allocation was assigned after all the treatment steps were completed, including insertion of the acupuncture needles, with the exception of the final step of applying the electro-stimulation current. After placement of the acupuncture needles by the clinician (JJ), a third person who was not involved in this study was called to the treatment room to witness the completion of needling and the randomization process by pressing a button on a computer using the REDCAP software.

Baseline and outcome measurements

Prior to receiving treatment, participants' demographic information, the level of pain and functional disability (PRTEE questionnaire), and the level of pain-related fear of movement (TSK-11 questionnaire), were recorded independently by the participants.

PFGS of unaffected and affected arms with LE were taken by a third, blinded investigator (EB) at baseline, immediately after treatment, and 24 and 72 h after the treatment. For PGFS (and the other outcome measures), 72 h was selected based on the expected duration of analgesia as observed by Molsberger and Hille [36]. Each measurement was repeated three times at 30-s intervals starting with the unaffected arm. Effort to get three consistent readings with less than 10% discrepancy between measurements was made by measuring PFGS more than three times if needed. To avoid bias, encouragement was not given at any time during PFGS measurements and participants were blinded to their PFGS readings. PFGS was measured with an electronic digital grip dynamometer (MIE Medical research, UK). Participants were in the supine position with the arm at the side (slight abduction), elbow extended, forearm pronated, and wrist extended. When testing PFGS, we ensured that the dynamometer and forearm were fully supported on the table top. For measurements in the affected arm, participants were instructed to apply force gradually on the grip and stop squeezing as soon as pain was felt; if participants had pain at rest, they were asked to squeeze until the point where their pain first increased; and for measurement of the unaffected arm, they were asked to squeeze the grip maximally.

Perceived pain level was recorded on an 11-point numeric rating scale (NRS) by a third investigator (EB). Participants were instructed to squeeze their fist as tightly as possible, and rate their resulting pain from 0 to 10, with 10 being the worst imaginable pain. This method of rating pain during a provocative maneuver was selected because (a) many people with LE do not have any resting pain, (b) the method avoids any manipulation or palpation of the elbow by an assessor, and (c) the method avoids any recall bias associated with rating average or worst pain during the previous week. The NRS has shown to a reliable tool for measuring pain in patients with musculoskeletal disorders of upper limb [48].

Acupuncture treatment, measurement of PFGS, and numeric rating of pain were all conducted in the same (supine) position. Before and after acupuncture treatment, PFGS was evaluated followed by pain rating.

Participants were provided with pain diaries to fill out after leaving the research centre, and asked to rate their pain 3 times a day (morning immediately on waking, midday, bedtime) for 72 h following treatment. For self-measurement, participants were instructed to stand straight and position their arms hanging at the side of their body, with their elbow extended, forearm pronated, and wrist extended, make a fist as tightly as possible, then rate their pain. Verbal instructions were given with demonstrations to participants onsite, and the written and visual instructions were listed on the first page of their pain diary.

The GROC scale is a reliable and valid measure of patient's perceived level of change in their condition over a period of time, commonly used in clinical research and practice [49]. Although we considered it unlikely that there would be any significant clinical improvement over the brief course of our experiments, at the 24 h time point participants were asked "Over the past 24 h since you received acupuncture treatment, how has your condition changed with respect to your elbow pain?" and were asked to rate their condition on a seven-point Likert type scale—much better, moderately better, slightly better, unchanged, slightly worse, moderately worse, and much worse.

At the conclusion of the study, participants were asked to guess their group allocation and report their confidence level with the answer. They had choices of 'Not confident at all', 'Somewhat confident', 'Neutral', 'Confident' and 'Very confident'. In addition, they were questioned: (1) whether they needed to take NSAIDS or any other pain killers for pain control; (2) whether they avoided receiving any therapy; and (3) whether they avoided any activities that aggravate their elbow pain during their participation period.

Statistical analysis

Linear mixed-effects models (repeat measures ANOVA) were used to determine whether there were changes in pain-free grip strength and perceived pain level over a 72-h period after one treatment of either EA or MA, and whether this change differed between the two treatment groups. Pain levels measured on site and at home (via diaries) were considered as separate outcomes (due to the variation in testing position necessitated by the experimental design), and were therefore analyzed in separate models. The independent variables were time (within-participants) and treatment (between-participants). Although this was not the primary goal of the study, the impact of potential covariates (hand dominance, age, sex, duration of LE, TSK score, PRTEE total score and subscores) were included in the statistical model to determine their potential influence on the change in pain or change in PFGS. P values were adjusted using the Bonferroni method, and P values of less than 0.05 were considered statistically significant. Analysis was performed by an independent statistician at UBC.

Results

Recruitment, allocation, and drop-outs

During the period May to December 2015, twenty-one participants were enrolled in the study. All participants received the treatment according to their group allocation. Twenty out of 21 (95%) participants completed the study and one participant dropped out after the first visit due to a family matter (Fig. 1).

Because of the low recruitment rate of male participants during the first half of the recruitment period, our initial plan of recruiting an equal number of male (10) and female (10) participants was revised to recruit a total of 20 participants regardless of sex. During the study period, an additional randomization list of 20 equally weighted allocations was generated and uploaded to REDCAP in order to have enough group allocations for female participants.

Protocol deviations

Pressure pain threshold was abandoned prior to the start of the study due to concerns during preparatory pilot testing that this additional testing might influence participants' pain levels. Therefore this outcome was not assessed or collected for any participants. There were no other changes to the protocol, which was completed as described in the trial registry.

Missing data

Data imputation was not performed for any missing values. Other than the missing data from the participant who dropped out after 24 h, all data were present and analyzed with the following exceptions: missing PFGS measure for one participant (EA group) due to hard-drive crash, several missing entries for pain rating from pain diaries (9 missing out of 180, randomly distributed among participants and time points), and 2 missing entries on caffeine intake during the follow-up period.

Participant characteristics

The baseline characteristics of the participants are summarized in Table 1. Random, sex-stratified allocation resulted in two groups with equivalent characteristics for all measured parameters.

Adverse effects

The study was completed without any significant adverse or side effects. Six participants (five in EA; one in MA) reported post-treatment soreness at 24 h follow up. Post treatment-soreness gradually disappeared in all participants by their second follow up at 72 h. One participant in the MA group reported a mild bruising in the needling region.

Non-protocol treatments

All participants answered that they did not take NSAIDS or any other painkillers for pain control nor receive any therapy during the study period. All participants in the EA group and all but one in the MA group reported that they avoided any activities that aggravated their elbow pain.

Outcome measures

There were no differences in pain (NRS) or pain threshold (PFGS) between the EA and MA groups at any time point, either before or after acupuncture treatment. In the entire group of 20 participants, 11 experienced an immediate reduction in pain, 8 stayed the same, and 1 participant's pain worsened. There was no apparent trend toward improvements being experienced in one group or the other (EA vs. MA). Of the 11 who experienced a reduction in pain, the reduction was at least 2 points on the NRS for 7 participants.

There was a statistically significant change in the perceived pain level over time, reflected both in onsite measurements (Fig. 2a, b) and in the pain diary (Fig. 2c).

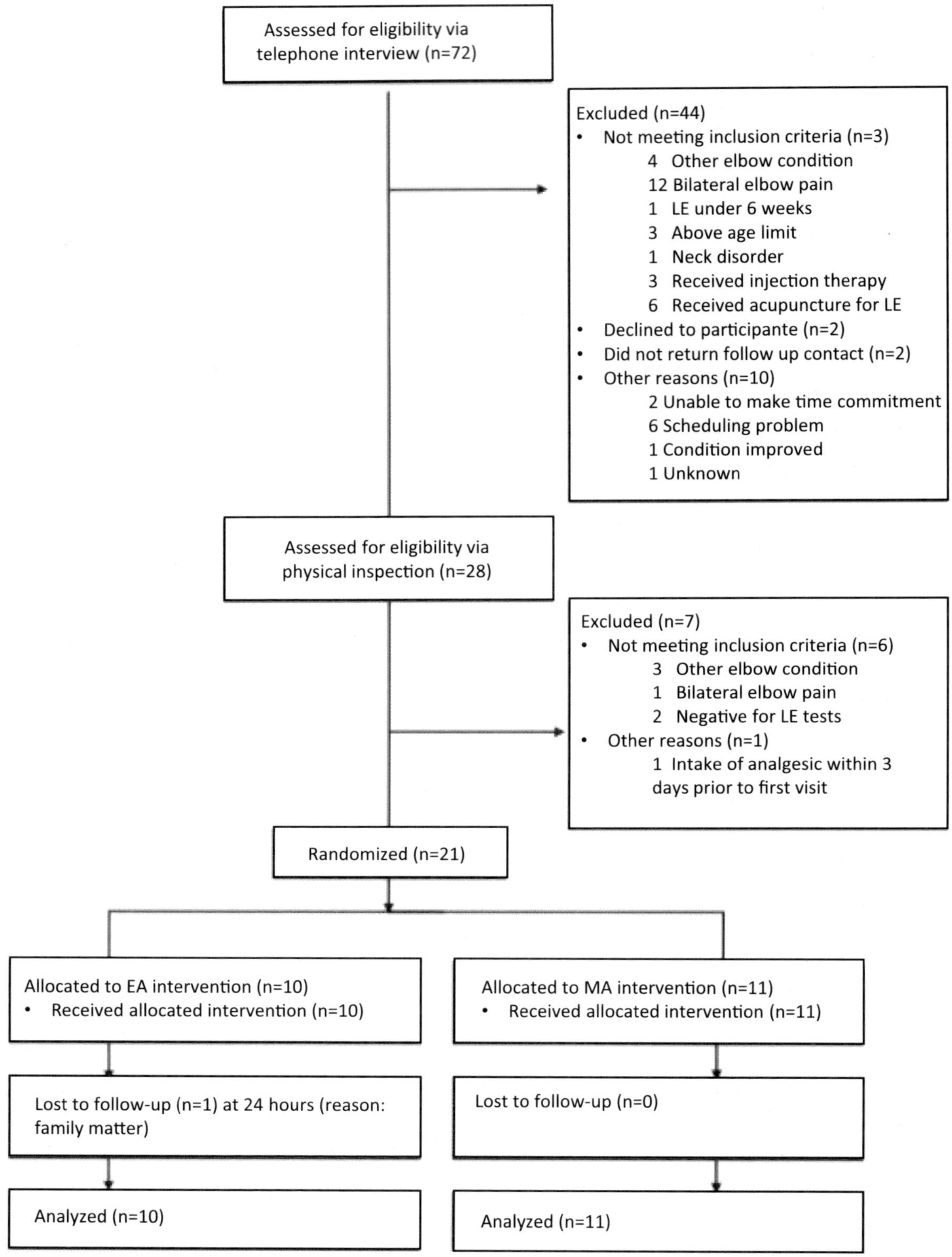

Fig. 1 Flow of participants

Onsite measurements showed that this reduction in pain occurred immediately after treatment (i.e. while the participant was still lying on the treatment plinth), and it appeared to be maintained, on average but with some intra-individual variation, throughout the 72-h follow-up period (Fig. 2c). The diary ratings of pain intensity

Table 1 Baseline demographic and clinical characteristics

Baseline	EA group	MA group
Age (years)	46 (9.2)	47 (7.5)
Sex (male/female)	5/5	4/7
Duration (months)	6 (29)[a]	5.2 (3.2)
Location of LE (dominant/non-dominant arm)	6/4	11/0
Employment (employed/not employed)	8/2	7/4
Employment involves repeated wrist/arm movements (yes/no)	5/3	5/2
Heavy lifting & carrying (yes/no)	1/7	2/5
Sports (yes/no)	7/3	8/3
TSK-11 (out of 44)	28 (6.3)	26 (6.1)
PRTEE (total) (out of 100)	52 (21)	50 (20)
PRTEE (subscale: pain)	27 (9.9)	27 (10)
PRTEE (subscale: specific activities)	31 (15)	19 (29)[a]
PRTEE (subscale: usual activities)	20 (9.7)	17 (8.6)
PFGS of unaffected arm (N)	340 (130)	310 (120)
PFGS of affected arm (N)	110 (130)[a]	76 (100)[a]
NRS	4.7 (3.6)	4.1 (1.5)

Values are expressed as mean (standard deviation) except[a], expressed as median (interquartile range) due to asymmetrical distribution of data. N = 21, 20 and 20 for the three time points shown. Error bars represent 95% CI

NRS numeric rating scale

indicated that from day 1 midday (after treatment), average pain severity continued (unexpectedly) to decrease during the follow-up period.

Unlike pain, there was no consistent change in PFGS immediately following treatment (Fig. 3a, b). However, a pattern of a gradual increase in PFGS was observed over the 72-h follow-up period (Fig. 3b), and a significant improvement of PFGS was demonstrated by 72 h follow-up.

With regard to the participants' global rating of change, 24 h after treatment the majority of participants reported feeling at least 'slightly better' (67% in EA and 54% in MA), and one subject (MA) reported feeling much better.

Efficacy of blinding

Ten out of eleven participants in the MA group answered that they received EA treatment with confidence levels of 'very confident' (60%), 'neutral' (30%) and 'somewhat confident' (10%), indicating that allocation blinding was successful in 91% of the participants. None of these ten participants had previously experienced EA or electro-stimulation. One participant in the MA group who guessed her treatment allocation correctly (with a confidence level of 'neutral') had previous experience with electro-stimulation treatments. Thus, the method of sham EA used in the current study was effective as long as the participants did not have previous experience with electroacupuncture or electro-stimulation treatment before. All participants who were allocated to EA guessed correctly that they had received EA with confidence levels of 'very confident' (67%) and 'confident' (33%).

The assessor guessed the participants' group allocations correctly 45% of the time (with two 'somewhat confident' and seven 'not confident at all'). Therefore, it can be concluded that the assessor (EB) was successfully blinded to the participants' group allocation.

Discussion

This is the first study investigating the simultaneous time course of pain relief and pain-free grip strength in patients with LE after a single acupuncture treatment (MA or EA). It is only the second study, to our knowledge, which has examined the acute time course of LE pain relief following a single acupuncture treatment [36]. Our study was completed without any significant change in methods & procedure, or significant adverse effects. We found that, although there was a small but noticeable improvement in perceived pain immediately following acupuncture treatment, there was not a simultaneous improvement in PFGS. Therefore, acupuncture cannot be recommended as a method to improve pain threshold during gripping for people with LE. Although this is a small study, it nevertheless may have implications for clinical reasoning when prescribing rehabilitation exercises in conjunction with acupuncture.

Our results are consistent with many other trials which have demonstrated that, on average, the acute effects of acupuncture typically result in a small reduction of pain—in our study the mean improvement was 1.2, 95% CI 0.45–1.9, which is very similar to the magnitude of effect observed in recent systematic review including 3025 participants in 13 clinical trials [50]. Mechanistic studies have shown that this effect, at least in a model of experimental pain, is dependent on an expectation of benefit by the recipient, and is of similar magnitude to the placebo response [31]. At an individual level, one third (7 of 21) participants in our study experienced an immediate reduction in pain intensity of at least 30%, which has been proposed as a provisional benchmark for a moderately important clinical change [51].

While our experimental study was not intended to assess the clinical importance of acupuncture in the management of LE, we are intrigued that our results are so divergent from Molsberger et al. [36], a widely cited study which reaches very different conclusions than the current study. In that study, 19 out of 24 who received a *verum* treatment (needling of a non-segmental point, GB34, on the leg for 5 min) obtained significant pain relief ($\geq$50% reduction) immediately after treatment compared to only 6/21 participants in our study who received needling on the same point, GB 34, during the

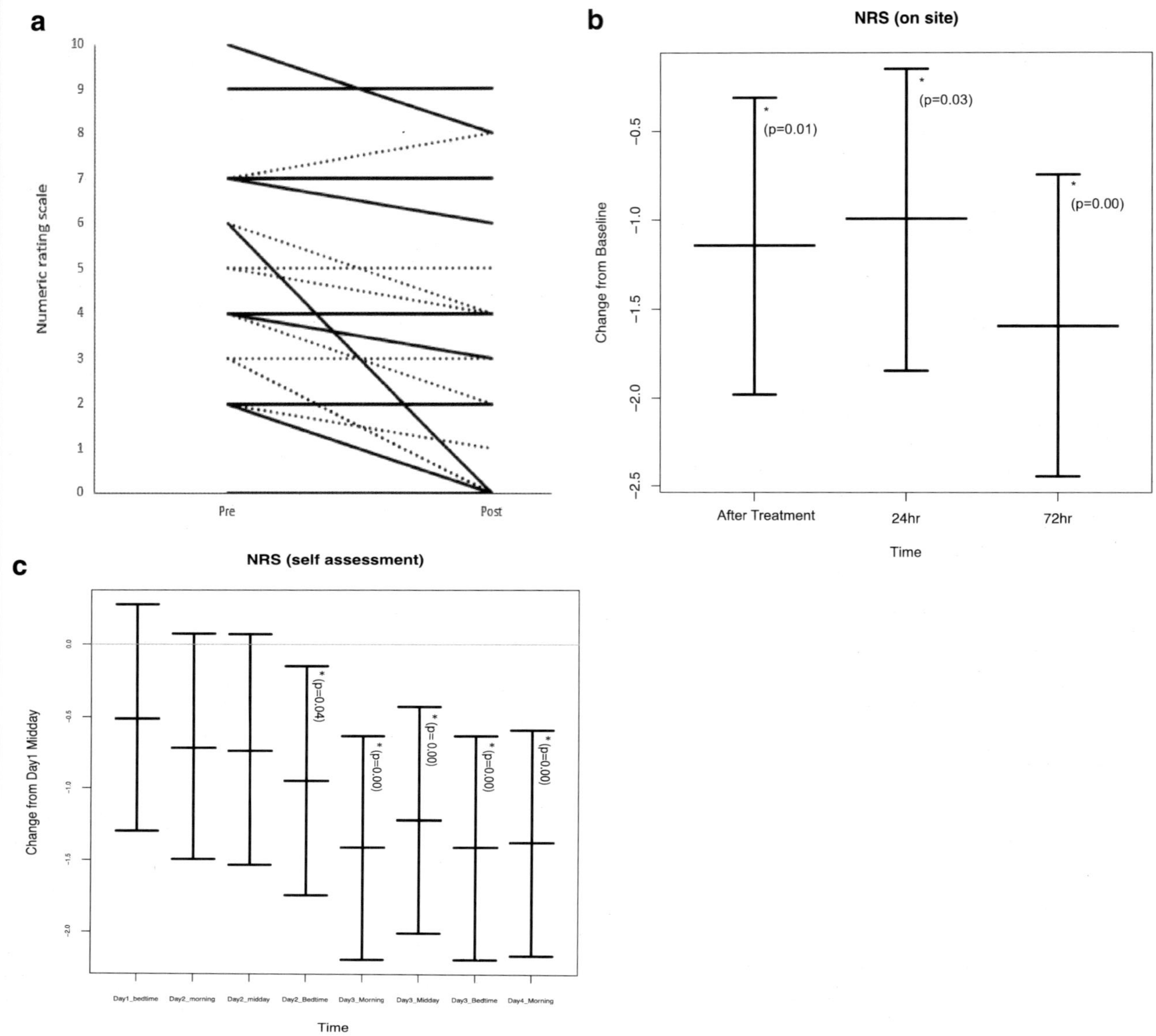

Fig. 2 Changes in LE pain over time. **a** Participant-reported pain level before (pre) and after (post) treatment with manual acupuncture (*dotted line*) or electroacupuncture (*solid line*). There was a consistent trend for pain to lessen immediately after treatment, regardless of type of acupuncture. **b** The change in pain from baseline is indicated, with negative numbers indicating a lessening of pain. *Asterisks* indicate statistically significant improvements in pain compared to baseline. *NRS* numeric rating scale. N = 21, 20 and 20 for the three time points shown. *Error bars* represent 95% CI. **c** The pain diary measures demonstrated that, unexpectedly and for unknown reasons, pain levels continued to decline during the 72-h follow-up period. Changes are shown relative to day 1 midday, which was the first diary entry following acupuncture treatment, which took place in the morning of day 1. NRS: Numeric rating scale. N = 20 for all time points shown. *Error bars* represent 95% CI

treatment. While there are many differences between our study and that by Molsberger et al. perhaps the most salient is the method of pain assessment: In the trial by Molsberger et al. an examiner "assisted the patient in evaluating his or her personal pain level by physical assessment of the elbow with respect to pressure, load, or movements of the forearm which were causing elbow pain." In comparison, we simply asked participants to make a fist and rate the level of pain, without any need for assistance by the examiner—this method was successful at provoking pain in 20 of the 21 participants, and the internal consistency of the magnitude of provoked pain can be observed in Fig. 2, as can the consistent occurrence of a small hypoalgesic effect. We suggest that the methods of pain assessment used in the current study are less prone to bias, and may be providing more accurate results than the methods used in the Molsberger et al. trial [36].

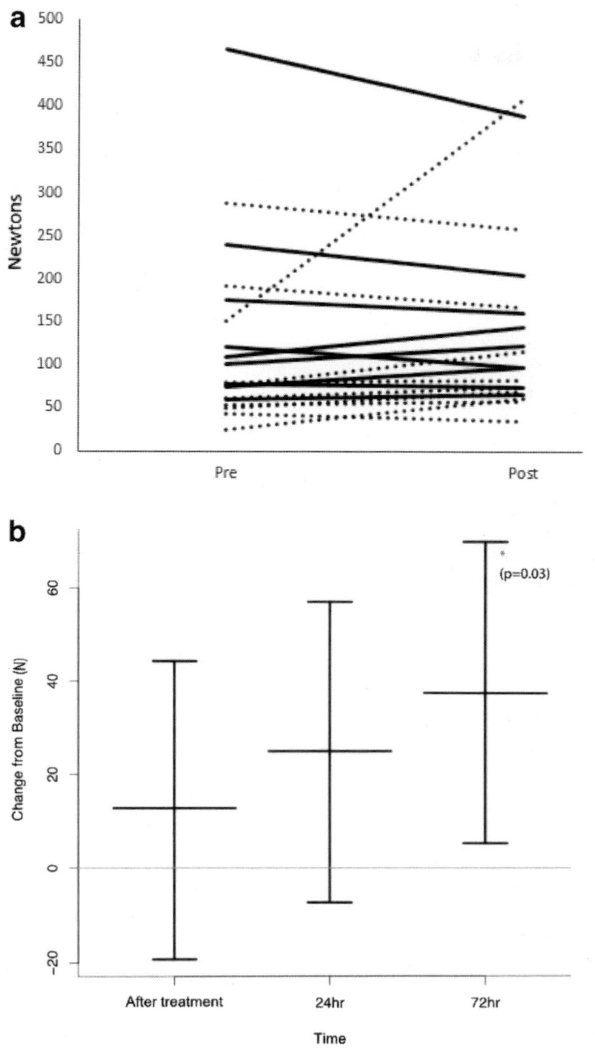

Fig. 3 Changes in pain free grip strength (PFGS) over time. **a** The sensory threshold at which point participants report the onset of pain during gripping, before (pre) and after (post) treatment with manual acupuncture (*dotted line*) or electroacupuncture (*solid line*). There was no consistent trend observed for either type of acupuncture, and no difference between the two treatment groups. **b** The change in PFGS from baseline is indicated for all participants (both treatment groups), with positive numbers indicating an improved (raised) pain threshold. Unexpectedly and for unknown reasons, PFGS improved during the 72-h follow-up period. *Asterisk* indicates a statistically significant improvement in PFGS compared to baseline, but this occurred too late in the experiment to be confidently attributed to the effects of acupuncture. N = 21, 20 and 20 for the three time points shown. *Error bars* represent 95% CI

In this double-blind, randomized pilot experiment, no significant difference was detected between two types of acupuncture at any time point during a 72-h period, for any outcome measure. This result is similar to a previous study conducted in people with OA of the knee [52] in which the effect of a single treatment of EA vs. MA on pain and strength was examined. As in the current study, both EA and MA provided a similar, significant improvement in pain intensity after a single treatment, but no difference in strength. Similar to our findings, there were no significant differences between EA and MA with regard to pain or strength [52]. It could be speculated that a longer course of treatment may provide different results, as was suggested by Leung and Tsui [53], who investigated the effect of EA and MA on patients with LE after a course of treatments (6 treatments over 2 weeks) and concluded that EA produced significantly greater pain relief and improvement of PFGS compared to MA. However, that study did not report the confidence intervals for the effect size—visual inspection of the published results of that study indicates that a meaningful difference between the EA and MA groups, in terms of change in pain or PFGS, is unlikely. In addition, that study failed to describe the randomization method and did not blind the clinician or the participants. Based on the findings of our study as well as the previous study by Tsui et al. [53], it is unlikely that a single treatment of EA will provide any additional benefit over MA.

Statistically significant improvements in PFGS and perceived pain level were observed in both groups over a 72-h period after one treatment of EA or MA. This was unexpected, because a previous study reported maximum pain relief immediately after needling, followed by a gradual reduction in the therapeutic effect over the ensuring 72 h [36]—the exact opposite of what was observed here. The divergent time course in the two main outcomes (immediate pain relief, followed by more gradual improvement in PFGS) suggests that there may be more than one mechanism underlying these changes. It is likely that, because our participants were instructed to refrain from aggravating activities during the follow-up period, their tendon became gradually less irritable during the follow-up period.

Unlike the pain ratings, significant changes were not observed in the GROC scale. For GROC, 'much better' and 'moderately better' were considered as success; despite anticipating a small improvement in pain levels, we did not expect that a single needling treatment would result in clinical success. At 24 h follow-up, only one participant reported feeling 'much better' and none 'moderately better', therefore it can be concluded that a single acupuncture treatment is unlikely to provide substantial improvements for most patients 24 h following treatment. Also, 25% of participants reported feeling worse after the treatment at 24 h follow up for unexplained reasons, perhaps due to the fluctuating nature of LE pain.

A variety of factors can influence individuals' pain and disability experiences. Although kinesiophobia did not significantly influence the outcomes of this study, previous studies have suggested that anxiety and depression might influence an individual's pain perception [54, 55]. Considering that patients with LE have shown significantly increased levels of anxiety and depression due to pain and functional disability of the arm [56], the results of this study might have been influenced by participants' psychosocial status. In addition to controlling for various elements of the placebo response, future studies may wish to examine the impact of anxiety and depression levels on acupuncture-induced hypoalgesia in LE.

There were some limitations in this study: (1) There was no 'no treatment' control group in this study. However, given that there was no immediate change in PFGS following needling, we can nevertheless be confident that acupuncture does not have an immediate impact on this outcome, and therefore reject this part of the hypothesis. (2) Over a 72-h period, a pattern of gradual increase in PFGS was seen. Whether PFGS would further increase or decline after a 72-h period is not known as the study ended at 72 h follow up. (3) This study provided one treatment only, and did not include a placebo control (i.e. sham needling). Given that LE is a chronic condition that typically requires several weeks to demonstrate improvement with conservative treatment, the results of this study do not address the relative effectiveness of EA or MA in treatment of LE as it is typically provided (several times a week for several weeks). Nevertheless, the results of this study do suggest that there is no substantial difference between EA and MA with regard to the time course of pain relief and improvement of PFGS after one treatment, which was the hypothesis being tested in this experiment.

Conclusions

Although acupuncture resulted in noticeable improvements in pain immediately following treatment, this was not accompanied by a simultaneous change in PFGS. The use of acupuncture or electroacupuncture, as administered in the current study, is unlikely to acutely enhance the ability of people with LE to engage in pain-free rehabilitation exercise (Additional file 2: Table S1).

Abbreviations

EA: electro-acupuncture; GROC: global rating of change; LE: lateral epicondylalgia; MA: manual acupuncture (no electricity); NRS: numeric rating scale; NSAIDs: non-steroidal anti-inflammatory drugs; PFGS: pain-free grip strength; PRP: platelet rich plasma; TSK: Tampa Scale of Kinesiophobia.

Authors' contributions

JJ and AS drafted the study protocol. EB and JJ piloted study procedures. JJ recruited and consented participants and carried out interventions. JJ and EB collected data. JJ and AS, contributed to the statistical analysis, and drafted the manuscript. All authors read and approved the final manuscript.

Acknowledgements

The authors acknowledge the valuable contributions of all the staff at the Centre for Hip Health and Mobility, Vancouver.

Competing interests

All authors have completed the ICMJE uniform disclosure form at www.icmje.org/coi_disclosure.pdf and declare: no support from any organisation for the submitted work; no financial relationships with any organisations that might have an interest in the submitted work in the previous three years; no other relationships or activities that could appear to have influenced the submitted work.

Consent for publication

Not applicable.

Funding

This research received no specific grant from any funding agency in the public, commercial or not-for-profit sectors. Dr. Scott was supported in part by the Michael Smith Foundation of Health Research. Erin Bussin was supported in part by a Graduate Student Incentive award from the University of British Columbia. Jaewon Jeon was self-funded. The facility usage for the Centre for Hip Health and Mobility was paid through internal (UBC) unrestricted research funds allocated to Dr. Scott's tendinopathy research program.

References

1. du Toit C, Stieler M, Saunders R, et al. Diagnostic accuracy of power Doppler ultrasound in patients with chronic tennis elbow. Br J Sports Med. 2008;42:872–6.
2. Jespersen A, Amris K, Graven-Nielsen T, et al. Assessment of pressure-pain thresholds and central sensitization of pain in lateral epicondylalgia. Pain Med. 2013;14:297–304.
3. Kraushaar BS, Nirschl RP. Tendinosis of the elbow (tennis elbow). Clinical features and findings of histological, immunohistochemical, and electron microscopy studies. J Bone Joint Surg Am. 1999;81:259–78.
4. Peterson M, Svardsudd K, Appel L, et al. PET-scan shows peripherally increased neurokinin 1 receptor availability in chronic tennis elbow: visualizing neurogenic inflammation? PLoS ONE. 2013;8:e75859.
5. Scott A, Backman LJ, Speed C. Tendinopathy: update on pathophysiology. J Orthop Sports Phys Ther. 2015;45:833–41.
6. Coombes BK, Bisset L, Vicenzino B. Thermal hyperalgesia distinguishes those with severe pain and disability in unilateral lateral epicondylalgia. Clin J Pain. 2012;28:595–601.
7. Pitzer ME, Seidenberg PH, Bader DA. Elbow tendinopathy. Med Clin North Am. 2014;98:833–49.
8. Nirschl RP. Elbow tendinosis/tennis elbow. Clin Sports Med. 1992;11:851–70.
9. Coombes BK, Bisset L, Vicenzino B. A new integrative model of lateral epicondylalgia. Br J Sports Med. 2009;43:252–8.
10. Bisset L, Beller E, Jull G, et al. Mobilisation with movement and exercise, corticosteroid injection, or wait and see for tennis elbow: randomised trial. BMJ. 2006;333:939.
11. Raman J, MacDermid JC, Grewal R. Effectiveness of different methods of resistance exercises in lateral epicondylosis—a systematic review. J Hand Ther. 2012;25:5–25.
12. Coombes BK, Bisset L, Brooks P, et al. Effect of corticosteroid injection, physiotherapy, or both on clinical outcomes in patients with unilateral lateral epicondylalgia: a randomized controlled trial. JAMA. 2013;309:461–9.
13. De Das S, Vranceanu AM, Ring DC. Contribution of kinesophobia and catastrophic thinking to upper-extremity-specific disability. J Bone Joint Surg Am. 2013;95:76–81.
14. Vicenzino B. Lateral epicondylalgia: a musculoskeletal physiotherapy perspective. Man Ther. 2003;8:66–79.
15. Vicenzino B, Scott A, Bell S, et al. Elbow and arm pain. In: Brukner P, Kahn K, editors. Clinical sports medicine. 5th ed. Sydney: McGraw Hill; 2017. p. 439–62.

16. Deare JC, Zheng Z, Xue CC, et al. Acupuncture for treating fibromyalgia. Cochrane Database Syst Rev. 2013;5:CD007070.
17. Paley CA, Johnson MI, Tashani OA, et al. Acupuncture for cancer pain in adults. Cochrane Database Syst Rev. 2015;10:CD007753.
18. Manheimer E, Cheng K, Linde K, et al. Acupuncture for peripheral joint osteoarthritis. Cochrane Database Syst Rev. 2010;1:CD001977.
19. Manheimer E, Cheng K, Wieland LS, et al. Acupuncture for treatment of irritable bowel syndrome. Cochrane Database Syst Rev. 2012;5:CD005111.
20. Kim TH, Lee MS, Kim KH, et al. Acupuncture for treating acute ankle sprains in adults. Cochrane Database Syst Rev. 2014;6:CD009065.
21. Boldt I, Eriks-Hoogland I, Brinkhof MW, et al. Non-pharmacological interventions for chronic pain in people with spinal cord injury. Cochrane Database Syst Rev. 2014;17:CD009177.
22. Linde K, Allais G, Brinkhaus B, et al. Acupuncture for the prevention of episodic migraine. Cochrane Database Syst Rev. 2016;6:CD001218.
23. Green S, Buchbinder R, Hetrick S. Acupuncture for shoulder pain. Cochrane Database Syst Rev. 2005;2:CD005319.
24. Casimiro L, Barnsley L, Brosseau L, et al. Acupuncture and electroacupuncture for the treatment of rheumatoid arthritis. Cochrane Database Syst Rev. 2005;4:CD003788.
25. Furlan AD, van Tulder MW, Cherkin DC, et al. Acupuncture and dry-needling for low back pain. Cochrane Database Syst Rev. 2005;25:CD001351.
26. Smith CA, Collins CT, Crowther CA, et al. Acupuncture or acupressure for pain management in labour. Cochrane Database Syst Rev. 2011;7:CD009232.
27. Green S, Buchbinder R, Barnsley L, et al. Acupuncture for lateral elbow pain. Cochrane Database Syst Rev. 2002;1:CD003527.
28. Bisset L, Paungmali A, Vicenzino B, et al. A systematic review and meta-analysis of clinical trials on physical interventions for lateral epicondylalgia. Br J Sports Med. 2005;39:411–22.
29. Webster-Harrison P, White A, Rae J. Acupuncture for tennis elbow: an E-mail consensus study to define a standardised treatment in a GPs' surgery. Acupunct Med. 2002;20:181–5.
30. Guowei L, Rongzhao L, Jingqiang X, et al. Role of peripheral afferent nerve fiber in acupuncture analgesia elicited by needling point zusanli. Sci Sin. 1979;22:680–92.
31. Kong J, Kaptchuk TJ, Polich G, et al. Expectancy and treatment interactions: a dissociation between acupuncture analgesia and expectancy evoked placebo analgesia. Neuroimage. 2009;45:940–9.
32. Mayer DJ, Price DD, Rafii A. Antagonism of acupuncture analgesia in man by the narcotic antagonist naloxone. Brain Res. 1977;121:368–72.
33. Moret V, Forster A, Laverriere MC, et al. Mechanism of analgesia induced by hypnosis and acupuncture: is there a difference? Pain. 1991;45:135–40.
34. Chapman CR, Benedetti C, Colpitts YH, et al. Naloxone fails to reverse pain thresholds elevated by acupuncture: acupuncture analgesia reconsidered. Pain. 1983;16:13–31.
35. Cheng LL, Ding MX, Xiong C, et al. Effects of electroacupuncture of different frequencies on the release profile of endogenous opioid peptides in the central nerve system of goats. Evid Based Complement Alternat Med. 2012;2012:476457.
36. Molsberger A, Hille E. The analgesic effect of acupuncture in chronic tennis elbow pain. Br J Rheumatol. 1994;33:1162–5.
37. Lim EC. Pain free grip strength test. J Physiother. 2013;59:59.
38. Baeumler PI, Fleckenstein J, Takayama S, et al. Effects of acupuncture on sensory perception: a systematic review and meta-analysis. PLoS ONE. 2014;9:e113731.
39. Bisset LM, Collins NJ, Offord SS. Immediate effects of 2 types of braces on pain and grip strength in people with lateral epicondylalgia: a randomized controlled trial. J Orthop Sports Phys Ther. 2014;44:120–8.
40. Vicenzino B, Brooksbank J, Minto J, et al. Initial effects of elbow taping on pain-free grip strength and pressure pain threshold. J Orthop Sports Phys Ther. 2003;33:400–7.
41. McLean S, Naish R, Reed L, et al. A pilot study of the manual force levels required to produce manipulation induced hypoalgesia. Clin Biomech. 2002;17:304–8.
42. Davidson J, Vandervoort A, Lessard L, et al. The effect of acupuncture versus ultrasound on pain level, grip strength and disability in individuals with lateral epicondylitis: a pilot study. Physiother Can. 2001;53:195–202.
43. Fink M, Wolkenstein E, Luennemann M, et al. Chronic epicondylitis: effects of real and sham acupuncture treatment: a randomised controlled patient- and examiner-blinded long-term trial. Forsch Komplementarmed Klass Naturheilkd. 2002;9:210–5.
44. Haker E, Lundeberg T. Acupuncture treatment in epicondylalgia: a comparative study of two acupuncture techniques. Clin J Pain. 1990;6:221–6.
45. Bowsher D. Mechanisms of acupuncture. In: Filshie J, White A, editors. Medical acupuncture: a Western scientific approach. Edinburgh: Churchill-Livinstone; 1998.
46. Ghoname ES, Craig WF, White PF, et al. The effect of stimulus frequency on the analgesic response to percutaneous electrical nerve stimulation in patients with chronic low back pain. Anesth Analg. 1999;88:841–6.
47. White PF, Li S, Chiu JW. Electroanalgesia: its role in acute and chronic pain management. Anesth Analg. 2001;92:505–13.
48. Stratford P, Spadoni G. The reliability, consistency, and clinical application of a numeric pain rating scale. Physiother Can. 2001;53:88–91.
49. Preston CC, Colman AM. Optimal number of response categories in rating scales: reliability, validity, discriminating power, and respondent preferences. Acta Psychol. 2000;104:1–15.
50. Madsen MV, Gotzsche PC, Hrobjartsson A. Acupuncture treatment for pain: systematic review of randomised clinical trials with acupuncture, placebo acupuncture, and no acupuncture groups. BMJ. 2009;338:a3115.
51. Dworkin RH, Turk DC, Wyrwich KW, et al. Interpreting the clinical importance of treatment outcomes in chronic pain clinical trials: IMMPACT recommendations. J Pain. 2008;9:105–21.
52. Plaster R, Vieira WB, Alencar FA, et al. Immediate effects of electroacupuncture and manual acupuncture on pain, mobility and muscle strength in patients with knee osteoarthritis: a randomised controlled trial. Acupunct Med. 2014;32:236–41.
53. Tsui P, Leung MC. Comparison of the effectiveness between manual acupuncture and electro-acupuncture on patients with tennis elbow. Acupunct Electrother Res. 2002;27:107–17.
54. Kivrak Y, Kose-Ozlece H, Ustundag MF, et al. Pain perception: predictive value of sex, depression, anxiety, somatosensory amplification, obesity, and age. Neuropsychiatr Dis Treat. 2016;12:1913–8.
55. Thompson T, Correll CU, Gallop K, et al. Is pain perception altered in people with depression? a systematic review and meta-analysis of experimental pain research. J Pain. 2016;17:1257–72.
56. Alizadehkhaiyat O, Fisher AC, Kemp GJ, et al. Pain, functional disability, and psychologic status in tennis elbow. Clin J Pain. 2007;23:482–9.

17

Blood and urinary metabolomic evidence validating traditional Chinese medicine diagnostic classification of major depressive disorder

Lan-Ying Liu[1], Hong-Jian Zhang[2], Li-Yuan Luo[1], Jin-Bao Pu[2], Wei-Qing Liang[2], Chun-Qin Zhu[1], Ya-Ping Li[3], Pei-Rong Wang[1], Yuan-Yuan Zhang[1], Chun-Yu Yang[1] and Zhang-Jin Zhang[4*]

Abstract

Background: Major depressive disorder (MDD) is a highly heterogeneous disease. Further classification may characterize its heterogeneity. The purpose of this study was to examine whether metabolomic variables could differentiate traditional Chinese medicine (TCM) diagnostic subtypes of MDD.

Methods: Fifty medication-free patients who were experiencing a recurrent depressive episode were classified into Liver Qi Stagnation (LQS, n = 30) and Heart and Spleen Deficiency (HSD, n = 20) subtypes according to TCM diagnosis. Healthy volunteers (n = 28) were included as controls. Gas chromatography-mass spectrometry (GC–MS) was used to examine serum and urinary metabolomic profiles.

Results: Twenty-eight metabolites were identified for good separations between TCM subtypes and healthy controls in serum samples. Both TCM subtypes had similar profiles in proteinogenic branched-chain amino acids (BCAAs) (valine, leucine, and isoleucine) and energy metabolism-related metabolites that were differentiated from healthy controls. The LQS subtype additionally differed from healthy controls in multiple amino acid metabolites that are involved in biosynthesis of monoamine and amino acid neurotransmitters, including phenylalanine, 3-hydroxybutric acid, *o*-tyrosine, glycine, L-tryptophan, and *N*-acetyl-L-aspartic acid. Threonic acid, methionine, stearic acid, and isobutyric acid are differentially associated with the two subtypes.

Conclusions: While both TCM subtypes are associated with aberrant BCAA and energy metabolism, the LQS subtype may represent an MDD subpopulation characterized by abnormalities in the biosynthesis of monoamine and amino acid neurotransmitters and closer associations with stress-related pathophysiology. The metabolites differentially associated with the two subtypes are promising biomarkers for predicting TCM subtype-specific antidepressant response [registered at http://www.clinicaltrials.gov (NCT02346682) on January 27, 2015].

Keywords: Major depressive disorder, Traditional Chinese medicine, Classification, Metabolomics

*Correspondence: zhangzj@hku.hk
[4] School of Chinese Medicine, LKS Faculty of Medicine, The University of Hong Kong, 10 Sassoon Road, Pokfulam, Hong Kong, China
Full list of author information is available at the end of the article

Background

Major depressive disorder (MDD) is a highly heterogeneous mental illness with a wide range of clinical manifestations and multi-system etiopathogenesis. The core symptoms of low mood and loss of interest and pleasure are often accompanied by somatic and other psychiatric symptoms, such as pain, sleep disturbance, anxiety, and neurocognitive dysfunction [1]. Although a great attempt has been made to characterize its heterogeneity by subdividing MDD based on its clinical features, severity, and polygenic features, convincing evidence for the existence of depressive symptom dimensions and symptomatic subtypes is lacking, mainly due to symptomatic diversity and the absence of patterns [2–5]. Therefore, a novel classification system that could improve clinical applicability and more precisely identify pathological heterogeneity of MDD is highly desirable.

As an ancient medical practice, traditional Chinese medicine (TCM) has an established distinct diagnostic system. One key approach to diagnosis is the differentiation of etiopathological pattern which is generally defined by a comprehensive analysis of clinical symptoms and signs collected through inspection, auscultation, olfaction, interrogation, and palpation of the pulses [6]. Over the past decade, several large-scale studies have revealed 12 different TCM patterns of MDD on the basis of the modern psychiatric diagnostic instruments and analysis tools, such as latent tree model analysis [7–12]. Despite disagreements on some patterns, a consensus on clinical diagnostic criteria for the two most common and opposing patterns, Liver Qi Stagnation (LQS) and Heart and Spleen Deficiency (HSD), which account for approximately 2/3 of depressed patients, have been reached as shown in Table 1 [7, 9, 10].

Differential profiles of functional brain connectivity has been observed between "deficiency" and "excessive" patterns of MDD [13]. One recent study has further revealed differences between patients with liver-depression and spleen-deficiency syndrome and healthy volunteers in multiple serum metabolic pathways associated with amino acid and energy metabolism [14]. On the other hand, aberrant amino acid metabolism that is involved in protein synthesis, energy metabolism, monoamine and amino acid neurotransmitter biosynthesis has been suggested in the pathogenesis of MDD and antidepressant response [15]. Differential metabolomic profiles are

Table 1 Clinical manifestations and diagnostic criteria of TCM-based subtypes of MDD

	Liver Qi Stagnation (LQS)	Heart and Spleen Deficiency (HSD)
Mood symptom characters	Depressed mood with frustration, nervousness, and/or irritability	Depressed mood with excessive pensiveness, suspicion, and/or timorousness
Somatic symptoms	A. Frequently sighing (0 = absent, 1 = slight, 2 = mild, 3 = moderate, 4 = severe) B. Chest distension and/or hypochondriac pain (0 = absent, 1 = slight, 2 = mild, 3 = moderate, 4 = severe) C. Abdominal bloating (0 = absent, 1 = slight, 2 = mild, 3 = moderate, 4 = severe) D. Decreased appetite (0 = absent, 1 = mild, 2 = moderate, 3 = severe) E. Loose stool (0 = absent, 1 = mild, 2 = moderate, 3 = severe) F. Breast tenderness (0 = absent, 1 = slight, 2 = mild, 3 = moderate, 4 = severe) G. Irregular menstruation (0 = normal, 1 = seldom, 2 = sometimes, 3 = frequent)[a] H. Menstrual pain (0 = absent, 1 = mild, 2 = moderate, 3 = severe)[a]	A. Palpitation (0 = normal, 1 = seldom, 2 = sometimes, 3 = most times, 4 = all times) B. Forgetfulness (0 = absent, 1 = slight, 2 = mild, 3 = moderate, 4 = severe) C. Insomnia or dream-disturbed sleep (0 = absent, 1 = sometimes, 3 = most times) D. Decreased appetite (0 = absent, 1 = slight, 2 = mild, 3 = moderate, 4 = severe) E. Abdominal fullness (0 = absent, 1 = sometimes, 3 = most times) F. Loose stool or dysfunctional diarrhea (0 = absent, 1 = slight, 2 = mild, 3 = moderate, 4 = severe) G. Pale and sallow complexion (0 = normal, 1 = slightly apparent, 2 = mildly apparent; 3 = moderately apparent, 4 = very apparent) H. Tiredness (0 = absent, 1 = mild, 2 = moderate, 3 = severe)
Tongue and pulse	I. Red tongue body with thin and white coating (0 = normal, 1 = mildly apparent, 2 = moderately apparent, 3 = very apparent) J. Wiry pulse (0 = normal, 1 = slightly apparent, 2 = mildly apparent; 3 = moderately apparent, 4 = very apparent)	I. Pale and tender or watery tongue body with white coating (0 = normal, 1 = slightly apparent, 2 = mildly apparent; 3 = moderately apparent, 4 = very apparent) J. Weak and thin pulse (0 = normal, 1 = slightly apparent, 2 = mildly apparent; 3 = moderately apparent, 4 = very apparent)
Diagnostic criteria[b]	[1]. Must have A, B, I, and J; at least one of D and E; and at least one of F, G, and H for women [2]. Total score of physical symptoms and tongue and pulse signs is not less than 10	[1]. Must have at least two of A, B and C; at least two of D, E and F; at least one of G and H; I and J [2]. Total score of physical symptoms and tongue and pulse signs is not less than 10

The diagnostic criteria are modified based on Ref. [7, 9, 10]

[a] F, G, and H items are only applied for women

[b] Those who fail to meet either LQS or HSD subtype are classified as Other Subtypes

also associated with the severity of MDD and whether the patients had early life stress and suicidal ideation [16–20]. These studies have led to the hypothesis that certain metabolic pathways particularly associated with protein synthesis, energy metabolism, and biosynthesis of monoamine and amino acid neurotransmitters could serve valid biomarkers for differentiating TCM diagnostic subtypes of MDD.

To test this hypothesis, this study was designed to examine whether blood and urinary metabolomic profiles were different between the LQS and HSD subtypes of MDD with the inclusion of healthy volunteers as controls.

Materials and methods

Setting and participants

This study was conducted at Tongde Hospital of Zhejiang Province in Hangzhou, China between April 2015 and March 2017. The study protocol was approved by the Medical Ethical Committee [equivalent to the Institutional Review Board (IRB)] of Tongde Hospital of Zhejiang Province on March 11, 2014 (The approved document is attached in Additional file 1) and registered at http://www.clinicaltrials.gov (NCT02346682) on January 27, 2015 (https://clinicaltrials.gov/ct2/show/NCT02346682). All participants gave voluntary, written, informed consent before entering the study. We reported this study according to the Minimum Standards of Reporting Checklist (see Additional file 2).

Participants were sought from out-inpatients. Subjects were eligible for this study if they: (a) were aged 18–65 years; (b) were currently experiencing a recurrent, moderate or severe depressive episode according to the Diagnostic and Statistical Manual of Mental Disorders, Fifth Edition (DSM-5), as evidenced by a score of at least 21 on the 24-item Hamilton Rating Scale for Depression (HAMD-24) [21]; (c) met the diagnostic criteria of the LQS or HSD subtype as defined in Table 1 with representative tongue manifestations as shown in Fig. 1; and (d) had received no treatment with antidepressants and other psychotropic drugs in the previous 3 months. Tongue diagnosis is a critical diagnostic approach in discriminating different TCM patterns according to manifestations of the tongue coating and body [22].

Patients were excluded from this study if they: (a) were experiencing their first episode of depression; (b) had serious comorbid cardiac, hepatic, or renal conditions; (c) had a history of brain injury or surgery; (d) had a history of manic, hypomanic, or mixed episodes; (e) had received investigational drug treatment within the previous 6 months; (f) had experienced alcohol or drug abuse within the previous 12 months; or (g) were pregnant or breastfeeding.

A group of healthy volunteers who had no personal or family history of significant mental and physical illness was recruited from Tongde Hospital and local community to serve as controls.

Screening, assessment, and TCM diagnosis

The screening of patients and healthy volunteers was done by a psychiatrist and a TCM practitioner. The severity of the depression symptoms of the patients and healthy controls was assessed using HAMD-24 [21]. The assessment was conducted by a trained rater (L.Y.L., C.Q.Z.). TCM subtypes diagnoses were made by at least two senior TCM practitioners (Y.P.L., C.Q.Z.) and a third TCM practitioner (L.Y.L.) was involved in the diagnosis process if the first two practitioners could not reach an agreement.

To ensure consistency of assessment and diagnosis, a manual was provided and a training workshop was

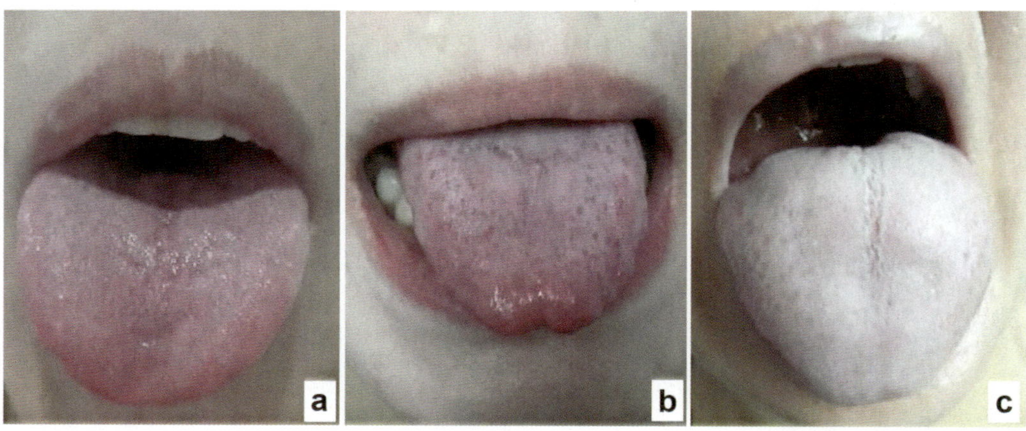

Fig. 1 Representative tongue pictures taken from a healthy volunteer (**a**), depressed patients with Liver Qi Stagnation (**b**) and Heart Spleen Deficiency (**c**) subtypes

carried out on videotaped patients with different TCM subtypes before the study was initiated. An inter-rater reliability coefficient of > 0.85 was achieved after the completion of the training workshop.

Collection and preparation of serum and urine samples

Blood and urine sample for each were collected within 2 days after the completion of clinical assessment. Following the sample collection, patients immediately received antidepressant and other psychotropic treatment at psychiatrists' discretion based on their clinical condition, with routine subsequent monitoring.

In the morning (09:00–10:00) after an overnight fasting, 10 ml of midstream urine were collected; 15 ml of blood were drawn and sera were immediately separated. Samples were further prepared for metabolomic measurement as described previously [17, 23]. Briefly, 500 μl of urine or sera was mixed with 50 μl heptanoic acid and 10 mg/ml para-chlorophenylalanine as the internal standard solution. 500 μl methanol was added to precipitate protein, mixed for 5 min, and then centrifuged at 12,000 rpm/min for 15 min at 4 °C. A 500-μl aliquot of supernatant was transferred to a clean Eppendorf tube and dried under a low temperature vacuum drier. The residue was derivatized by adding 100 μl methoxyamine hydrochloride (15 mg/ml in pyridine) at 30 °C for 90 min. For each sample, 100 μl BSTFA (1% TMCS) was added and the mixture was heated at 70 °C for 60 min. The derivative was cooled and filtered in 0.45 μm membrane prior to GC–MS analysis. Quality control samples and the reference standard were processed as done for experimental samples.

GC–MS acquisition

One μl aliquot of derivatized sample was injected into a Varian 450-GC/240-MS equipped with 19091 N-113 capillary column (30 m × 0.32 mm × 0.25 μm, Agilent J & W Scientific, USA) at a split ratio of 10:1. Helium was used as the carrier gas with a constant flow rate of 1 ml/min. The initial temperature was set at 70 °C for 4 min, elevated to 300 °C at a rate of 8°C/min, and then maintained for 3 min. Temperature for the injector, transfer line, and ion source was set at 280 °C, 250 °C, and 220 °C, respectively. The mass range (50–800 m/z) in a full-scan mode for electron impact ionization (1.0 kV) was applied. The solvent delay time was set to 6 min.

Statistical analysis

There were no studies detecting metabolomic effects in TCM subtypes of MDD. Sample size estimation was based on one previous study that has revealed differential metabolomic profiles between MDD patients with and without early life stress [17]. As the LQS and HSD subtypes are appear to be differentially associated with stress-related (reactive) and endogenous (melancholic) depression [2, 9], we assumed that metabolomic differences between the two TCM subtypes was similar to that of MDD patients with and without early life stress [17]. The study has shown an averaged 36% difference in plasma level of major metabolites between MDD patients with and without early life stress with an averaged standard deviation of 41% [17]. A sample size of 22 each group would be sufficient to yield an 80% power at a statistical level of 0.05.

For baseline data, one-way analysis of variance (ANOVA) was used to detect differences in continuous variables among healthy controls and the two TCM subtypes. Student's *t*-test was used to detect differences in continuous variables between the two TCM subtypes. Categorical baseline variables were analyzed using Chi square (χ^2) test.

For metabolomic data, the pretreatment process was performed, including novel nonlinear retention time alignment, baseline filtration, peak identification, matching, and integration. The resulting data matrix consisting of variables, sample code, and peak area was further processed using Microsoft Excel program. The original spectral data obtained from GC-MS spectroscopy were scaled to unit variance (z), which was calculated from the formula $z=(x-y)/s$, where x, y, and s represent the level of the particular metabolite in one subject, the mean level and the standard deviation of this metabolite across all subjects, respectively.

Nonparametric Mann–Whitney U test was used to detect significantly differential metabolites. All metabolites were determined by standard samples and/or a similarity of > 70% that was obtained by comparing with the mass spectral database of the US National Institute for Standards and Technology (NIST).

Metabolites were determined using variable importance in the projection (VIP) which value was defined as > 1 and *t*-test was set at a level of 95%. The principal component analysis (PCA) was used to discriminate metabolic patterns among the three groups. The orthogonal projection to latent structures-discriminant analysis (OPLS-DA) model was further constructed to identify meaningful metabolites that could differentiate between the three groups using SIMCA-P 13.0 program. A regression method was applied to establish the optimal discriminant model with controlling gender as a confounding factor. The quality of the model was tested with cross-validation and R^2X, R^2Y, and Q^2 values were obtained. OPLS-DA models which all R^2X, R^2Y, and Q^2 values were ≥ 0.5 were acceptable. Hierarchical clustering patterns were further established with heatmap analysis using R i386 3.3.0 software for visual verification of

OPLS-DA models. The impact pathway was determined using MetaboAnalyst 3.0 (http://www.metaboanalyst.ca), a web-based tool for pathway analysis, with the criteria as *p*-value < 0.05, false discovery rate (FDR) < 0.05, and impact value > 0. Visualization of metabolomic correlation network was drawn with CytoScape 3.3.0. The receiver operating characteristic (ROC) curve analysis was conducted to determine the optimal metabolite combination patterns that could well dichotomize the subtypes and healthy controls at acceptable sensitivity and specificity (defined as greater than 80% for both).

Statistical analysis was conducted using SPSS 18.0 (SPSS Inc., Chicago, IL, USA) and, unless otherwise indicated, significance level was set at a two-tailed $P < 0.05$.

Results

Participant characteristics

Flowchart of screening and recruitment is shown in Fig. 2. Of 243 depressed patients screened, 189 met the diagnostic criteria of LQS (n = 102) and SHD (n = 87) subtype; 27.0% (51/189) rejected to participate the study; 30 LQS subtypes and 20 SHD subtypes who met the inclusion criteria but did not meet any exclusion criteria were recruited. Twenty-eight healthy volunteers were recruited to serve as controls. The proportion of female participants of the LQS subtype was significantly higher than that of the HSD subtype ($\chi^2 = 6.696$, $p = 0.035$) (Table 2). Other demographic and clinical variables were not different among the three groups.

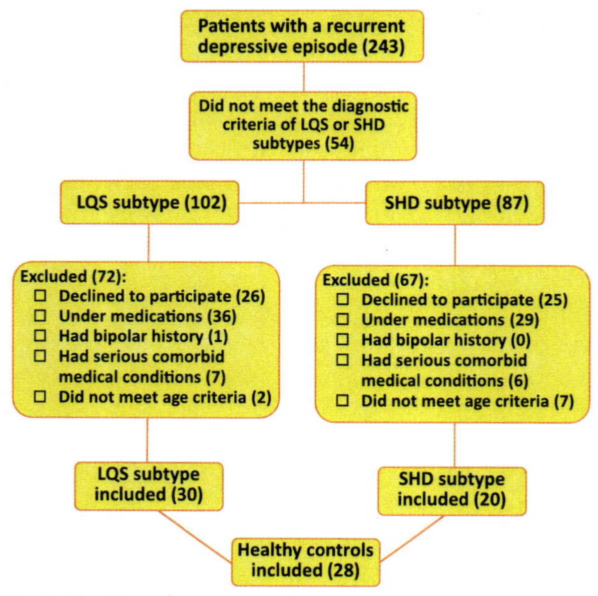

Fig. 2 Flowchart of screening and recruitment. *LQS* Liver Qi Stagnation, *HSD* Heart and Spleen Deficiency

Clustering patterns of differential metabolite profiles

A total of 28 metabolites were identified to well differentiate the two TCM subtypes from healthy controls (Table 3); 8 of them were present in both serum and urine samples and/or in the two subtypes. The OPLS-DA models revealed that serum metabolite profiles of both subtypes were clearly separated from healthy controls with R^2X values of ≥ 0.842, R^2Y values of ≥ 0.670, and Q^2 values of ≥ 0.502 (Fig. 3a, b). Urinary metabolite profiles of the two subtypes were not well separated from healthy controls, with considerable overlaps and low R^2Y and Q^2 values (Fig. 2d, e). The two subtypes showed large overlaps in serum and urinary metabolite profiles with low R^2Y and Q^2 values (Fig. 2c, f). Hierarchical clustering analysis displayed remarkable differences in mentalism between the three groups, visually validating OPLS-DA models in serum and urine samples (Figs. 4 and 5).

Differential metabolites of TCM subtypes

Between LQS subtype and healthy controls

24 metabolites were valid in discriminating the LQS subtype from healthy controls (Fig. 6, Table 3). In serum samples, levels of L-valine, L-phenylalanine, L-lysine, L-proline, L-leucine, and isobutyric acid were markedly higher than those of healthy controls and positively correlated with the LQS subtype. L-lactic acid level of the LQS subtype was greater than that of healthy subjects with negative correlation with the subtype. Levels of glycine and threonic acid were significantly lower than those of healthy controls and negatively correlated with the LQS subtype.

In urine samples, levels of L-sorbose, diacetyl, *N*-acetyl-D-glucosamine, L-methionine, 3-hydroxybutyric acid, pyruvic acid, stearic acid, trans-aconitic acid, glycine, *N*-acetyl-L-aspartic acid, and threonic acid were significantly higher than those of healthy subjects and positively correlated with the LQS subtype. Levels of L-tryptophan, α-lactose, L-lactic acid, palmitic acid, indoxyl sulfate, and o-tyrosine were significantly greater than those of healthy subjects but negatively correlated with the LQS subtype. Levels of *p*-hydroxyphenylacetic acid and citric acid were significantly lower higher than those of healthy subjects and negatively correlated with the LQS subtype.

Between HSD subtype and healthy controls

13 metabolites were identified to be effective in distinguishing the HSD subtype from healthy controls (Fig. 6, Table 3). In serum samples, levels of L-valine, L-leucine, and L-lysine were remarkably higher than those of healthy subjects and positively correlated with the HSD subtype. Levels of L-threonine, D-chiro-Inositol,

Table 2 Demographic and clinical characteristics of participants

Variables	Healthy controls (n = 28)	LQS subtype[a] (n = 30)	HSD subtype[a] (n = 20)	*p* value[b,c]
Female, n (%)[b]	17 (60.7)	25 (83.3)	10 (50.0)	0.035
Age (y)[c]	34.1 ± 8.1	38.1 ± 13.4	41.5 ± 13.7	0.107
Educational level, n (%)[b]				0.331
Primary	2 (7.1)	6 (20.0)	5 (25.0)	
Middle	5 (17.9)	4 (13.3)	5 (25.0)	
High[d]	21 (75.0)	20 (66.7)	10 (50.0)	
Marital status, n (%)[b]				0.734
Married	23 (82.1)	26 (86.7)	18 (90.0)	
Single/divorced/widowed	5 (17.9)	4 (13.3)	2 (10.0)	
Income level, n (%)[b,e]				0.775
Low	4 (14.3)	7 (23.3)	3 (15.0)	
Middle	17 (60.7)	18 (60.0)	14 (70.0)	
High	7 (25.0)	5 (16.7)	3 (15.0)	
Family history with severe mental diseases, n (%)[b,f]	3 (10.7)	4 (13.3)	0	0.250
Comorbid conditions, n (%)[b,g]		3 (10)	4 (20)	0.560
Medication history, n (%)[b,h]				0.803
SSRIs/SNRIs[a]		25 (83.3)	18 (90.0)	
Antipsychotics		5 (16.7)	2 (10.0)	
Previous depressive episode, n (%)[b]				0.684
Single		18 (60.0)	10 (50.0)	
Multiple		12 (40.0)	10 (50.0)	
Duration of the illness (months)[c,i]		39.5 ± 60.9	33.6 ± 47.8	0.716
HAMD-24 score[a,c]		32.5 ± 8.5	30.1 ± 6.5	0.286

[a] *LQS* Liver Qi Stagnation, *HSD* Heart and Spleen Deficiency, *SSRIs* selective serotonin reuptake inhibitors, *SNRIs* serotonin–norepinephrine reuptake inhibitors, *HAMD-24* 24-item Hamilton Rating Scale for Depression

[b] Categorical data was analyzed using Chi square (χ^2) test

[c] Continuous data are expressed mean ± SD and analyzed using one-way analysis of variance (ANOVA) for the three groups and Student t-test for LQS and HSD subtypes

[d] High levels included high school, college, and postgraduate education

[e] Compared to average local household incomes

[f] Severe mental diseases mainly included schizophrenia, bipolar disorders, and severe depression

[g] Most comorbid conditions were cardiovascular and diabetic diseases

[h] SSRIs mainly included paroxetine, sertraline, citalopram, and fluoxetine. SNRIs mainly include venlafaxine and duloxetine. Antipsychotics mainly include quetiapine, olanzapine, and risperidone. All medications were taken earlier than 3 months ago at screening

[i] Duration of the illness was calculated from the first episode of depression

L-methionine, and L-lactic acid were significantly lower than those of healthy subjects and negatively correlated with the HSD subtype.

In urine samples, levels of L-Isoleucine, isobutyric acid, threonic acid, and *N*-acetyl-D-glucosamine were considerably higher than those of healthy subjects and positively correlated with the HSD subtype. Level of stearic acid was also significantly higher than that of healthy controls but negatively correlated with the HSD subtype. Level of α-lactose was significantly lower than that of healthy controls and negatively correlated with the HSD subtype.

Between LQS and HSD subtypes

10 metabolites showed correlations with both subtypes (Fig. 6). They are urine α-lactose, *N*-acetyl-D-glucosamine, and stearic acid; serum L-lactic acid, L-lysine, L-valine, and L-leucine; and isobutyric acid, threonic acid, and L-methionine in both serum and urine samples. Most metabolite correlates with the two subtypes were consistent. Serum threonic acid correlate was negative with the LQS subtype but positive with the HSD subtype. Urine stearic acid correlate was positive with the LQS subtype but negative with the HSD subtype. L-Methionine correlate was positive with the LQS subtype in urine

Table 3 Differential metabolites identified from MDD patients with TCM subtypes and healthy controls [a]

Group samples	Metabolites	Formula	r^b	*p*-value[c]	FC (MDD/HC)[a]	Pathway
Serum: LQS vs. HC[a]						
1[d]	L-Valine	$C_5H_{11}NO_2$	0.236	0.009	0.930	Aminoacyl-tRNA biosynthesis
2[d]	L-Phenylalanine	$C_9H_{11}NO_2$	0.199	0.237	0.350	Aminoacyl-tRNA biosynthesis
3[d]	L-Lysine	$C_6H_{14}N_2O_2$	0.150	0.761	0.459	Aminoacyl-tRNA biosynthesis
4	L-Proline	$C_5H_9NO_2$	0.143	0.447	0.182	Aminoacyl-tRNA biosynthesis
5[d]	L-Leucine	$C_6H_{13}NO_2$	0.124	0.000	1.047	Aminoacyl-tRNA biosynthesis
6[e]	Isobutyric acid	$C_4H_8O_2$	0.103	0.565	0.702	Protein digestion and absorption
7	L-Lactic acid	$C_3H_6O_3$	−0.147	0.370	0.013	Propanoate metabolism
8	Glycine	$C_2H_5NO_2$	−0.151	0.279	−0.954	Aminoacyl-tRNA biosynthesis
9	Threonic acid	$C_4H_8O_5$	−0.175	0.250	−1.080	Ascorbate and aldarate metabolism
Urine: LQS vs. HC[a]						
1	L-Sorbose	$C_6H_{12}O_6$	0.149	0.624	0.661	Unknown
2	Diacetyl	$C_4H_6O_2$	0.147	0.120	0.825	Butanoate metabolism
3	*N*-Acetyl-D-glucosamine	$C_8H_{15}NO_6$	0.146	0.748	0.304	Amino sugar and nucleotide sugar metabolism
4[d]	L-Methionine	$C_5H_{11}NO_2S$	0.144	0.417	0.546	Cysteine and methionine metabolism
5[d]	3-Hydroxybutyric acid	$C_4H_8O_3$	0.139	0.088	0.819	Butanoate metabolism
6[d]	Pyruvic acid	$C_3H_4O_3$	0.125	0.116	1.085	Citrate cycle (TCA cycle)
7[d]	Stearic acid	$C_{18}H_{36}O_2$	0.117	0.327	0.490	Fatty acid biosynthesis
8	trans-Aconitic acid	$C_6H_6O_6$	0.115	0.648	0.444	C5-Branched dibasic acid metabolism
9[d]	Glycine	$C_2H_5NO_2$	0.111	0.685	0.441	Aminoacyl-tRNA biosynthesis
10[d]	*N*-Acetyl-L-aspartic acid	$C_6H_9NO_5$	0.107	0.176	0.680	Alanine, aspartate and glutamate metabolism
11	Threonic acid	$C_4H_8O_5$	0.101	0.906	0.428	Ascorbate and aldarate metabolism
12[d]	L-Tryptophan	$C_{11}H_{12}N_2O_2$	−0.108	0.054	0.186	Glycine, serine and threonine metabolism
13	α-Lactose	$C_{12}H_{22}O_{11}$	−0.114	0.116	0.259	Galactose metabolism
14[d]	L-Lactic acid	$C_3H_6O_3$	−0.129	0.735	0.263	Propanoate metabolism
15[d]	Palmitic acid	$C_{16}H_{32}O_2$	−0.149	0.005	0.303	Fatty acid metabolism
16	Indoxyl sulfate	$C_8H_7NO_4S$	−0.164	0.673	0.583	Unknown
17[d]	*o*-Tyrosine	$C_9H_{11}NO_3$	−0.203	0.217	0.080	Unknown
18	*p*-Hydroxyphenylacetic acid	$C_9H_8O_3$	−0.122	0.673	−0.120	Tyrosine metabolism
19[d]	Citric acid	$C_6H_8O_7$	−0.156	0.015	−0.265	Citrate cycle (TCA cycle)
Serum: HSD vs. HC[a]						
1[d]	L-Valine	$C_5H_{11}NO_2$	0.226	0.079	0.689	Aminoacyl-tRNA biosynthesis
2[d]	L-Leucine	$C_6H_{13}NO_2$	0.161	0.000	1.120	Aminoacyl-tRNA biosynthesis
3[d]	L-Lysine	$C_6H_{14}N_2O_2$	0.148	0.337	0.722	Aminoacyl-tRNA biosynthesis
4	L-Threonine	$C_4H_9NO_3$	−0.105	0.000	−0.191	Glycine, serine and threonine metabolism
5	D-chiro-Inositol	$C_6H_{12}O_6$	−0.135	0.138	−0.200	Inositol phosphate metabolism
6[d]	L-Methionine	$C_5H_{11}NO_2S$	−0.140	0.009	−0.299	Cysteine and methionine metabolism
7	L-Lactic acid	$C_3H_6O_3$	−0.170	0.253	−0.183	Propanoate metabolism
Urine: HSD vs. HC[a]						
1[d]	L-Isoleucine	$C_6H_{13}NO_2$	0.161	0.007	0.681	Valine, leucine and isoleucine degradation
2	Threonic acid	$C_4H_8O_5$	0.113	0.349	0.687	Ascorbate and aldarate metabolism
3	*N*-Acetyl-D-glucosamine	$C_8H_{15}NO_6$	0.109	0.283	0.432	Amino sugar and nucleotide sugar metabolism
4[d]	Stearic acid	$C_{18}H_{36}O_2$	−0.104	0.002	0.019	Fatty acid biosynthesis
5	α-Lactose	$C_{12}H_{22}O_{11}$	−0.116	0.000	−0.126	Galactose metabolism
Urine: LQS vs. HSD[a]						
1	Isobutyric acid	$C_4H_8O_2$	0.127	0.304	1.114[e]	Protein digestion and absorption

[a] *FC* fold change, *MDD* major depressive disorder, *HC* healthy controls, *LQS* Liver Qi Stagnation, *HSD* Heart and Spleen Deficiency

[b] Correlation coefficients (*r*) were obtained from OPLC-DA with a threshold of 3.010. Positive and negative coefficients respectively indicate higher and lower levels of metabolites compared to healthy controls

[c] *p*-values were obtained from Wilcoxon-Mann–Whitney test between TCM subtypes and healthy controls

[d] Metabolites were determined using standard samples

[e] FC value represents LQS/HSD

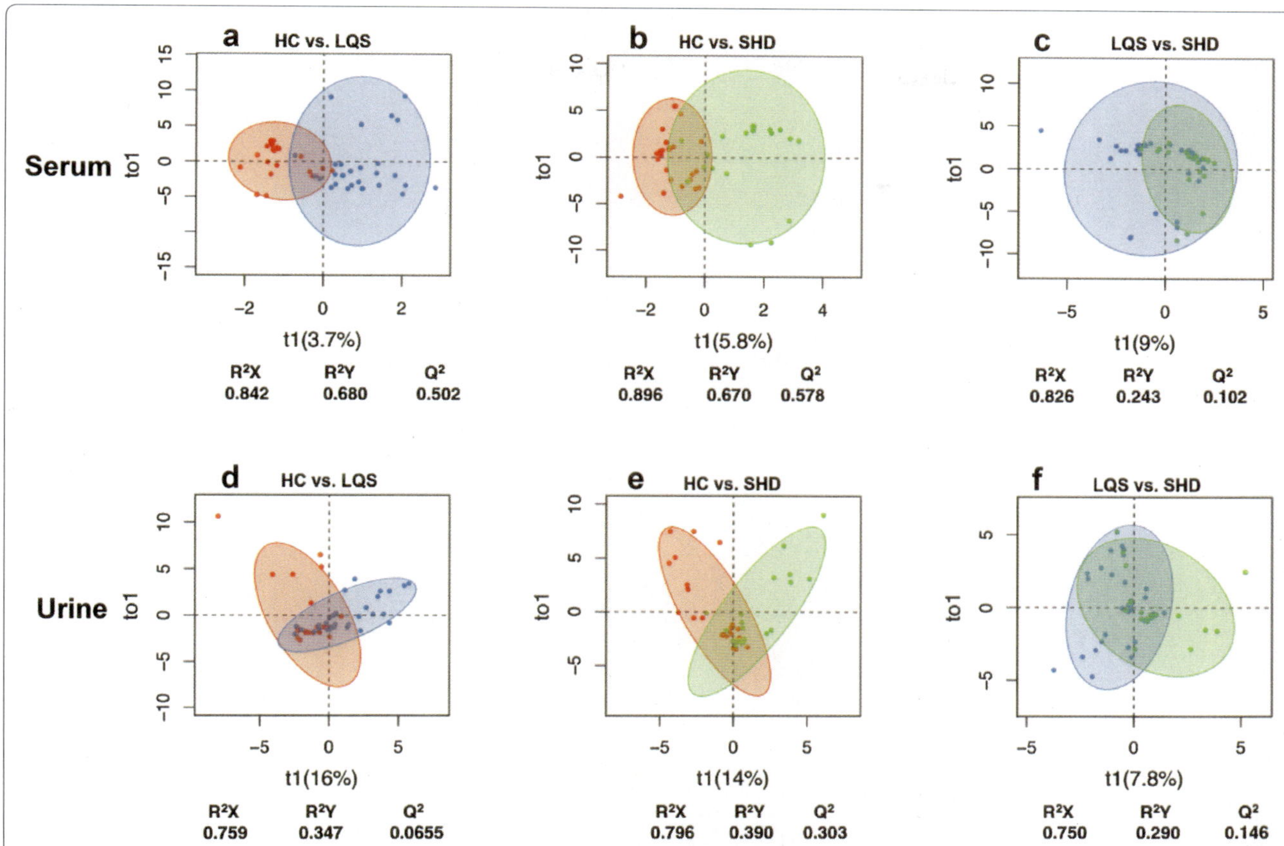

Fig. 3 Clustering analysis of serum (**a**, **b**, **c**) and urine (**d**, **e**, **f**) metabolomic profiles. OPLS-DA models were built in patients with Liver Qi Stagnation (LQS) and Heart and Spleen Deficiency (HSD) subtypes of MDD and healthy controls (HC). Acceptable criteria for the models were defined as all R^2X, R^2Y, and Q^2 values of ≥ 0.5. Comparisons were conducted between HC and LQS (**a**, **d**), HC and HSD (**b**, **e**), and LQS and HSD (**c**, **f**)

samples but negative with the HSD subtype in serum samples. The LQS subtype had a markedly lower urinary level of isobutyric acid than the HSD subtype ($P=0.047$).

Metabolite-associated biochemical pathways

The impact pathway analysis revealed that the differential metabolites of the LQS subtype were significantly associated with aminoacyl-tRNA biosynthesis; valine, leucine and isoleucine biosynthesis; butanoate metabolism; phenylalanine metabolism; and glycine, serine and threonine metabolism (Fig. 7a). The differential metabolites of the HSD subtype were heavily involved in aminoacyl-tRNA biosynthesis; valine, leucine and isoleucine biosynthesis; and valine, leucine and isoleucine degradation (Fig. 7b).

The optimal metabolite profiles for separating TCM subtypes and healthy controls

ROC analysis showed that the optimal metabolite profile with a combination of five serum metabolites (leucine, valine, phenylalanine, threonic acid, and glycine) well separated the LQS subtype and healthy controls with a sensitivity of 0.87 and a specificity of 0.80 (Fig. 8a). A combination of five serum metabolites (leucine, valine, threonine, methionine, and inositol) optimally dichotomized the HSD subtype and healthy controls with a sensitivity of 0.95 and a specificity of 0.88 (Fig. 8b). There were no optimal urinary metabolite profiles that could separate TCM subtypes and healthy controls at the acceptable sensitivity and specificity (data not shown).

Discussion

This study represents the first attempt to introduce TCM-based diagnostic subtypes into the modern classification of depressive disorders. It not only could improve personalized treatment of depression, but also promote the integration of TCM theoretical concepts into the modern biomedical knowledge system. The sample recruited in this study was representative of MDD patients seen in China [7, 9, 11, 16].

The purpose of this study was to explore blood and urinary metabolomic evidence that could validate TCM diagnostic classification of MDD. A total of 28 meaningful metabolites were identified as potential biomarkers for differentiating MDD and healthy subjects. These

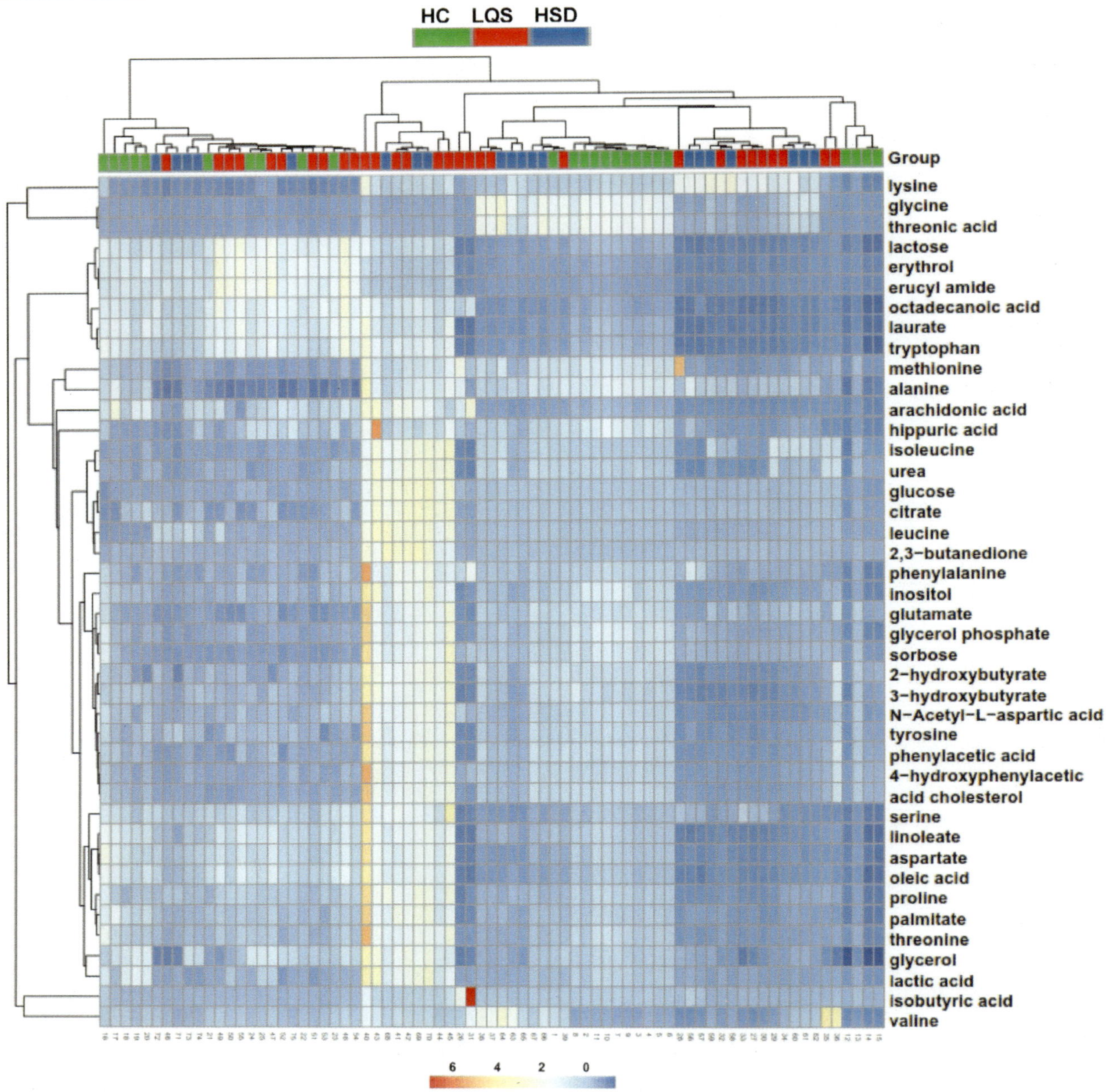

Fig. 4 Heat maps generated from hierarchical Pearson clustering show metabolites in serum samples obtained from Liver Qi Stagnation (LQS) and Heart and Spleen Deficiency (HSD) subtypes of MDD and healthy controls (HC)

metabolites mainly included amino acid metabolites involved in the synthesis of monoamine and amino acid neurotransmitters (L-tryptophan, phenylalanine, *o*-tyrosine, glycine, 3-hydroxybutric acid, and *N*-acetyl-L-aspartic acid), proteinogenic branched-chain amino acids (BCAAs) (valine, leucine, and isoleucine), oxaloacetate-derived amino acids (L-lysine, L-threonine and L-methionine) which are mainly involved in the biosynthesis of proteins and energy production via gluconeogenesis, and energy metabolism-related metabolites (L-lactic acid, palmitic acid, citric acid, stearic acid, pyruvic acid, and α-lactose) [24].

Clustering analyses revealed that the two TCM subtypes of MDD were well separated from healthy controls on serum metabolic profiles, but not on the urinary profiles. Likewise, ROC analysis displayed that the two optimal metabolite combination patterns for dichotomizing the TCM subtypes of MDD and healthy subjects

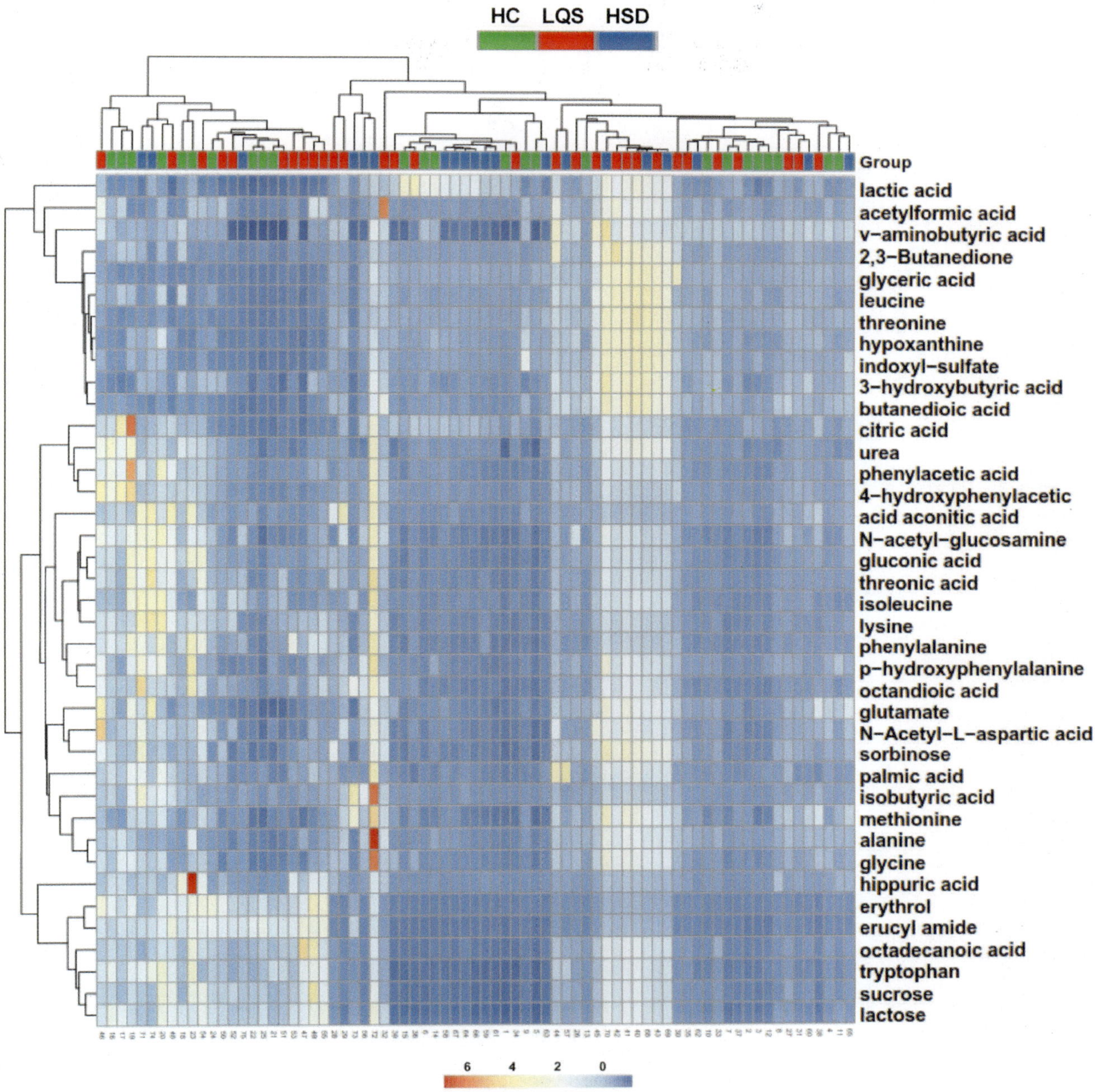

Fig. 5 Heat maps generated from hierarchical Pearson clustering show metabolites in urine samples obtained from Liver Qi Stagnation (LQS) and Heart and Spleen Deficiency (HSD) subtypes of MDD and healthy controls (HC)

were identified from serum samples, but not from urine samples. Similar results also have been observed in previous studies that attempted to identify blood and urine metabolic biomarkers for the severity of MDD [16, 20]. Blood metabolites seem to be more sensitive than urinary metabolites in distinguishing MDD from healthy subjects. This may be largely because blood metabolites can be maintained at a relatively constant state compared to urinary metabolites [25].

Although clustering analyses showed large overlaps in serum and urinary metabolite patterns between the two TCM subtypes of MDD, the LQS subtype had strong mixed correlations with multiple amino acid metabolites involved in the biosynthesis of monoamine and

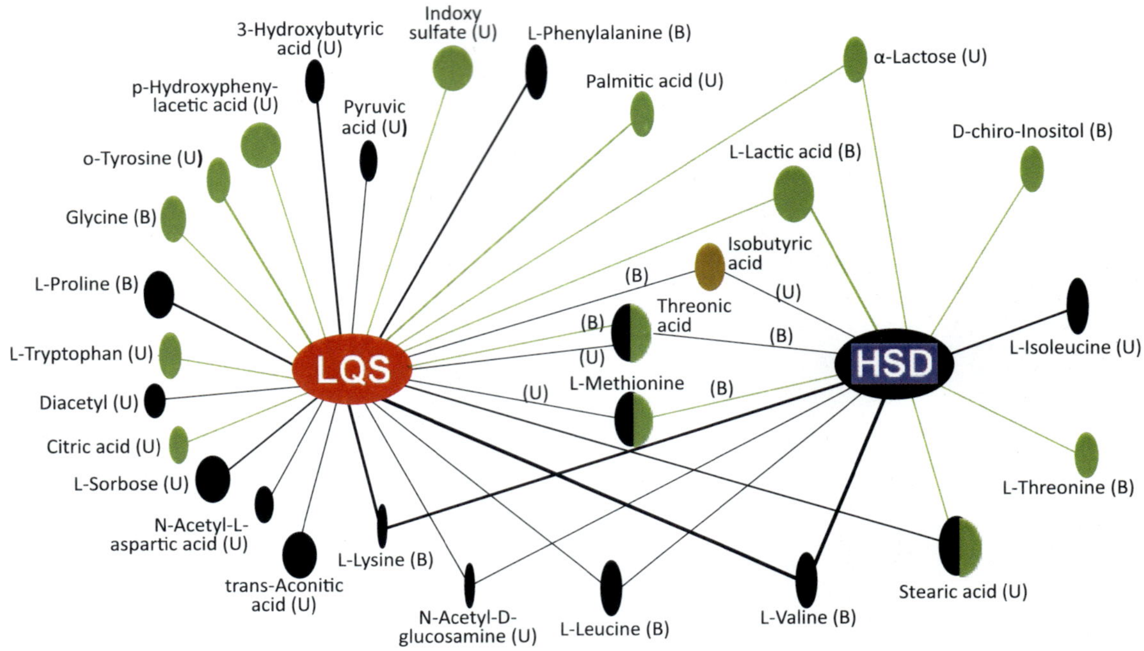

Fig. 6 Correlation network analysis of 28 differential metabolites among Liver Qi Stagnation (LQS) and Heart and Spleen Deficiency (HSD) subtypes of MDD versus healthy controls. Green and red lines with ovals indicates negative and positive correlation, respectively. The ovals with half green and half red colors indicate mixed correlations. The oval size represents *p* value compared with healthy controls. Isobutyric acid (dark brown oral) has a significant difference between the two subtypes. *B* blood samples, *U* urine samples

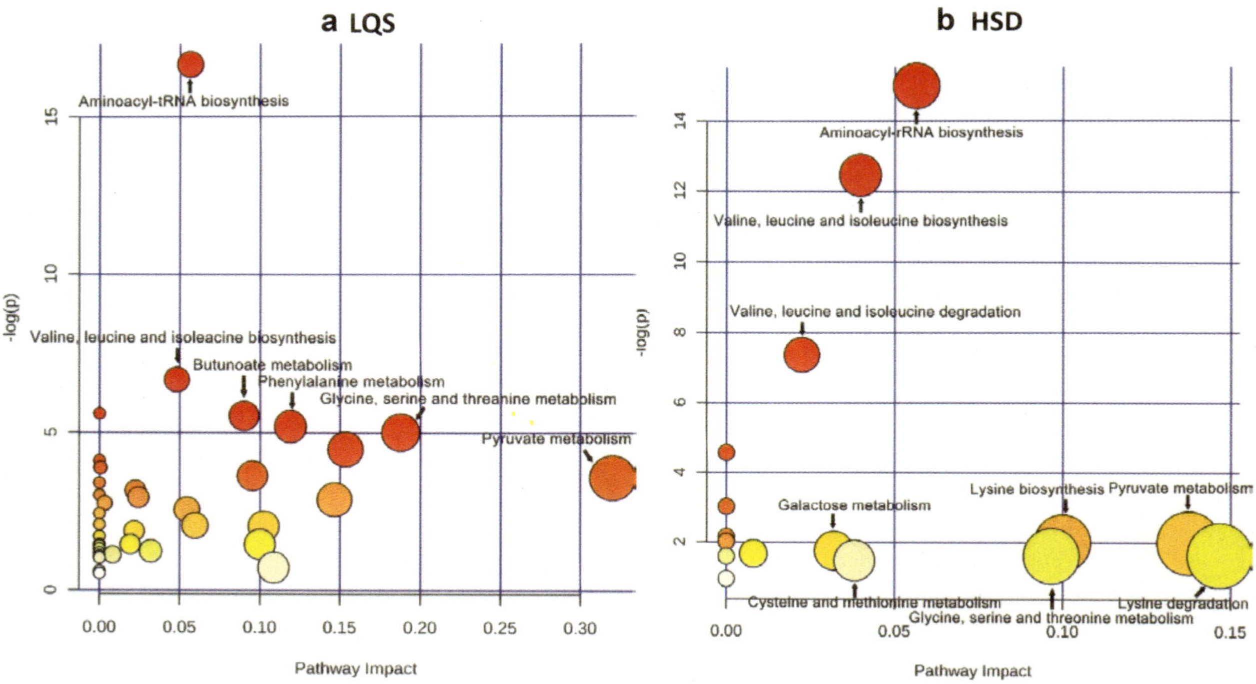

Fig. 7 Biochemical pathway analysis shows biological impacts in differentiating Liver Qi Stagnation (LQS, **a**) and Heart and Spleen Deficiency (HSD, **b**) subtypes of MDD from healthy controls. X- and Y-axis indicates the magnitude of the impact and *p* value compared with healthy controls, respectively. Aminoacyl-tRNA biosynthesis and valine, leucine and isoleucine biosynthesis pathways are most closely associated with the two subtypes. The HSD subtype was additionally associated with valine, leucine and isoleucine degradation

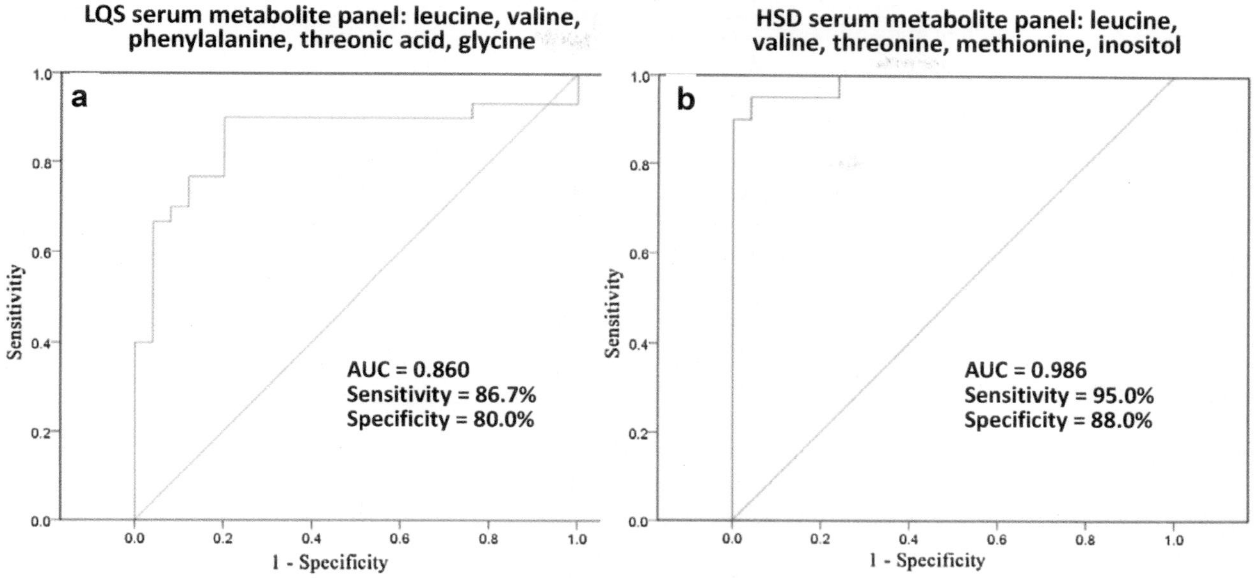

Fig. 8 Receiver operating curve (ROC) analysis show the optimal serum metabolite panels that well differentiate Liver Qi Stagnation (LQS, **a**) and Heart and Spleen Deficiency (HSD, **b**) subtype from healthy controls

amino acid neurotransmitters, including phenylalanine, 3-hydroxybutric acid, *o*-tyrosine, glycine, L-tryptophan, and *N*-acetyl-L-aspartic acid; but the HSD subtype did not. ROC analysis further indicated that phenylalanine and glycine were among the optimal metabolite combination pattern for discriminating the LQS subtype and healthy controls. A preliminary study also has observed differences in multiple brain monoamine neurotransmission among TCM subtypes of MDD [26]. According to the presence and absence of stress prior to its onset, MDD can be classified as reactive and endogenous (melancholic) subtypes [2]. Stress-associated depression has been suggested to be more closely associated with dysfunction of brain catecholamine and amino acid neurotransmitters, in particular norepinephrine, glutamate and γ-aminobutyric acid systems [27, 28]. Clinically, the LQS subtype patients often exhibit stress-related comorbid symptoms and signs, such as nervousness, irritability, agitation, and a wiry pulse [2, 10]. It thus appears that the LQS subtype may represent a subpopulation of MDD characterized by abnormal biosynthesis of monoamine and amino acid neurotransmitters and closer associations with stress-related pathophysiology.

Moreover, both subtypes had opposing correlations with serum threonic acid, serum/urine L-methionine, and urine stearic acid. Serum threonic acid and L-methionine were also among the optimal metabolite combination patterns for respectively discriminating the LQS and HSD subtype from healthy controls. Threonic acid is a metabolite of ascorbic acid (vitamin C) and methionine is an essential amino acid in humans [24]. Dietary treatment with threonic acid- and methionine-derived supplements (e.g., magnesium-L-threonate (MgT) and S-adenosyl-methionine (SAMe)) had the benefits in improving multiple brain functions, in particular memory, depression, and anxiety [29–31]. Stearic acid is a saturated fatty acid which plasma concentrations have been found to be abnormally altered in patients with winter episode of MDD [32] and in the superior temporal gyrus and orbitofrontal cortex of bipolar patients [33, 34]. We further found that the LQS subtype had a markedly lower urinary level of isobutyric acid, a short-chain fatty acid than the HSD subtype. Plasma level of β-amino-isobutyric acid of autistic children has been shown to be significantly higher than that of healthy children [35]. These results suggest that threonic acid, methionine, stearic acid, and isobutyric acid are differentially associated with the two TCM subtypes and may be promising biomarkers for TCM classification of MDD.

However, the present study revealed that both subtypes had large overlaps in serum and urinary metabolite panels and shared several similar profiles, in particular proteinogenic BCAAs (valine and leucine) and energy metabolism-related metabolites (α-lactose and L-lactic acid), manifesting as consistent positive correlations with serum levels of valine and leucine, and negative correlations with levels of urine α-lactose and serum L-lactic acid. Biochemical pathway analysis displayed that both subtypes had consistent and closer links with valine, leucine, and isoleucine biosynthesis and aminoacyl-tRNA biosynthesis. ROC analysis also revealed that valine and leucine were involved in the two optimal metabolite combination patterns identified for discriminating the two subtypes and healthy controls. BCAAs and energy metabolism dysfunction is related to the pathogenesis of multiple psychiatric disorders and a common comorbidity in depressive disorders [36, 37]. The BCAAs play a key role in maintaining the supply of the neurotransmitters glutamate and γ-aminobutyric acid (GABA) [38]. Our study suggests that aberrant BCAA and energy metabolism seems to be distinct biochemical profiles in the pathophysiology of MDD and the BCAA-glutamate/GABA metabolic cycle in the brain may be potential biomarkers and therapeutic targets for MDD [36, 38, 39].

Several limitations of this study should be noted. First, there are 12 subtypes according to TCM classification of MDD [7–11], but we only examined the two most common and opposing subtypes of MDD. Whether other subtypes also have differential profiles needs further investigation. Second, the TCM diagnostic procedure was conducted mainly based on empirical practice and subjective assessments. Objective and precise TCM diagnostic approaches should be sought. Third, the sample size was relatively small with medication-free participant and gender imbalance. This may limit the applicability of the findings of this study. Whether similar results could be achieved in first-episode and treatment-resistant depressed populations needs further determination. Finally, we did not examine the differential response of the two subtypes to antidepressant treatment. Whether metabolomic biomarkers identified are effective in predicting TCM subtype-specific treatment outcomes deserves further examination.

Conclusions

While the two subtypes are associated with aberrant BCAA and energy metabolism, the LQS subtype may represent a subpopulation of MDD characterized by abnormal biosynthesis of monoamine and amino acid neurotransmitters and closer associations with stress-related pathophysiology. Threonic acid, methionine, stearic acid, and isobutyric acid are differentially associated with the two subtypes and may be promising biomarkers for TCM classification of MDD. This study suggests that the TCM diagnostic subtypes could serve a valid classification of MDD.

Abbreviations

ANOVA: analysis of variance; BCAAs: proteinogenic branched-chain amino acids; DSM-5: Statistical Manual of Mental Disorders, Fifth Edition; GABA: γ-aminobutyric acid; GC–MS: gas chromatography-mass spectrometry; HAMD-24: 24-item Hamilton Rating Scale for Depression; HSD: Heart and Spleen Deficiency; LQS: Liver Qi Stagnation; MDD: major depressive disorder; OPLS-DA: latent structures-discriminant analysis; PCA: principal component analysis; ROC: receiver operating characteristic; TCM: traditional Chinese medicine; VIP: variable importance in the projection.

Authors' contributions

LYL and ZZJ were involved in conception and design of the study, data analysis, and preparation of the manuscript. HJZ, JBP, and WQL were responsible for metabolomic experiments and data analysis. LYLuo, CQZ, YPL, PRW, YYZ, and CYY recruited subjects, conducted clinical assessment, and collected clinical data. All authors read and approved the final manuscript.

Author details

[1] Department of Psychiatry, Tongde Hospital of Zhejiang Province, Hangzhou 310012, Zhejiang, China. [2] Zhejiang Academy of Traditional Chinese Medicine, Hangzhou 310007, Zhejiang, China. [3] Department of Internal Chinese Medicine, Tongde Hospital of Zhejiang Province, Hangzhou 310012, Zhejiang, China. [4] School of Chinese Medicine, LKS Faculty of Medicine, The University of Hong Kong, 10 Sassoon Road, Pokfulam, Hong Kong, China.

Acknowledgements

Not applicable.

Competing interests

The authors declare that they have no competing interests.

Consent for publication

All authors have provided consent for publication in the journal of Chinese Medicine.

Funding

This study was supported by the National Natural Science Foundation of China (81403502, L.Y.L.) and Research Grant Council of Hong Kong (17115017, 17124119, Z.J.Z.).

References

1. Kennedy SH. Core symptoms of major depressive disorder: relevance to diagnosis and treatment. Dialogues Clin Neurosci. 2008;10:271–7.
2. Malki K, Keers R, Tosto MG, et al. The endogenous and reactive depression subtypes revisited: integrative animal and human studies implicate multiple distinct molecular mechanisms underlying major depressive disorder. BMC Med. 2014;12:73.
3. van Loo HM, de Jonge P, Romeijn JW, Kessler RC, Schoevers RA. Data-driven subtypes of major depressive disorder: a systematic review. BMC Med. 2012;10:156.
4. Ilgen MA, Downing K, Zivin K, Hoggatt KJ, Kim HM, Ganoczy D, Austin KL, McCarthy JF, Patel JM, Valenstein M. Exploratory data mining analysis identifying subgroups of patients with depression who are at high risk for suicide. J Clin Psychiatry. 2009;70:1495–500.
5. Milaneschi Y, Lamers F, Peyrot WJ, Abdellaoui A, Willemsen G, Hottenga JJ, Jansen R, Mbarek H, Dehghan A, Lu C, CHARGE inflammation working group, Boomsma DI, Penninx BW. Polygenic dissection of major depression clinical heterogeneity. Mol Psychiatry. 2016;21:516–22.
6. Cheung F. Modern TCM: enter the clinic. Nature. 2011;480:S94–5.

7. Chen Z, Hu S, Zhang H, Zhang H, Zheng L, Li X. Study on criteria for commonly seen TCM syndrome of depression. JTCM. 2005;46:47–9.
8. Guo R, Yu M, Wang JL, et al. Establishing a TCM pattern element identification scale for depression. J Beijing Univ TCM. 2015;38:561–5.
9. Hu SY, Wang SE, Zhang CH. Relationship between symptom stratification and syndrome differentiation of traditional Chinese medicine for depressive episode. Zhong Xi Yi Jie He Xue Bao. 2011;9:933–6.
10. China Academy of Chinese Medical Sciences and China Association for Acupuncture and Moxibustion. Evidence-based guidelines of clinical practice in Chinese medicine: acupuncture. Beijing: China Traditional Chinese Medicine Publishing House; 2011. p. 107.
11. Zhou L, Chen WK, Mei XY. Study on the characteristics of population distribution of TCM syndromes and its related factors in patients of depression. Zhongguo Zhong Xi Yi Jie He Za Zhi. 2006;26:106–9.
12. Yeung WF, Chung KF, Zhang NL, Zhang SP, Yung KP, Chen PX, Ho YY. Identification of Chinese medicine syndromes in persistent insomnia associated with major depressive disorder: a latent tree analysis. Chin Med. 2016;11:4.
13. Zhang YF, Han Y, Wang YZ, et al. Characterization of resting-state fMRI-derived functional connectivity in patients with deficiency versus excess patterns of major depression. Complement Ther Med. 2015;23:7–13.
14. Fu S, Xie ZY, Yu CJ, Gao XY. Methods to establishment of serum induced syndrome of liver-depression and spleen-deficiency cell model. Zhongguo Zhong Yao Za Zhi. 2018;43:2999–3005.
15. Peng GJ, Tian JS, Gao XX, Zhou YZ, Qin XM. Research on the pathological mechanism and drug treatment mechanism of depression. Curr Neuropharmacol. 2015;13:514–23.
16. Chen JJ, Zhou CJ, Zheng P, et al. Differential urinary metabolites related with the severity of major depressive disorder. Behav Brain Res. 2017;332:280–7.
17. Ding X, Yang S, Li W, et al. The potential biomarker panels for identification of Major Depressive Disorder (MDD) patients with and without early life stress (ELS) by metabonomic analysis. PLoS ONE. 2014;9:e97479.
18. Liu X, Zheng P, Zhao X, et al. Discovery and validation of plasma biomarkers for major depressive disorder classification based on liquid chromatography-mass spectrometry. J Proteome Res. 2015;14:2322–30.
19. Liu Y, Yieh L, Yang T, et al. Metabolomic biosignature differentiates melancholic depressive patients from healthy controls. BMC Genomics. 2016;17:669.
20. Setoyama D, Kato TA, Hashimoto R, et al. Plasma metabolites predict severity of depression and suicidal ideation in psychiatric patients—a multicenter pilot analysis. PLoS ONE. 2016;11:e0165267.
21. Hamilton M. A rating scale for depression. J Neurol Neurosurg Psychiatry. 1960;23:56–62.
22. Ye J, Cai X, Cao P. Problems and prospects of current studies on the microecology of tongue coating. Chin Med. 2014;9:9.
23. Zheng P, Chen JJ, Huang T, et al. A novel urinary metabolite signature for diagnosing major depressive disorder. J Proteome Res. 2013;12:5904–11.
24. Nelson DL, Cox MM. Principles of Biochemistry. 4th ed. New York: W. H. Freeman; 2005.
25. Barrios C, Spector TD, Menni C. Blood, urine and faecal metabolite profiles in the study of adult renal disease. Arch Biochem Biophys. 2016;589:81–92.
26. Kim KN, Li YH, Xiang TY. TCM syndrome differentiation of depression and the clinical S-Et analysis. Chin J Exp Tradit Med Formulae. 2010;16:215–8.
27. Gao SF, Bao AM. Corticotropin-releasing hormone, glutamate, and γ-aminobutyric acid in depression. Neuroscientist. 2011;17:124–44.
28. Moret C, Briley M. The importance of norepinephrine in depression. Neuropsychiatr Dis Treat. 2011;7(Suppl 1):9–13.
29. Huang Y, Huang X, Zhang L, et al. Magnesium boosts the memory restorative effect of environmental enrichment in Alzheimer's disease mice. CNS Neurosci Ther. 2018;24:70–9.
30. Sharma A, Gerbarg P, Bottiglieri T, et al. S-Adenosylmethionine (SAMe) for neuropsychiatric disorders: a clinician-oriented review of research. J Clin Psychiatry. 2017;78:e656–67.
31. Slutsky I, Abumaria N, Wu LJ, et al. Enhancement of learning and memory by elevating brain magnesium. Neuron. 2010;65:165–77.
32. Otoki Y, Hennebelle M, Levitt AJ, et al. Plasma phosphatidylethanolamine and triacylglycerol fatty acid concentrations are altered in major depressive disorder patients with seasonal pattern. Lipids. 2017;52:559–71.
33. McNamara RK, Jandacek R, Rider T, et al. Deficits in docosahexaenoic acid and associated elevations in the metabolism of arachidonic acid and saturated fatty acids in the postmortem orbitofrontal cortex of patients with bipolar disorder. Psychiatry Res. 2008;160:285–99.
34. McNamara RK, Rider T, Jandacek R, Tso P. Abnormal fatty acid pattern in the superior temporal gyrus distinguishes bipolar disorder from major depression and schizophrenia and resembles multiple sclerosis. Psychiatry Res. 2014;215:560–7.
35. Zaki MM, Abdel-Al H, Al-Sawi M. Assessment of plasma amino acid profile in autism using cation-exchange chromatography with postcolumn derivatization by ninhydrin. Turk J Med Sci. 2017;47:260–7.
36. Baranyi A, Amouzadeh-Ghadikolai O, von Lewinski D, et al. Branched-chain amino acids as new biomarkers of major depression—a novel neurobiology of mood disorder. PLoS ONE. 2016;11:e0160542.
37. Zuccoli GS, Saia-Cereda VM, Nascimento JM, Martins-de-Souza D. The energy metabolism dysfunction in psychiatric disorders postmortem brains: focus on proteomic evidence. Front Neurosci. 2017;11:493.
38. Cole JT, Sweatt AJ, Hutson SM. Expression of mitochondrial branched-chain aminotransferase and α-keto-acid dehydrogenase in rat brain: implications for neurotransmitter metabolism. Front Neuroanat. 2012;6:18.
39. Mathews DC, Henter ID, Zarate CA. Targeting the glutamatergic system to treat major depressive disorder: rationale and progress to date. Drugs. 2012;72:1313–33.

Permissions

All chapters in this book were first published in CM, by BioMed Central; hereby published with permission under the Creative Commons Attribution License or equivalent. Every chapter published in this book has been scrutinized by our experts. Their significance has been extensively debated. The topics covered herein carry significant findings which will fuel the growth of the discipline. They may even be implemented as practical applications or may be referred to as a beginning point for another development.

The contributors of this book come from diverse backgrounds, making this book a truly international effort. This book will bring forth new frontiers with its revolutionizing research information and detailed analysis of the nascent developments around the world.

We would like to thank all the contributing authors for lending their expertise to make the book truly unique. They have played a crucial role in the development of this book. Without their invaluable contributions this book wouldn't have been possible. They have made vital efforts to compile up to date information on the varied aspects of this subject to make this book a valuable addition to the collection of many professionals and students.

This book was conceptualized with the vision of imparting up-to-date information and advanced data in this field. To ensure the same, a matchless editorial board was set up. Every individual on the board went through rigorous rounds of assessment to prove their worth. After which they invested a large part of their time researching and compiling the most relevant data for our readers.

The editorial board has been involved in producing this book since its inception. They have spent rigorous hours researching and exploring the diverse topics which have resulted in the successful publishing of this book. They have passed on their knowledge of decades through this book. To expedite this challenging task, the publisher supported the team at every step. A small team of assistant editors was also appointed to further simplify the editing procedure and attain best results for the readers.

Apart from the editorial board, the designing team has also invested a significant amount of their time in understanding the subject and creating the most relevant covers. They scrutinized every image to scout for the most suitable representation of the subject and create an appropriate cover for the book.

The publishing team has been an ardent support to the editorial, designing and production team. Their endless efforts to recruit the best for this project, has resulted in the accomplishment of this book. They are a veteran in the field of academics and their pool of knowledge is as vast as their experience in printing. Their expertise and guidance has proved useful at every step. Their uncompromising quality standards have made this book an exceptional effort. Their encouragement from time to time has been an inspiration for everyone.

The publisher and the editorial board hope that this book will prove to be a valuable piece of knowledge for researchers, students, practitioners and scholars across the globe.

List of Contributors

Meng-yue Liu, Cheng-wei Wang and Ning Li
Department of Integrated Traditional Chinese and Western Medicine, West China Hospital of Si-chuan University, Chengdu, Sichuan, China

Zhou-peng Wu
Department of Liver and Vascular Surgery, West China Hospital of Si-chuan University, Chengdu, Sichuan, China

Li Li, Hong Meng and Yin-mao Dong
Key Laboratory of Cosmetic, China National Light Industry, Beijing Technology and Business University, No. 11/33, Fucheng Road, Haidian District, Beijing 100048, People's Republic of China
Beijing Key Laboratory of Plant Resources Research and Development, Beijing Technology and Business University, No. 11/33, Fucheng Road, Haidian District, Beijing 100048, People's Republic of China

Fan Yi
Key Laboratory of Cosmetic, China National Light Industry, Beijing Technology and Business University, No. 11/33, Fucheng Road, Haidian District, Beijing 100048, People's Republic of China
Beijing Key Laboratory of Plant Resources Research and Development, Beijing Technology and Business University, No. 11/33, Fucheng Road, Haidian District, Beijing 100048, People's Republic of China
Institute of Medicinal Plant Development, Chinese Academy of Medical Sciences, Peking Union Medical College, Beijing, 151 Malianwa NNorth Road, Haidian District, Beijing 100193, People's Republic of China

Li-jia Xu, Hai-bo Liu and Pei-gen Xiao
Institute of Medicinal Plant Development, Chinese Academy of Medical Sciences, Peking Union Medical College, Beijing, 151 Malianwa NNorth Road, Haidian District, Beijing 100193, People's Republic of China

Zhixue Ou, Yueping Chen, Tao Chen, Xiangbin Rong, Feipan Long, Xiaoyun Zhang, Qinghua Liang and Zhe Feng
Department of Traumatic Orthopedics and Hand Surgery, Ruikang Hospital Affiliated to Guangxi University of Chinese Medicine, Block B, No 10 Huadong Road, Nanning 530011, Guangxi, China

Qi Cheng
Department of Traumatic Orthopedics, Daye Hospital of Traditional Chinese Medicine, Daye 435100, Hubei, China

Chaoyun Zhang and Cuiyue Zhang
Zhang Zhongjing College of Chinese Medicine, Nanyang Institute of Technology, Changjiang Road 80, Nanyang 473004, Henan, China

Qian Wang, Wenhua Zang, Li Han, Lei Yang, Songshan Ye and Hua Bian
Zhang Zhongjing College of Chinese Medicine, Nanyang Institute of Technology, Changjiang Road 80, Nanyang 473004, Henan, China
Henan Key Laboratory of Zhang Zhongjing Formulae and Herbs for Immunoregulation, Nanyang Institute of Technology, Nanyang, Henan, China

Jingfeng Ouyang
Experimental Research Center, China Academy of Chinese Medical Sciences, Beijing, China

Yuefeng Bi
School of Pharmaceutical Sciences, Zhengzhou University, Zhengzhou, Henan, China

Carla Marrassini, Ignacio Peralta and Claudia Anesini
Facultad de Farmacia y Bioquímica, Instituto de la Química y Metabolismo del Fármaco (IQUIMEFA), Consejo Nacional de Investigaciones Científicas y Técnicas, Universidad de Buenos Aires, Buenos Aires, Argentina

Hong-yu Jin, Ming-juan Wang, Li-na Liu, Tian-tian Zuo and Shuang-cheng Ma
National Institutes for Food and Drug Control, No. 2 Tiantan Xili, Dongcheng District, Beijing 100050, People's Republic of China

Lei Sun
National Institutes for Food and Drug Control, No. 2 Tiantan Xili, Dongcheng District, Beijing 100050, People's Republic of China
Xinjiang Institute for Food and Drug Control, Urumqi 830004, China

Run-tao Tian
Chemmind Technologies Co., Ltd., Beijing 100085, China

Liu-ping Ye
Huainan Food and Drug Inspection Center, Huainan 232007, China

Sheng Wang, Qingxiu Hao, Liping Kang, Chuanzhi Kang, Jian Yang, Wanzhen Yang, Jingyi Jiang and Lu-Qi Huang
National Resource Center for Chinese Materia Medica, State Key Laboratory Breeding Base of Dao-di Herbs, China Academy of Chinese Medical Sciences, Beijing 100700, People's Republic of China

Li Zhou and Lanping Guo
National Resource Center for Chinese Materia Medica, State Key Laboratory Breeding Base of Dao-di Herbs, China Academy of Chinese Medical Sciences, Beijing 100700, People's Republic of China
College of Traditional Chinese Medicine, Guangdong Pharmaceutical University, Guangdong 510006, China

Yuan Wei, Dujun Wang, Zhen Ouyang and Shuo Wang
School of Pharmacy, Jiangsu University, 301 Xuefu Road, Zhenjiang, Jiangsu, People's Republic of China

Meng Chen
Department of Molecular, Cellular and Biomedical Sciences, University of New Hampshire, Durham, NH, USA

Jun Gu
Wadsworth Center, New York State Department of Health, 1400 Washington Ave, Albany, NY, USA
School of Public Health, State University of New York at Albany, Albany, NY, USA

Ai-Ren Zuo
State Key Laboratory of Food Science and Technology, Nanchang University, Nanchang 330047, Jiangxi, China
Jiangxi University of Traditional Chinese Medicine, Nanchang, Jiangxi, China

Shu-Wen Cao
State Key Laboratory of Food Science and Technology, Nanchang University, Nanchang 330047, Jiangxi, China
Department of Chemistry, Nanchang University, Nanchang, Jiangxi, China

Huan-Huan Dong, Qing-Long Shu, Li-Xiang Zheng and Xiong-Ying Yu
Jiangxi University of Traditional Chinese Medicine, Nanchang, Jiangxi, China

Yan-Ying Yu
Department of Chemistry, Nanchang University, Nanchang, Jiangxi, China

Ping Wang
College of Pharmaceutical Science, Hubei University of Chinese Medicine, Wuhan 430065, China

Chao Xiong and Shi-Lin Chen
College of Pharmaceutical Science, Hubei University of Chinese Medicine, Wuhan 430065, China
Institute of Chinese Materia Medica, China Academy of Chinese Medical Sciences, Beijing 100700, China

Bao-Zhong Duan
College of Pharmaceutical Science, Hubei University of Chinese Medicine, Wuhan 430065, China
Institute of Chinese Materia Medica, China Academy of Chinese Medical Sciences, Beijing 100700, China
College of Pharmaceutical Science, Dali University, Dali 671000, China

Xi-Wen Li
Institute of Chinese Materia Medica, China Academy of Chinese Medical Sciences, Beijing 100700, China

Hai-Lan Fang
Institute of Chinese Materia Medica, China Academy of Chinese Medical Sciences, Beijing 100700, China
College of Pharmaceutical Science, Dali University, Dali 671000, China

Ya-Ping Wang
Centre for Cancer and Inflammation Research, School of Chinese Medicine, Hong Kong Baptist University, Hong Kong, China

Ji Yeon Seo, Ju Yong Lee, Pham Ha Thanh Tung, Sang Hyun Sung and Won Keun Oh
Korea Bioactive Natural Material Bank, Research Institute of Pharmaceutical Sciences, College of Pharmacy, Seoul National University, Seoul 08826, Republic of Korea

Sang Kyum Kim
College of Pharmacy, Chungnam National University, Daejeon 34134, Republic of Korea

Phi Hung Nguyen
College of Pharmacy, Chosun University, Gwangju 61452, Republic of Korea

Fuhuan Fei, Huanmei Sun, Xixi Cheng, Jiajun Liu, Jing Wang, Qian Li and Yajun Zhang
Key Laboratory of Resource Biology and Biotechnology in Western China, Ministry of Education, College of Life Sciences, Northwest University, Xi'an 710069, China

Annie Xianghong Lin and Luwen Shi
International Research Center for Medicinal Administration, Peking University, Beijing, China

Hao Hu
International Research Center for Medicinal Administration, Peking University, Beijing, China
State Key Laboratory of Quality Research in TCM, Institute of Chinese Medical Sciences, University of Macau, Room 2057, Building N22, Avenida da Universidade, Taipa, Macao

Ging Chan, Yuanjia Hu, Defang Ouyang and Carolina Oi Lam Ung
State Key Laboratory of Quality Research in TCM, Institute of Chinese Medical Sciences, University of Macau, Room 2057, Building N22, Avenida da Universidade, Taipa, Macao

Ya-Jing Zhang, Hui-Juan Cao, Xin-Lin Li, Xiao-Ying Yang and Bao-Yong Lai
Centre for Evidence-Based Chinese Medicine, Beijing University of Chinese Medicine, 11 Bei San Huan Dong Lu, Beijing 100029, China

Jian-Ping Liu
Centre for Evidence-Based Chinese Medicine, Beijing University of Chinese Medicine, 11 Bei San Huan Dong Lu, Beijing 100029, China
The National Research Center in Complementary and Alternative Medicine (NAFKAM) Department of Community Medicine, Faculty of Health Science, UiT, The Arctic University of Norway, 9037 Tromsø, Norway

Guo-Yang Yang
National Institute of Complementary Medicine, Western Sydney University, Sydney, NSW 2751, Australia

Hui-Qin Li
School of Chinese Medicine, Faculty of Medicine, The Chinese University of Hong Kong, Hong Kong, SAR, People's Republic of China

Siu-Po Ip and Yan-Fang Xian
School of Chinese Medicine, Faculty of Medicine, The Chinese University of Hong Kong, Hong Kong, SAR, People's Republic of China
Brain Research Centre, School of Chinese Medicine, Faculty of Medicine, The Chinese University of Hong Kong, Hong Kong, SAR, People's Republic of China

Zhi-Xiu Lin
School of Chinese Medicine, Faculty of Medicine, The Chinese University of Hong Kong, Hong Kong, SAR, People's Republic of China
Brain Research Centre, School of Chinese Medicine, Faculty of Medicine, The Chinese University of Hong Kong, Hong Kong, SAR, People's Republic of China
Institute of Integrative Medicine, Faculty of Medicine, The Chinese University of Hong Kong, Hong Kong, SAR, People's Republic of China

Guo-Qing Zheng
Department of Neurology, The Second Affiliated Hospital and Yuying Children's Hospital of Wenzhou Medical University, Wenzhou, Zhejiang Province, People's Republic of China

Jaewon Jeon, Erin Bussin and Alex Scott
Centre for Hip Health and Mobility, Vancouver Coastal Health Research Institute and Department of Physical Therapy, University of British Columbia, 2635 Laurel Street, Vancouver, BC V5Z3M9, Canada

Lan-Ying Liu, Li-Yuan Luo, Chun-Qin Zhu, Pei-Rong Wang, Yuan-Yuan Zhang and Chun-Yu Yang
Department of Psychiatry, Tongde Hospital of Zhejiang Province, Hangzhou 310012, Zhejiang, China

Hong-Jian Zhang, Jin-Bao Pu and Wei-Qing Liang
Zhejiang Academy of Traditional Chinese Medicine, Hangzhou 310007, Zhejiang, China

Ya-Ping Li
Department of Internal Chinese Medicine, Tongde Hospital of Zhejiang Province, Hangzhou 310012, Zhejiang, China

Zhang-Jin Zhang
School of Chinese Medicine, LKS Faculty of Medicine, The University of Hong Kong, 10 Sassoon Road, Pokfulam, Hong Kong, China

Index